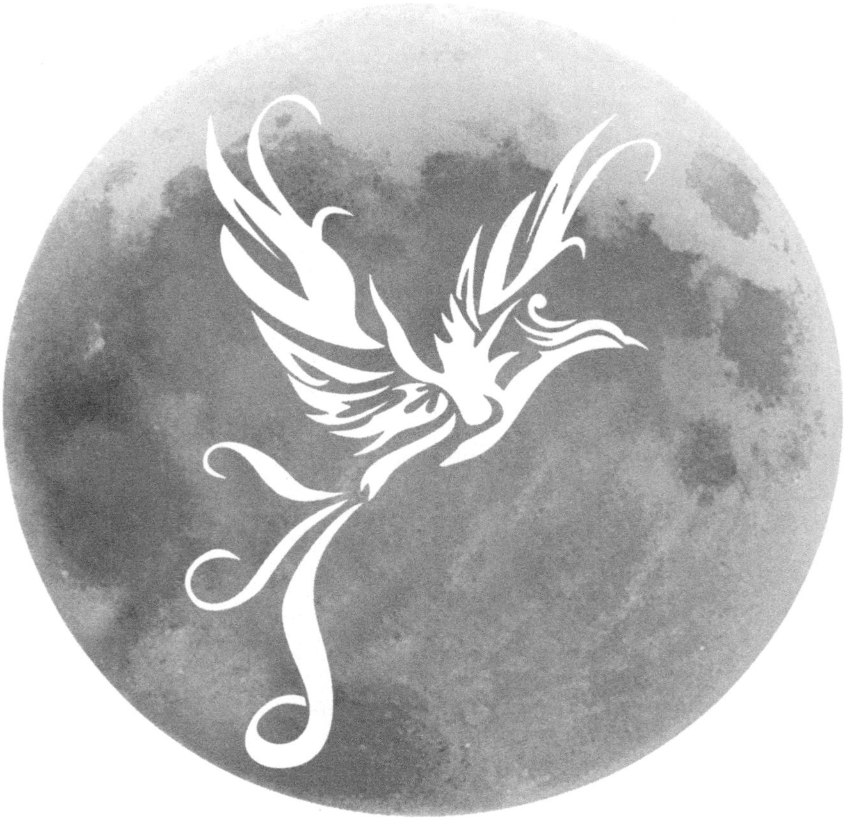

MENOPAUSE

A COMPREHENSIVE GUIDE FOR PRACTITIONERS

Katherine Berry and Natalie Chandra Saunders

With Suzanne Cochrane and Brian Grosam
Foreword by Honora Lee Wolfe

Book design by Adam Raes and Katherine Berry
Edited by Suzanne Cochrane (PhD)
Clinical Advisor Brian Grosam (PhD)
Graphic design by Adam Raes
Hardcopy (US spelling)

ISBN 978-1-7391308-0-0

First published in 2022
By Katherine Berry in partnership with the Journal of Chinese Medicine
Locale 5, 15 Carrer de Sant Vicent
Santa Eulária des Riu, Ibiza, Islas Baleares
Spain 07840
Treating Women Academy
TreatingWomen.com

The information in this book is intended as a resource and guide for practitioners who have trained in traditional Chinese and East Asian medicine (TCEAM). It is not intended to substitute for such training and should not be considered to supplant the clinical judgement derived from such training. Whilst every effort has been made to include cautions with regard to treatment, the authors cannot accept responsibility for any treatment advice offered.

Front cover
The moon represents cycles; not only the monthly cycles that occur throughout one's reproductive years but also the continual waxing and waning of yin and yang that exist throughout the natural world. It reminds us that there are no beginnings and no endings, only the infinite ebb and flow of life.

The phoenix is a symbol of rising from the ashes and being reborn with renewed vitality, hope, and optimism. The authors chose this image to represent the power of women transitioning through menopause and beyond.

Acknowledgements

Publishing a medical textbook, especially one of this scale, is a team effort. The authors would like to acknowledge the invaluable behind the scenes help from Margie Candy, a freelance virtual assistant in South Africa. In addition to our listed international experts, Suzanne Cochrane from Australia and US-based Brian Grosam were instrumental as our editors and clinical guides, sharing their gems of wisdom gleaned from years of practice. Elements of this book were inspired by Brian's publication: *Understanding and Treating Hot Flashes in Menopause with Chinese Medicine*. Graphic designer Adam Raes was delightful to work with and brought 'The Book' to life with his creative vision, while professional indexer Pilar Wyman did an outstanding job of making the text into a useable resource.

The authors are grateful for the support of Peter Deadman and Danny Maxwell from the Journal of Chinese Medicine, Jim Belcher and Charlene Payne from Balance Healthcare, and John O'Connor from Eastland Press. Honora Lee Wolfe played a unique role as a contributor by co-authoring a chapter, providing guidance on the publishing process, and writing a deeply moving foreword. We would also like to thank Angela Hicks and Debra Betts for their glowing endorsements, and Sebastian Maciocia for granting permission to use Giovanni's advanced training in the Treating Women Academy's Menopause Masterclass that inspired this book.

The International Menopause Society is an extraordinary clearinghouse of information and a wonderful resource to tap in to. Membership to the IMS opened up an avenue into our western medical colleagues' growing body of knowledge. One particularly valuable publication was *A Practitioner's Toolkit for Managing Menopause* by Jane and Davis, which has been reproduced with permission in Appendix 8.2.

In addition to professional support, the authors appreciate the love, encouragement, and guidance provided by their mentors, friends, and family. And finally, though wildly broad, we are grateful to the inspiring women all over the world who have contributed to making this a worthwhile project.

CONTENTS

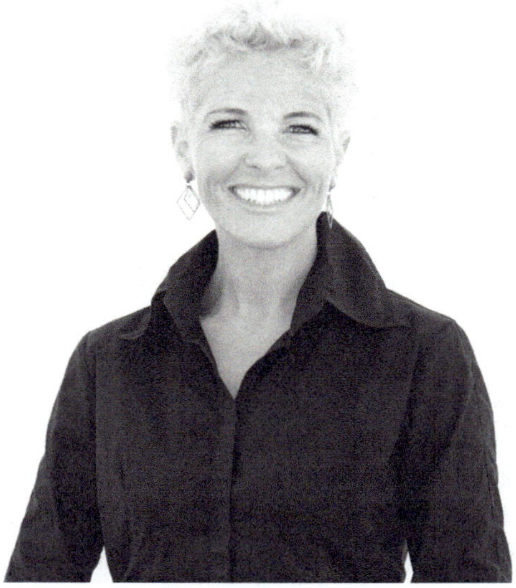

Katherine Berry

Katherine Berry, BHSc, MSc, is an acupuncture educator with over 25 years of clinical experience. Having commenced a Bachelor's degree in TCM in Australia in 1995, and graduating in 2000, Kath spent time working in several hospitals in China.

She then returned to Australia and completed a Master of Science Research degree (MSc) in drug and alcohol addiction medicine at the University of Technology Sydney (UTS). Her thesis was based on a clinical trial she set up between UTS and Sydney South West Area Health Service.

As Australia's first ever hospital-based acupuncture clinical trial, the study required two years of preparation across three ethics jurisdictions and paved the way for further collaboration between TCM university departments and hospitals.

Concurrently, Kath fueled her passion for enhancing the acupuncture profession through high quality education, networking, and mentoring by setting up a nonprofit organization, *The Acupuncture Network*. In 2007 she studied at the Lincoln Recovery Center in NYC with Dr.. Michael Smith and became a certified NADA ear acupuncture trainer.

From 2008 to 2010 she worked with *Balance Healthcare* and the *Journal of Chinese Medicine* in the UK before consulting with *Acupuncture Professional*. After moving to Ibiza in Spain in 2015, she was nominated Vice President of the *Acupuncture Now Foundation* and consultant to *Evidence Based Acupuncture*, two US non-profit advocacy organizations.

In 2018 she joined with pediatric expert Dr. Julian Scott to provide continuing professional development training for acupuncturists all over the world via TreatingChildren.com.

Then, in 2019 she developed fertility and menopause masterclasses with eminent acupuncture specialists; their teachings inspired this book and are shared through the Treating Women Academy at TreatingWomen.com.

Kath is a happily divorced mother of two and proud women's health advocate. She helps practitioners empower women to reach their full potential through courses on enhancing health, achieving balance, promoting confidence, and encouraging sexual vibrancy. Contact Kath for coaching to be an online *Menopause Mentor*.

Natalie Chandra Saunders

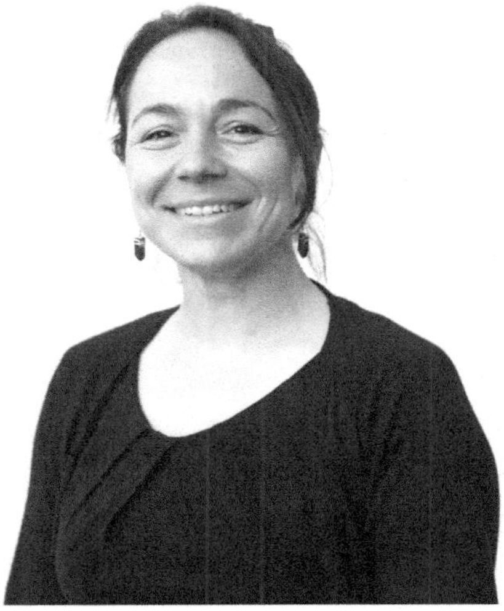

Natalie Chandra Saunders, BA(Hons), LicAc is a writer, translator, and educator specialising in the fields of acupuncture and East Asian medicine.

After completing her secondary education, she began work as a pharmacy technician, gaining a National Vocational Qualification in Pharmacy Services and a solid understanding of biomedicine.

However, she quickly became disillusioned with the pharmaceutical industry and decided to pursue a more holistic career.

She enrolled at the College of Traditional Acupuncture in her hometown of Leamington Spa, UK, graduating with an honors degree in Traditional Acupuncture in 2007.

Natalie set up her practice in Birmingham, concurrently working as a volunteer acupuncturist for Freshwinds, a charity offering therapies to people living with life-threatening and life-limiting illnesses.

Between 2011 and 2014, she also acted as Regional Group Coordinator (West Midlands) for the British Acupuncture Council. In 2012, Natalie won a scholarship to study traditional Chinese medicine at Heilongjiang University of Chinese Medicine in Harbin, China.

During her studies, she fell in love with Chinese culture and in 2014 she returned to the country on a more long-term basis. She lived in the northern coastal city of Dalian for over two years, self-studying herbal medicine, dietary therapy, and Mandarin.

It was during this period that she discovered her passion for writing and completed her first book, The Qi of Tea, a treatise on the history and use of tea in traditional Chinese medicine.
On returning to the UK, she began working closely with Katherine Berry at : TreatingWomen.com, and the concept for Menopause: A Comprehensive Guide for Practitioners was born.

Natalie has a special interest in menopause and healthy aging, particularly the concept of *yangsheng*, or "nourishing life." She currently lives in rural Wales where she works as a freelance writer and menopause coach, offering in-person and online consultations to people around the world.

Foreword by Honora Lee Wolfe

In the mid 1990s, I wrote a small book called *Managing Menopause Naturally with Chinese Medicine*. Though intended for laywomen and not as a clinical text, women practitioners of acupuncture and Chinese herbal medicine embraced it as a reference for helping menopausal patients navigate that life passage with more ease and comfort.

Since then, several other books on this subject, mostly clinical manuals, have been added to the English-language Chinese medical lexicon to help practitioners support patients effectively with acupuncture, herbal medicine, and other East Asian medical tools. So why is this new addition to the literature, *Menopause: A Comprehensive Guide for Practitioners*, useful and needed? Two things about this book have struck me as especially useful relative to other available literature on this subject.

First, the authors have woven together a clinical narrative that honors both Chinese, Western, and other natural or home care approaches without fear or favor. Though the text is *largely* about East Asian medicine, the authors clearly understand the importance of using whatever will work to help women maintain health. They have understood that women struggling with symptoms during menopause often do better when Western, naturopathic, East Asian, and possibly Ayurvedic, homeopathic, and psychologic approaches are skillfully combined to support them! No one approach has a monopoly on the truth.

Secondly, despite it being a full clinic manual on treating and preventing menopausal symptoms, the authors' narrative style is not burdened by excessive medical jargon. Its language is simple, straightforward, and uncondescending while at the same time being a thorough presentation of the clinical symptoms, the variety of treatment options, and self care tools for maintaining health through menopause and beyond. I applaud any technical book that is so easy to read and understand!

In a speech given at the Vancouver Peace Summit in 2009, the 14th Dalai Lama, Tenzin Gyatso, stated his emphatic belief that if the world was to be saved, it must be women, especially older women in the developed world, who could and would do it.

What a remarkable statement! What a noble idea, challenge, and responsibility. It is my belief that women can and must rise to this challenge. As practitioners of Chinese medical gynecology, we are in a singular position to respond by supporting, nourishing, and empowering our older women patients to become the "mothers of their communities" and the wise women who carry the mantle of leadership in difficult times.

Books such as *Menopause: A Comprehensive Guide for Practitioners* offer a source of information and inspiration to do that work more effectively.

~Honora Lee Wolfe
July, 2022

Menopause: More Than an Evolutionary Quirk?

Menopause is unique to just a handful of species; humans (*Homo sapiens*) and several aquatic mammals, including killer whales (*Orcinus orcas*), short-finned pilot whales (*Globicephala macrorhynchus*), beluga whales (*Delphinapterus leucas*), and narwhals (*Monodon monoceros*). While these sea creatures may initially appear to have little in common with humans, they are social animals and tend to live in groups, known as pods. These pods can consist of several families which are, in many cases, matrilineally related.

Experts have suggested that menopause is an evolutionary phenomenon that increases the chances of a mother passing on her genetics. It enables her to devote more energy to the family or pod's survival rather than continuing to reproduce.

Offspring born to older mothers have a lower survival rate than those born to younger individuals. Therefore, shutting off reproduction at middle age and assisting in the care of grandchildren preserves genetic lineage more efficiently than competing with younger descendants who are also reproducing.

This theory is known as the grandmother hypothesis of menopause. However, it is currently just that, a hypothesis. Although there is strong evidence to support it, some scientists argue that menopause is simply an evolutionary quirk that has persisted in our genes for no particular reason. However, if proven, the grandmother hypothesis would explain why humans and other species go through menopause, and why women's life spans can extend far beyond the reproductive years.

The authors highlight this evolutionary biology theory as it underpins one of the central themes of this book: reframing menopause as a positive experience. In both humans and killer whales, older females support the survival, wellbeing, and reproduction of their offspring and grand-offspring. In humans, this extends to society as a whole, meaning that even women who do not have children of their own can make valuable contributions to future generations by sharing their experience, love, and wisdom.

Figure 1. Shows 52 species of mammals and their average female life expectancy. The red bar indicates the reproductive years and the gray bar shows the number of years survived on average, after the reproductive years. An asterisk (*) indicates the species where postreproductive years are significant in comparison to reproductive years (killer whales, short-finned pilot whales, and humans).

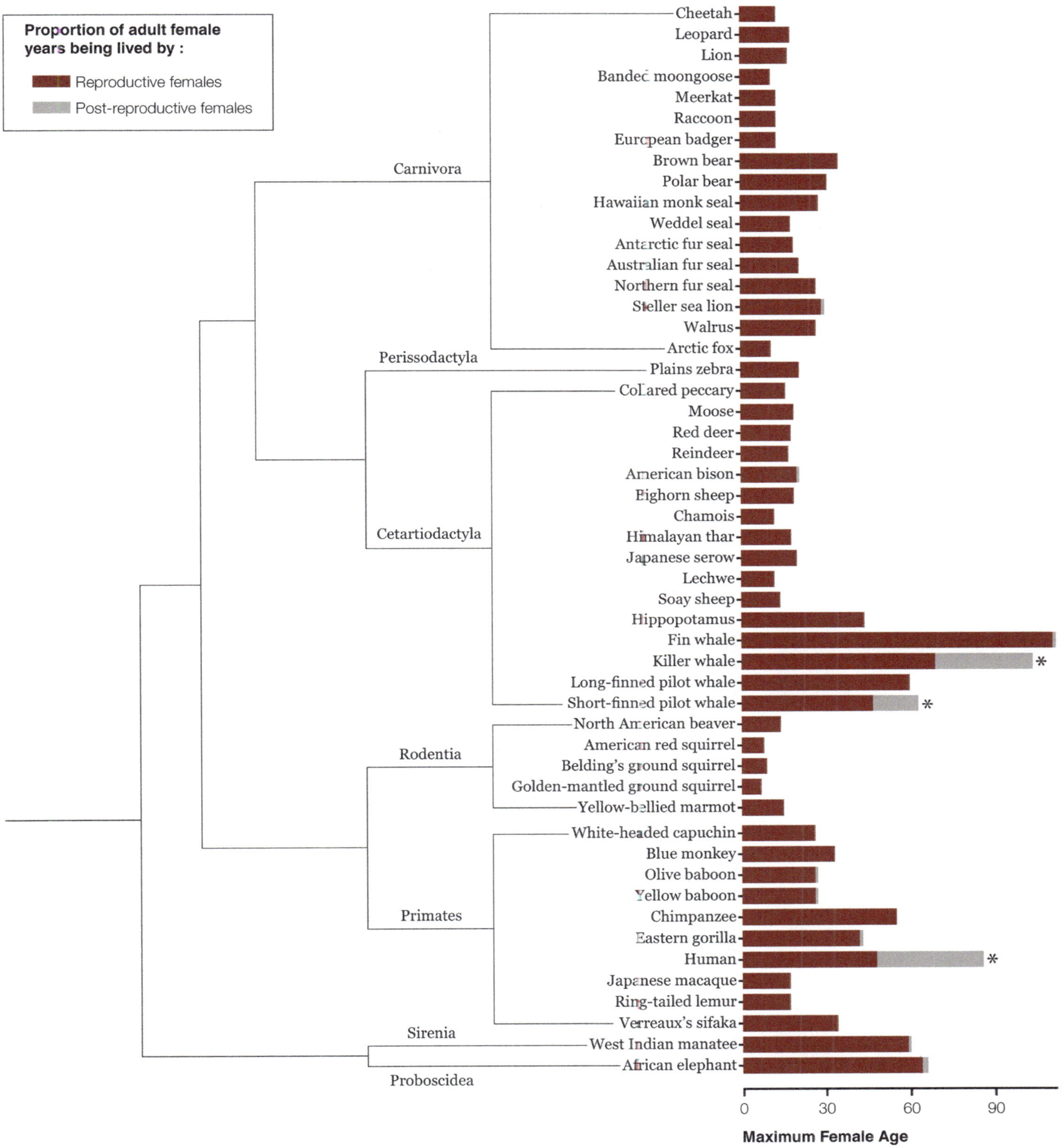

Figure 1: Postreproductive life expectancy in 52 mammals.[1]

[1]Ellis S, Franks DW, Nattrass S, et al. (2018). Postreproductive lifespans are rare in mammals. Ecol Evol. 2018;8:2482–2494. https://onlinelibrary.wiley.com/doi/epdf/10.1002/ece3.3856
https://doi.org/10.1002/ece3.3856

SECTION 1 - Introduction

1.1 Preface

Women's health is a burgeoning field of medicine that incorporates a wide variety of sub-specialties, and many Chinese and East Asian medicine practitioners dedicate their careers to gynecology, fertility, and obstetrics. However, fewer choose to specialize in the treatment of menopause and its related symptoms. There is also a lack of up-to-date, evidence-based information available on the subject of menopause in traditional Chinese and East Asian medicine (TCEAM).

This is perplexing, since vast numbers of women transition through menopause every year, sometimes experiencing significant deterioration in physical and mental health. Furthermore, with the average age of menopause in developed countries being 51, more and more women are spending over a third of their lives in the post-menopausal period, thus increasing their risk of chronic, age-related disease.

The aim of this book is to provide a comprehensive guide to menopause and the years that follow, bringing together modern biomedical research and ancient wisdom to provide practitioners with an integrated approach to treatment.

The text is largely based on the teachings of renowned and highly-experienced TCEAM practitioners, including, Suzanne Cochrane, Brian Grosam, Giovanni Maciocia, Honora Lee Wolfe, Bob Flaws, Peter Deadman, Julian Scott, Rebecca Avern, and Anastacïa White. It also includes information provided by experts in related fields, such as Professor Bruce Robinson M.D. and naturopathic nutritionist Susan Kath.

We discuss the physiology of menopause from both Eastern and Western perspectives, and pattern differentiation and treatment frameworks for some of the most common menopausal symptoms. We also cover a variety of conditions that frequently affect women following menopause.

Finally, we explore the concept of *yangsheng*, the ancient Chinese tradition of 'nourishing life,' and how to best advise patients on maintaining optimal wellbeing throughout menopause and beyond via good nutrition, stress and sleep management, and appropriate exercise.

We have assumed that readers have at least a basic understanding of TCEAM theory, although we have included a glossary of TCEAM terms for those with a background in medical acupuncture. Of course, while point prescriptions and formulas are suggested for numerous ailments, these should be viewed as a general guide and adapted to suit each patient's individual needs.

Acupuncture and Chinese herbal medicine hold significant potential to alleviate menopausal women's suffering, either as standalone treatments or in combination with other therapeutic approaches. Our hope is that this book will equip practitioners with the knowledge and confidence they require to become menopause specialists, or simply enhance their treatment of menopausal patients in general practice.

1.2 Menopause: Your Role as a Clinician

Menopause is a natural and inevitable phenomenon, yet its effects can be highly variable. Some individuals experience minimal disruption to their everyday lives, while others endure debilitating symptoms for years before and after the cessation of their menses.

With a limited range of medical treatments available, a growing number of people are turning to acupuncture and TCEAM to relieve their menopausal symptoms. So, how do we practice TCEAM with menopausal patients in a way that will facilitate their transition to a healthy older age?

This question could be truncated to: how do we practise TCEAM?

There are general guidelines for establishing a therapeutic relationship that focuses on promoting change to relieve our patients' suffering. It is this relationship that provides the foundations from which healing can emerge. In brief, this includes:

- Attending to the patient's needs with empathy, expressed through what has been described as "the art of doing nothing," i.e. listening, noticing, thinking, waiting, witnessing, and preventing harm.
- Undertaking the activity of attuning (*tiaohe*). This allows us to cooperate with the patient during a clinical encounter to determine the meaning of their presenting symptoms and their categorization within the discourse of TCEAM, and thus, a path to effective treatment.
- Developing a therapeutic alliance which enables the patient to become active in their own healing.
- Allowing space for both analytical and intuitive knowledge to emerge.
- Ensuring patients feel cared for during the consultation to promote treatment adherence.
- Reconfirming our knowledge that remedy and consultation are complementary. Acupuncture, herbs, massage, exercises, and diet (that is, the core of our practices) do work and are required ingredients for successful outcome(s). However, the 'therapeutic relationship' fostered by our consultations also plays a crucial role.
- Continually studying and revising to keep our knowledge up-to-date and better serve our patients.

If these principles need to be applied in any TCEAM encounter then do menopausal women require something more?

Indeed, there are strong arguments supporting more effort for, and a broader understanding of, these patients in our clinics. This is because a woman's attitude toward menopause, and aging in general, can significantly affect her experience.

We know that older women are located in our western societies in a particular way and face particular challenges. For example, we live in a world where great value is attached to youth and esthetic beauty, while aging is usually seen as something to fight against.

Older women also often have fewer financial and other resources to support themselves in their old age compared to men.

These factors directly correlate with health and the incidence of disease, meaning a woman's social position can significantly influence her physical and emotional wellbeing. We may not be able to remove these challenges for our patients but, as clinicians, we are uniquely placed to help them shift their attitudes.

Reframing the major physical and psychological change that menopause presents as a transformation rather than a pathology may make the process far more manageable. In fact, it is widely accepted that the 'medicalization' of menopause contributes to the occurrence of symptoms and that adopting a more positive viewpoint can ease the transition.

Of course, genetics, ethnicity, education, economic background, and lifestyle factors also have a significant impact. But helping our patients to change their perspectives is one way in which we can assist them in entering the next stage of their lives with optimism and confidence. We may even be able to utilize menopause as a healing opportunity and reduce or eliminate symptoms that have been troublesome earlier in life.

We can also offer advice that allows women to continue their healing journey beyond the treatment room. However, it is essential that this advice is presented in a sensitive, compassionate, and non-blaming manner.

For instance, women are the main target of the wellness industry. It is said to be an industry that offers a seductive distraction from the issues that are really impacting women's lives and glosses over the cultural and societal issues undermining their wellbeing.

So, how should TCEAM position itself within this industry?

When giving advice, we need to not only focus on what a woman 'should do' but also engage our understanding of why she is in this position today. To practice ethically, we need to support women to recognize the broader context of their situation and their efforts to transform their circumstances.

To become well, older menopausal women need allies who value them and can explain that it is not some failure on their part that has brought them to your door. Coming to the end of one's reproductive life is a chance to reassess what is really going on and how much influence one can have over one's situation. As TCEAM practitioners, we are in an ideal position to help our patients accept and understand their journey through menopause and enable them to enter later life with serenity, joy, and good health.

References

Saunders, N.C., Cochrane, S., Berry, K., (2022) The Great Transformation - Altering Attitudes Toward Menopause with Chinese Medicine, Journal of Chinese Medicine. Jun 2022, Vol. 129, (pp 17-22).

1.3 Terminology, Stages, and Definitions

There are many different ways to describe menopause and the years preceding and succeeding it. Many people erroneously use the word 'menopause' to describe the period prior to and following the cessation of menses, during which menopausal symptoms may occur. For the sake of simplicity, we have followed this convention throughout much of the text.

Terminology

Some of the terminologies most frequently used when discussing menopause and its related symptoms are listed below.

Adolescence
The transitional phase between the ages of 10 to 19 years old as a child develops into an adult.

Puberty
Occurring during adolescence, puberty in girls results from an increase of estrogen, progesterone, and other hormones. Physical changes such as the development of breasts and secondary sexual characteristics (e.g. underarm and pubic hair) occur. During this time her menstrual cycle begins (menarche).

Pre-menopause
The time period before menopause or perimenopause, during which a woman experiences regular or irregular menstrual periods. Sometimes referred to as "the fertile years" or "child-bearing age."

Perimenopause
The span of time between the onset of cycle irregularity and 12 months after the final menstrual period (FMP). The perimenopausal period may last as long as 10 years in total.

Menopause
The cessation of menstruation for a period of 12 months or more. The average age of menopause in economically developed countries is 51 although it can occur much earlier or later.

Early Menopause
Cessation of ovarian function between ages 40–45.

Post-menopause
The time from 12 months after the final menstrual period onwards.

Climacteric
Sometimes used interchangeably with the word 'menopause.' However, climacteric (from the Greek for 'steps') more accurately describes a gradual decrease in ovarian function from the pre to post-menopausal stages.

Climacteric Syndrome
A collection of symptoms that frequently occur during the climacteric period.

Induced or Iatrogenic 'Medical Menopause'
Menopause due to pharmaceutical drugs that cause premature ovarian insufficiency (POI).

Surgical Menopause
Cessation of menstruation due to surgical removal of the female reproductive organs and pelvic radiation therapy.

Premature Ovarian Insufficiency
Cessation of ovarian function before age 40. Sometimes referred to as premature menopause.

The Stages of Menopause

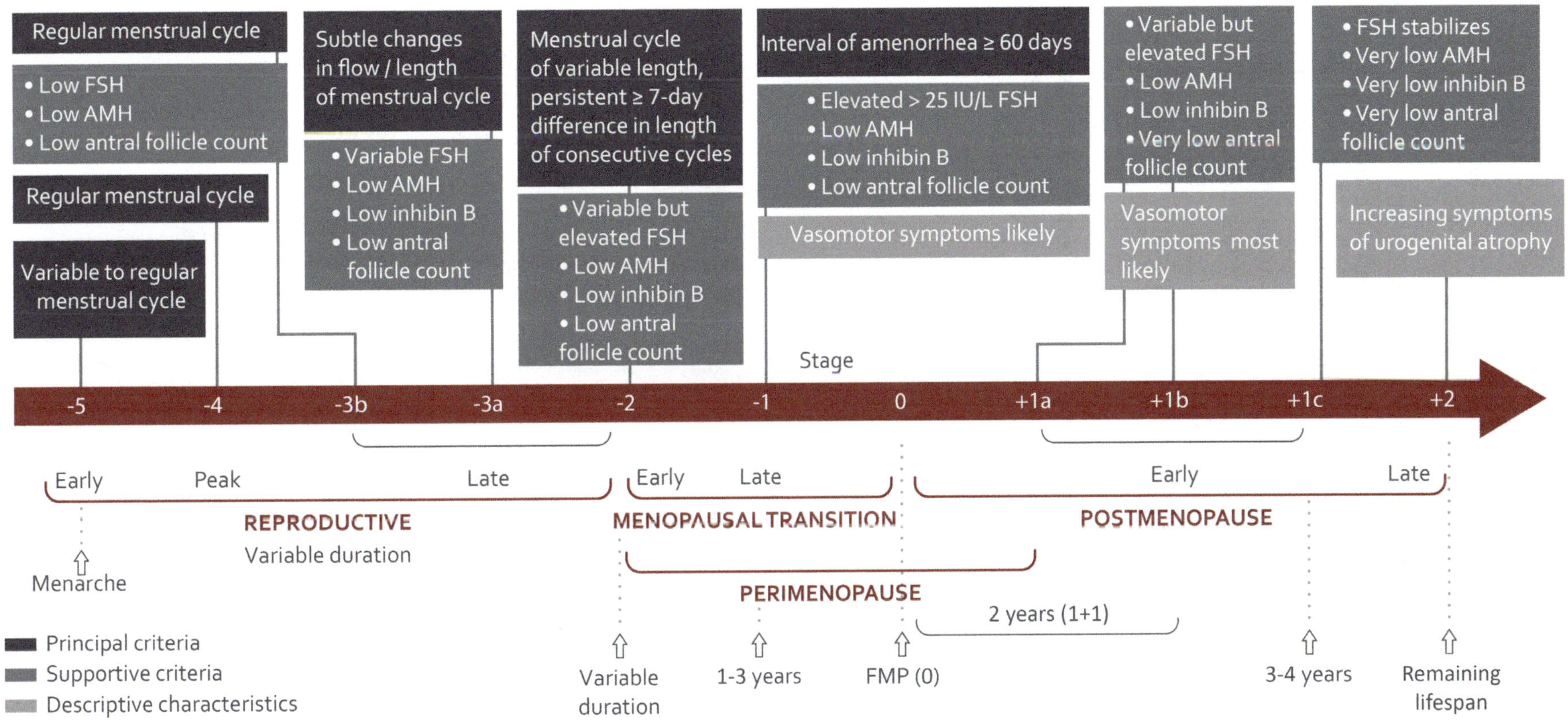

Figure 1.3a: The stages of reproductive aging in women. [2]

[2] Image source: Davis, S., Lambrinoudaki, I., Lumsden, M. et al. (2015). Menopause. Nature Reviews Disease Primers, Nat Rev Dis Primers 1, 15004 (2015). Sourced July 2022. https://www.nature.com/articles/nrdp20154

Definitions

Traditionally, the term 'menopause' has been used to define the end of the reproductive years in women. However, societal changes, such as increased awareness of gender dysphoria and a growing number of people identifying as LGBTQ+, have led to complexities regarding this definition. Trans men and non-binary individuals will also transition through menopause if they retain their ovaries, or if they undergo gender-affirming oophorectomy. Trans women can also experience menopause-like symptoms as a result of hormonal treatment withdrawal. We have attempted to use inclusive language wherever possible throughout the book, but have used the terms 'woman' and 'women' where it is appropriate in a medical, historical, or cultural context.

Finally, it is essential to recognize the significant differences between natural menopause, medically-induced menopause, and premature ovarian insufficiency. While they do share some similarities, they also present unique challenges and complications.

References

Blümel, JE., Lavín, P., Vallejo, MS., et al. (2013). Menopause or climacteric, just a semantic discussion or has it clinical implications?, NIH, National Library of Medicine, National Center for Biotechnology Information: Climacteric. 2014 Jun;17(3): (pp 235-41). Doi: 10.3109/13697137.2013.838948. https://pubmed.ncbi.nlm.nih.gov/23998690

Jane, FM., Davis, SR., (2014). A Practitioner's Toolkit for Managing the Menopause, Taylor Francis Online: Climacteric Volume 17, 2014 - Issue 5, doi.org/10.3109/13697137.2014.929651 https://www.tandfonline.com/doi/full/10.3109/13697137.2014.929651

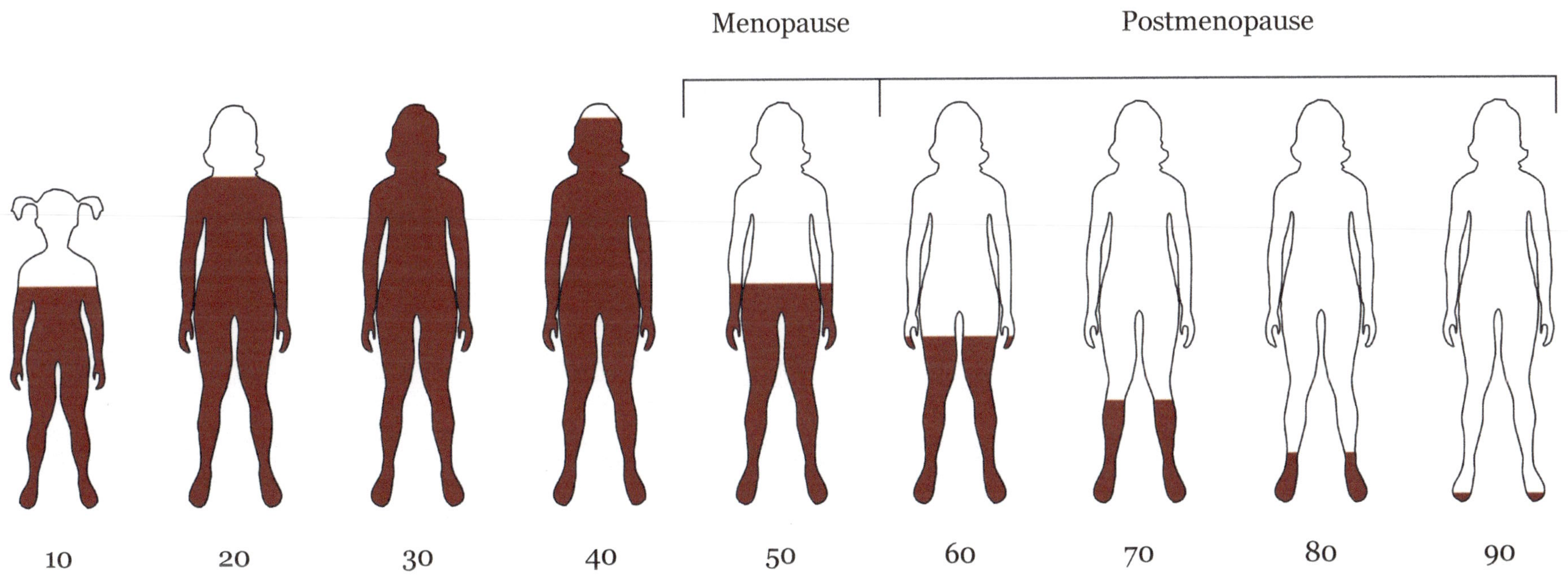

Figure 1.3b: Estrogen levels by age.

SECTION 2 - The Biology of Menopause

2.1 Female Anatomy and Physiology

The female reproductive and urogenital systems are complex, delicate, under-studied, and frequently misunderstood. As clinicians, it is essential to fully comprehend the anatomy and physiology of these systems in order to successfully diagnose and treat any gynecological issues, including those associated with menopause.

This chapter provides a brief overview of the internal and external genitalia, and associated musculature.

Internal Genitalia

Ovaries

The ovaries are the female gonads and are responsible for producing the reproductive hormones and oocytes, which develop into ova (eggs). They play an essential role in the menstrual cycle and maintenance of pregnancy, should it occur.

Fallopian Tubes

The fallopian tubes act as a passageway, allowing an ovum to travel from the ovaries to the uterus.

The portion of the fallopian tubes closest to the ovaries comprises finger-like structures called fimbriae that help the ovum move into the tube. The widest section of the tube is known as the ampulla. The section closest to the uterus is narrower and is known as the isthmus.

Uterus

The uterus includes the corpus (body) and the cervix. The upper section is known as the fundus, while the lower section is known as the isthmus or lower uterine segment.

The uterus comprises three distinct layers of tissue. The inner layer is the endometrium, which varies in thickness in response to hormonal changes throughout the menstrual cycle. In the absence of a pregnancy, the endometrium sheds, resulting in menstruation. The middle layer is the myometrium and is made up of smooth muscle fibers. The outermost layer is known as the serosa.

Cervix

The cervix is a tubular structure between the uterus and the vagina. It opens into the upper vagina at the cervical os. Its lining includes both columnar and squamous epithelial cells. The area where these two cell types meet is called the transformation zone, which is a common site for cervical dysplasia and malignancy.

Vagina

The vagina is a fibromuscular tube that changes with age and the decreased supply of estrogen. During and after the menopausal transition, it becomes shorter and narrower, with thinning and stiffening of the vaginal walls (known as Halban's fascia).

For many women, vaginal atrophy during and after menopause not only makes sexual intercourse painful but may also lead to various other uncomfortable or distressing symptoms. The term 'genitourinary syndrome of menopause' (GSM) describes a collection of genital, sexual, and urinary symptoms, and provides a more accurate description than previously used terms, such as vulvovaginal atrophy (VVA) and atrophic vaginitis. This condition is discussed in further detail in Chapter 4.4. Urogenital Symptoms.

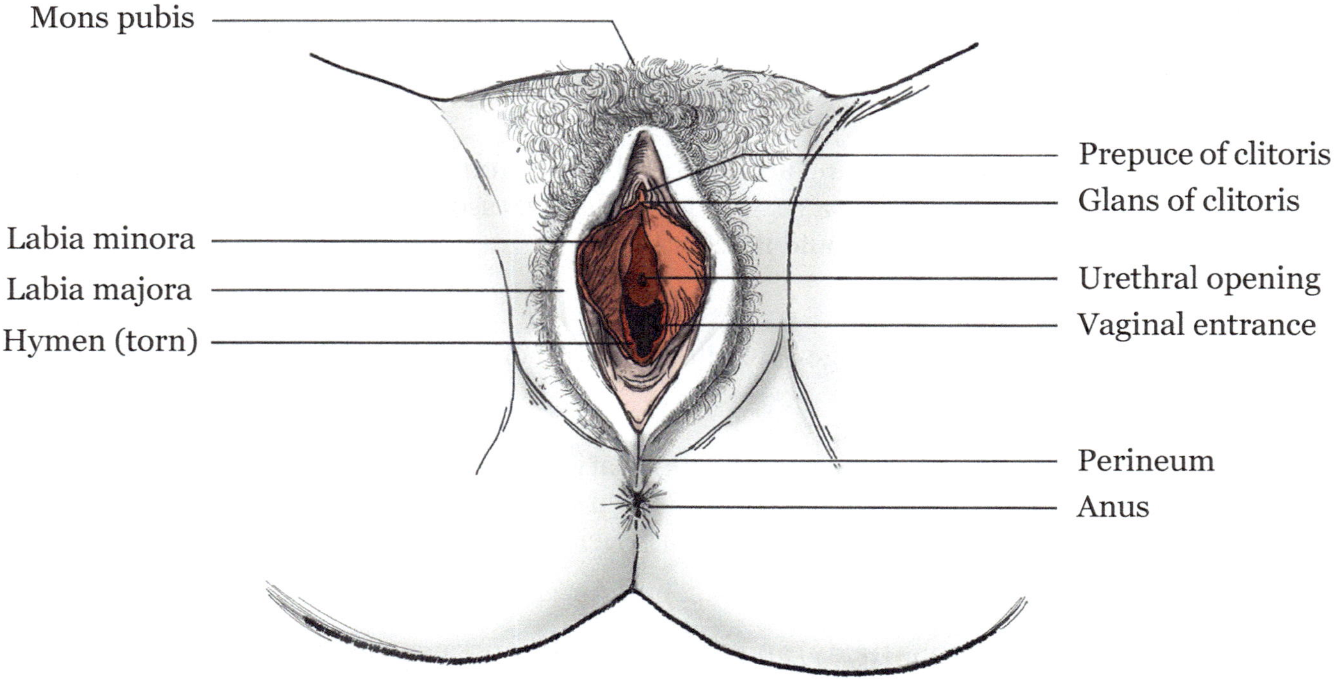

Figure 2.1a: Female external genitalia.

External Genitalia

Vulva

The vulva is the area of external genitalia comprising the:

• Mons pubis • Labia majora • Labia minora • Glans clitoris • Skene's glands • Urinary meatus *(opening to the urethra)* • Vaginal opening • Bartholin glands • Prior to penetrative sexual intercourse, the hymen.

Mons Pubis

A mound of fatty tissue that is covered with pubic hair. It acts as a cushion during sexual intercourse and contains pheromone-secreting glands, playing a role in sexual attraction.

Labia Majora

The labia majora are cutaneous folds that envelop the remaining external genital structures. They engorge with blood during arousal, giving them a swollen appearance.

Labia Minora

The labia minora is formed by two bodies (vestibular bulbs) of corpus spongiosum erectile tissue. They are rich in small blood vessels which engorge with blood during sexual arousal, becoming turgid and doubling or tripling in thickness. Rhythmic contraction of the bulbocavernosus muscles of the labia minora are responsible for what is referred to as 'vaginal orgasm.'

Clitoris

The clitoris is the primary source of female sexual pleasure. It is often mistaken to be the size of a pea because the erectile tissues of the clitoris are mostly internal. The external glans clitoris (what most people call 'the clitoris') is small and highly sensitive to touch due to the concentration of approximately 8,000 sensory nerve endings. However, the clitoris organ is the same size as the average-sized penis and works in the same way, engorging with blood to form an erection when aroused.

During sexual arousal, erectile tissue in the bulbs and crura swell with blood. Because of their location on either side of the vaginal canal, expansion of clitoral tissue causes pressure to be applied to the vagina muscles, increasing sexual stimulation and sensation.

Women can experience the same erection problems as men, although female erectile dysfunction is often labeled more broadly as 'sexual dysfunction.'

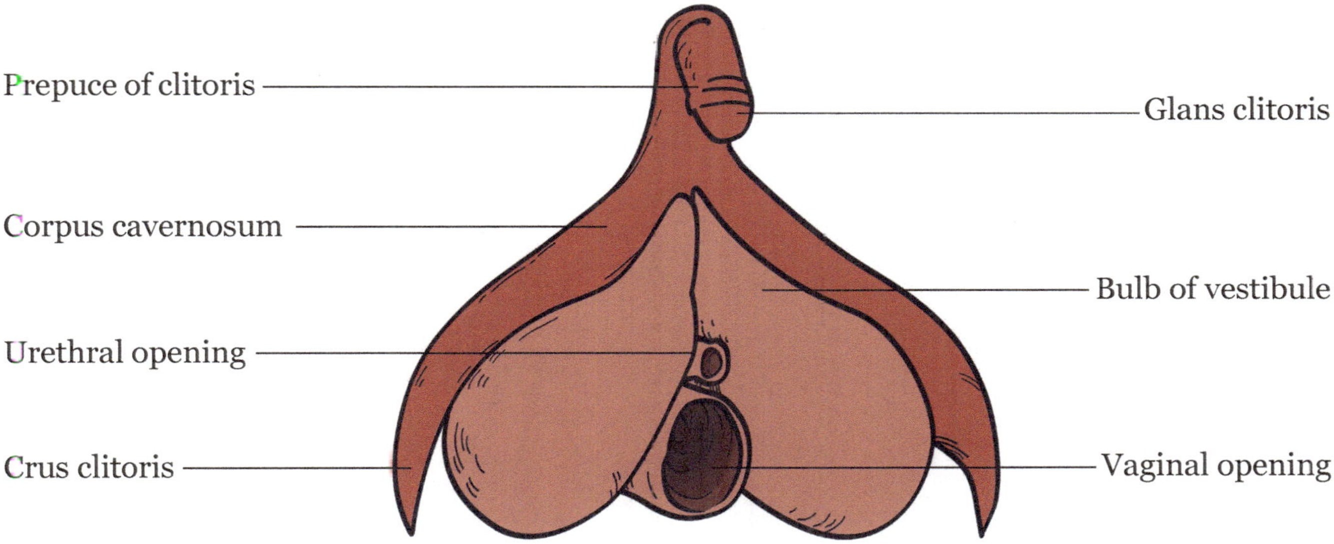

Figure 2.1b: Anatomy of the clitoris.

Bartholin Glands

The Bartholin glands are two pea-sized ducts at the entrance to the vagina which help keep the vagina lubricated. Like the vagina itself, they also shrink with age resulting in vaginal dryness.

Urethra

The urethra is an extension of the tube that allows urine to be excreted from the bladder. In females, its opening is located between the vagina and the clitoris.

Skene's Glands

Also known as the lower vestibular glands, the Skene's glands are two glands located on either side of the urethra. They produce a fluid that is believed to act as a lubricant and antimicrobial which may help prevent urinary tract infections (UTIs).

Stimulation of the Skene's glands results in the secretion of mucus-containing fluids, which help with lubrication during vaginal intercourse. Researchers also believe that fluid excretions from these glands may account for female ejaculation. Other names for Skene's glands include:
• Skene's ducts • Periurethral glands • Paraurethral gland • Female prostate[3]

The Pelvic Floor Muscles

The pelvic floor muscles are a hammock-like structure that stretches from back to front between the pubic bone and coccyx, and from left to right between the ischial tuberosities. Their primary function in female anatomy is supporting the uterus, bladder, bowel, and other pelvic organs.

The physiological changes that occur during menopause can cause these muscles to weaken, potentially leading to issues such as incontinence and prolapse. Weight gain, pregnancy, anal trauma during childbirth, surgery, and radiation treatment can also contribute to pelvic floor muscle dysfunction. Meanwhile, chronic conditions including diabetes and asthma can contribute to bowel and bladder dysfunction. Performing pelvic floor exercises (Kegel exercises) can be highly beneficial for pre and post-menopausal women. These are described in detail in chapter 4.4. Urogenital Symptoms.

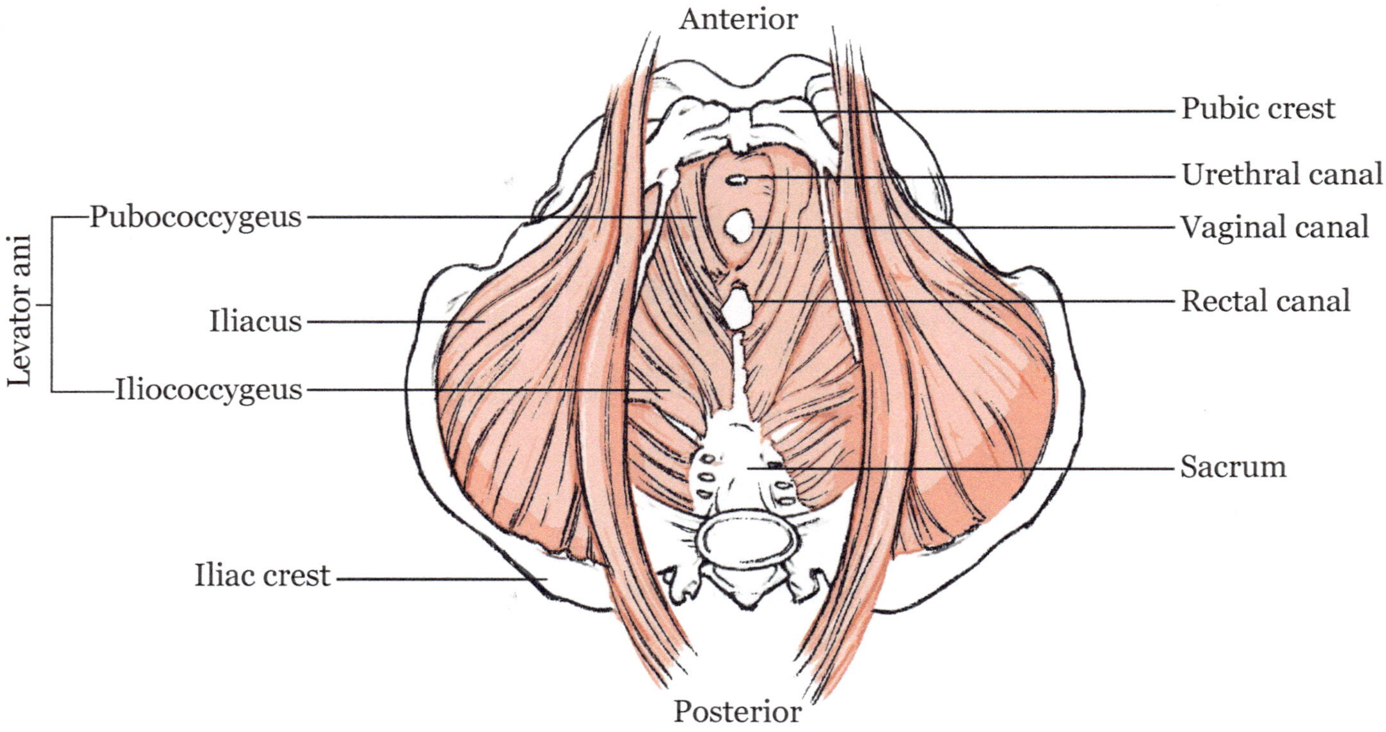

Figure 2.1c: Pelvic diaphragm (superior view).[4]

[3] The name 'female prostate' is due to similarities with the male prostate gland's ability to drain fluids into the urethra. However, Skene's glands are not identical to prostate glands in male anatomy.
[4] Image source: Betts, JG., Young, KA., Wise, JA. et al. OpenStax, Figure 11.19 Muscles of the Pelvic Floor, (2013), sourced July 2022.
https://openstax.org/books/anatomy-and-physiology/pages/11-4-axial-muscles-of-the-abdominal-wall-and-thorax

Summary

Female reproductive anatomy includes both internal and external structures that undergo significant changes during menopause. These changes can cause a variety of symptoms that may negatively impact a woman's overall quality of life. Fortunately, the majority of these symptoms are straightforward to treat and manage, providing that clinicians have a solid understanding of their underlying pathology. Further details can be found in Chapter 4.4. Urogenital Symptoms, and Chapter 4.6. Libido and Sexual Function.

References

Kim, H-K., Kang, S-Y., Chung, Y-L., et al. (2015). The Recent Review of the Genitourinary Syndrome of Menopause, PMC US National Library of Medicine, National Institutes of Health, Journal of Menopausal Medicine: J Menopausal Med. 2015 Aug; 21(2): (pp 65–71) Published online 2015 Aug 28. doi: 10.6118/jmm.2015.21.2.65
https://www.ncbi.nlm.nih.gov/pmc/articles/PMC4561742

Pfaus, JG., Quintana, GR., Cionnaith, CM., et al. (2016). The whole versus the sum of some of the parts: toward resolving the apparent controversy of clitoral versus vaginal orgasms, PMC US National Library of Medicine, National Institutes of Health, Taylor & Francis Group; Socioaffective Neuroscience & Psychology: Socioaffect Neurosci Psychol. 2016; 6: 10.3402/snp.v6.32578. Published online 2016 Oct 25. doi: 10.3402/snp.v6.32578.
https://www.ncbi.nlm.nih.gov/pmc/articles/PMC5084726

University of Rochester Medical Centre, (Sourced January 2021). Anatomy of the Vulva.
https://www.urmc.rochester.edu/encyclopedia/content.aspx?contenttypeid=34&contentid=19522-1

Rosner, J., Samardzic, T., Sarao, M.S., (2021). Physiology, Female Reproduction, NCBI, The National Center for Biotechnology Information: StatPearls [Internet].
https://www.ncbi.nlm.nih.gov/books/NBK537132

Nguyen, J., Duong, H., (2021). Anatomy, Abdomen and Pelvis, Female External Genitalia, NCBI, The National Center for Biotechnology Information: StatPearls [Internet].
https://www.ncbi.nlm.nih.gov/books/NBK547703

Biancardi, MF., Dos Santos, FCA., (2017), Female prostate: historical, developmental, and morphological perspectives.2017 - Wiley Online Library.: First published: 04 March 2017
https://doi.org/10.1002/cbin.10759
https://onlinelibrary.wiley.com/doi/abs/10.1002/cbin.10759

Continence Foundation of Australia, (sourced January 2021), Pelvic floor muscles in women,
https://www.continence.org.au/who-it-affects/women/female-pelvic-floor-muscles

MedlinePlus, (Sourced January 2021). Pelvic Floor Disorders Also called: Cystocele, Enterocele, Pelvic Prolapse, Rectocele,
https://medlineplus.gov/pelvicfloordisorders.html

Continence Foundation of Australia, (sourced January 2021). Menopause,
https://www.pelvicfloorfirst.org.au/pages/going-through-menopause-or-post-menopausal.html

2.2 Female Reproductive Hormones

Many of the key hormones involved in reproductive health (both androgens and estrogens) are steroid hormones. They derive from cholesterol, which is converted to pregnenolone, then progesterone, and finally to the reproductive hormones. Although these hormones all derive from the same source and have somewhat similar structures, the role that they play throughout the reproductive years and menopause are very different.

Steroid Hormones

Estrogen

Estrogen is a steroid hormone. It is responsible for the onset of puberty, regulating menstrual cycles, and maintaining pregnancy. It also has a protective role over the heart, liver, bones, brain, and skin.

There are three types of estrogen:

Estradiol
the most biologically active form of estrogen, produced by the ovaries in women of childbearing age.

Estriol
produced by the placenta during pregnancy.

Estrone
produced by the adrenal glands and adipose tissue after menopause.

As ovarian function declines, estradiol levels begin to fall resulting in menopausal symptoms and, eventually, the cessation of menstruation.

Progesterone

Progesterone is another steroid hormone. It is produced in the corpus luteum following ovulation and prepares the body for a potential pregnancy. It also plays a role in maintaining pregnancy, should it occur.

As with estrogen, progesterone levels decrease with age as ovarian function declines.

Androgens

Androgens are produced by the ovaries and adrenal cortex. They include the hormones dehydroepiandrosterone sulphate (DHEAS), dehydroepiandrosterone (DHEA), androstenedione, and testosterone.

Serum levels of DHEAS, DHEA, and testosterone begin to decline from the late reproductive years onwards. Although natural menopause is not associated with acute changes in androgen levels, medically-induced menopause has been linked with reduced testosterone, as has estrogen replacement therapy. Lower-than-average androgen levels have also been reported in premature ovarian insufficiency (see Chapter 2.6.).

Primary hormones (in CAPS) are made by organs by taking up cholesterol ★ and converting it locally to, for example, progesterone. Much less is made from circulating precursors like pregnenolone. For example, taking DHEA can create testosterone and estrogen, but far less than is made by the testes or ovaries, respectively.

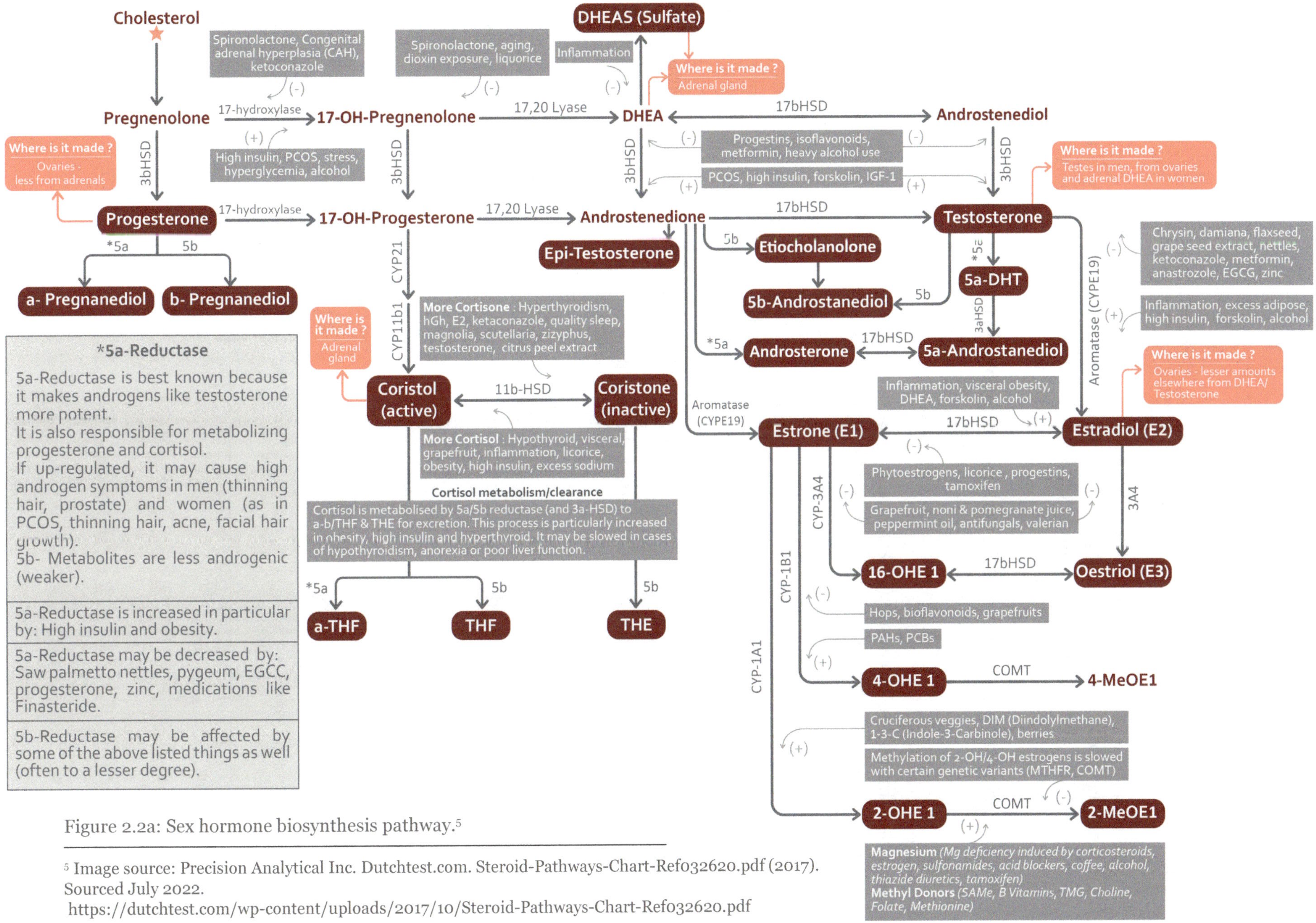

Figure 2.2a: Sex hormone biosynthesis pathway.[5]

[5] Image source: Precision Analytical Inc. Dutchtest.com. Steroid-Pathways-Chart-Ref032620.pdf (2017). Sourced July 2022. https://dutchtest.com/wp-content/uploads/2017/10/Steroid-Pathways-Chart-Ref032620.pdf

Other Hormones

Luteinising Hormone

Luteinising hormone (LH) is a glycoprotein produced by the pituitary gland. It triggers the release of the steroid hormones and regulates the menstrual cycle. It plays a role in both ovulation and egg implantation.

LH levels tend to increase three-fold in the years following menopause, or faster in women who have undergone medically-induced menopause.

Follicle Stimulating Hormone

Follicle stimulating hormone (FSH) is also produced by the pituitary gland. It works closely with LH to regulate the menstrual cycle. It plays a role in both estrogen production and follicle development.

FSH levels tend to increase dramatically (10–20 fold) following menopause. In premature ovarian insufficiency, FSH levels rise due to a lack of negative feedback from the ovaries.

Inhibin B

Inhibin B is a glycoprotein produced by the granulosa cells of the ovaries. It suppresses the synthesis and secretion of FSH, and its levels are associated with the number of developing follicles. Inhibin B levels become elevated during puberty and begin to fall from the late reproductive stage onwards.

Anti-Mullerian Hormone

Anti-mullerian hormone (AMH) is expressed in the granulosa cells of follicles. It plays a crucial role in follicle recruitment and development and is often used as a marker of ovarian reserve.

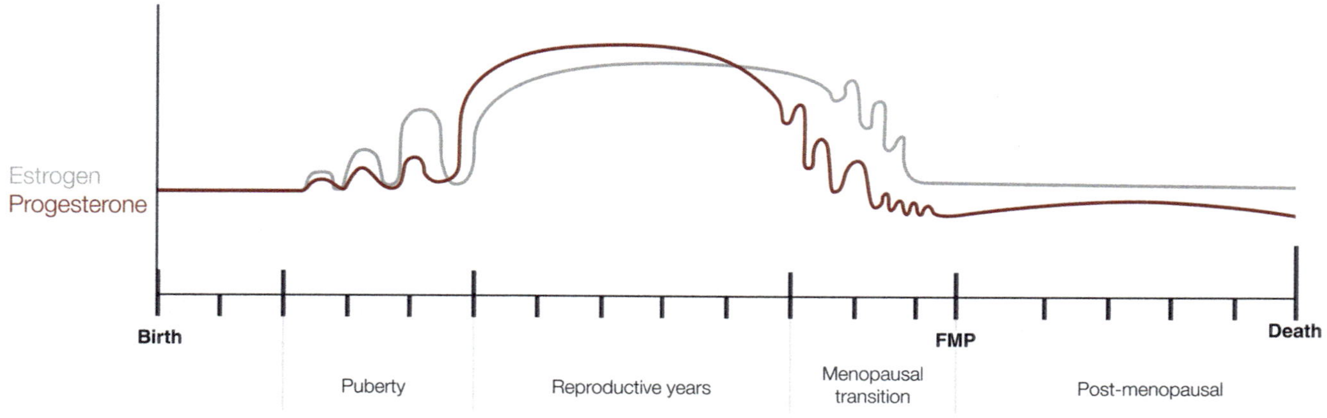

Figure 2.2b: Stages of the reproductive aging process.

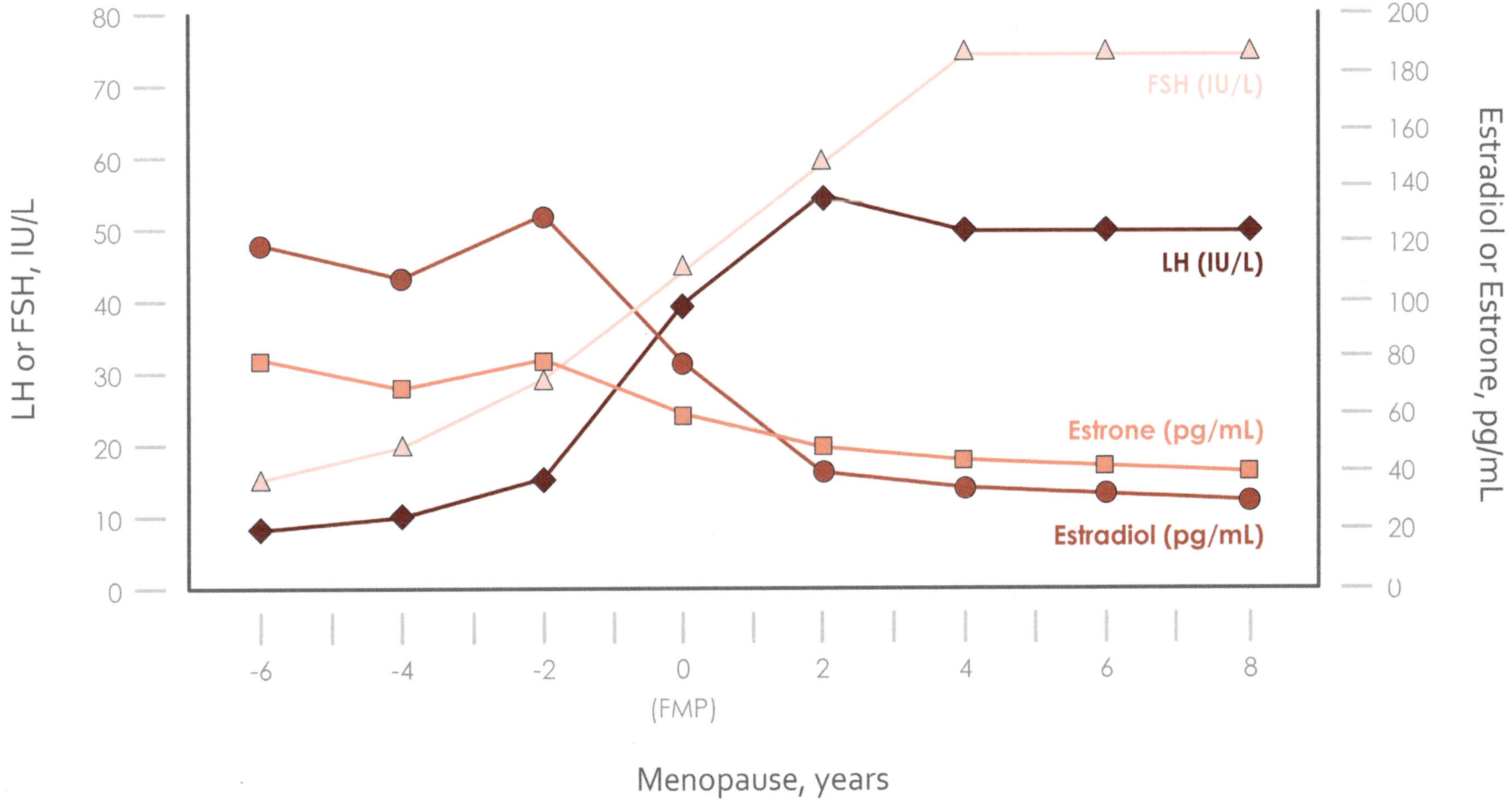

Figure 2.2c: Hormone changes during menopause.[6]

[6] Image source: Tang, J., (2014). Teleconference UKM, 27 August 2014, Slide 10. Sourced July 2022. https://www.slideshare.net/jvtglee/hormonal-replacement-therapy.

Hormones and the Stages of Menopause

There are three distinct stages to menopause; late reproductive, menopausal transition, and postmenopause. These stages are determined using the final or last menstrual period (FMP) as the reference point. The date of the FMP is determined retrospectively, since it is not known until 12 months after it occurs. Hence, although the average age of menopause in economically developed countries is 51, the FMP occurs at an average age of 50. Since everything hinges on a focal point that is not known until one year after the fact, it is challenging to use it clinically at the time.

Stage	-5	-4	-3b	-3a	-2	-1	+1a	+1b	+1c	+2
Terminology	**Reproductive**				**Menopausal transition**		**Postmenopause**			
	Early	Peak	Late		Early	Late	Early			Late
					Perimenopause					
Duration	Variable				Variable	1-3 years	2 years (1+1)		3-6 years	Remaining lifespan
Principal criteria										
Menstrual cycle	Variable to regular	Regular	Regular	Subtle changes in Flow/length	Variable length persistent ≥ 7 day difference in length of consecutive cycles	Interval of amenorrhea of ≥ 60 days				
Supportive criteria										
Endocrine FSH AMH Inhibin B			Low Low	Variable* Low Low	↑ Variable* Low Low	↑ > 25 IU/L** Low Low	↑ Variable Low Low		Stabilizes Very low Very low	
Antral follicle count			Low	Low	Low	Low	Very low		Very low	
Descriptive characteristics										
Symptoms						Vasomotor symptoms *Likely*	Vasomotor symptoms *Most likely*			*Increasing* symptoms of urogenital atrophy

*Blood draw on cycle days 2-5 ↑ Elevated
**Approximate expected level based on assays using current international pituitary standard

Figure 2.2d: The stages of reproductive aging.[7]

[7] Image Source: Harlow, SD., Gass, M., Hall, JE., (et al). (2012). The Stages of Reproductive Aging Workshop + 10 staging system for reproductive aging in women. (2012) J Clin Endocrinol Metab. 2012 Apr; 97(4): (pp 1150-1168) Published online 2012 Feb 16. doi: 10.1210/jc.2011-3362. Sourced July 2022. https://www.ncbi.nlm.nih.gov/pmc/articles/PMC3319184/figure/F2

Updated in 2011, the Stages of Reproductive Aging Workshop (STRAW+10) is considered the gold standard for characterising reproductive aging through menopause. Each stage is defined by various hormonal fluctuations and menstrual cycle changes:

Late Reproductive Phase (Stages -3b/-3a)

- FSH and estradiol levels become variable
- AMH and inhibin B levels are reduced
- Menstrual cycle is regular or slightly irregular
- Intermittent symptoms may occur

Menopausal Transition

Early Perimenopause (Stage -2)

- FSH and estradiol levels remain variable
- AMH and inhibin B remain low
- Increased menstrual irregularity
- Symptoms are more likely to occur

Late Perimenopause (Stage -1)

- FSH levels are elevated
- Estradiol levels decrease
- AMH and inhibin B remain low
- Menstrual cycle lengthens to 60 days or more
- Symptoms are more likely to occur
- Although fecundability is low at this stage, ovulation and pregnancy are still possible until one year after the final menstrual period

Final Menstrual Period (FMP = 0)

- The FMP is identified retrospectively and measured from the first day of the last menstrual period preceding 12 consecutive months of amenorrhea

Post Menopausal (Stage +1a, +1b, +1c, +2)

- FSH levels are elevated
- Estradiol, progesterone, AMH, and inhibin B are low
- Menstruation ceases for 12 months or more
- Symptoms are much more variable
- Increased risk of chronic disease

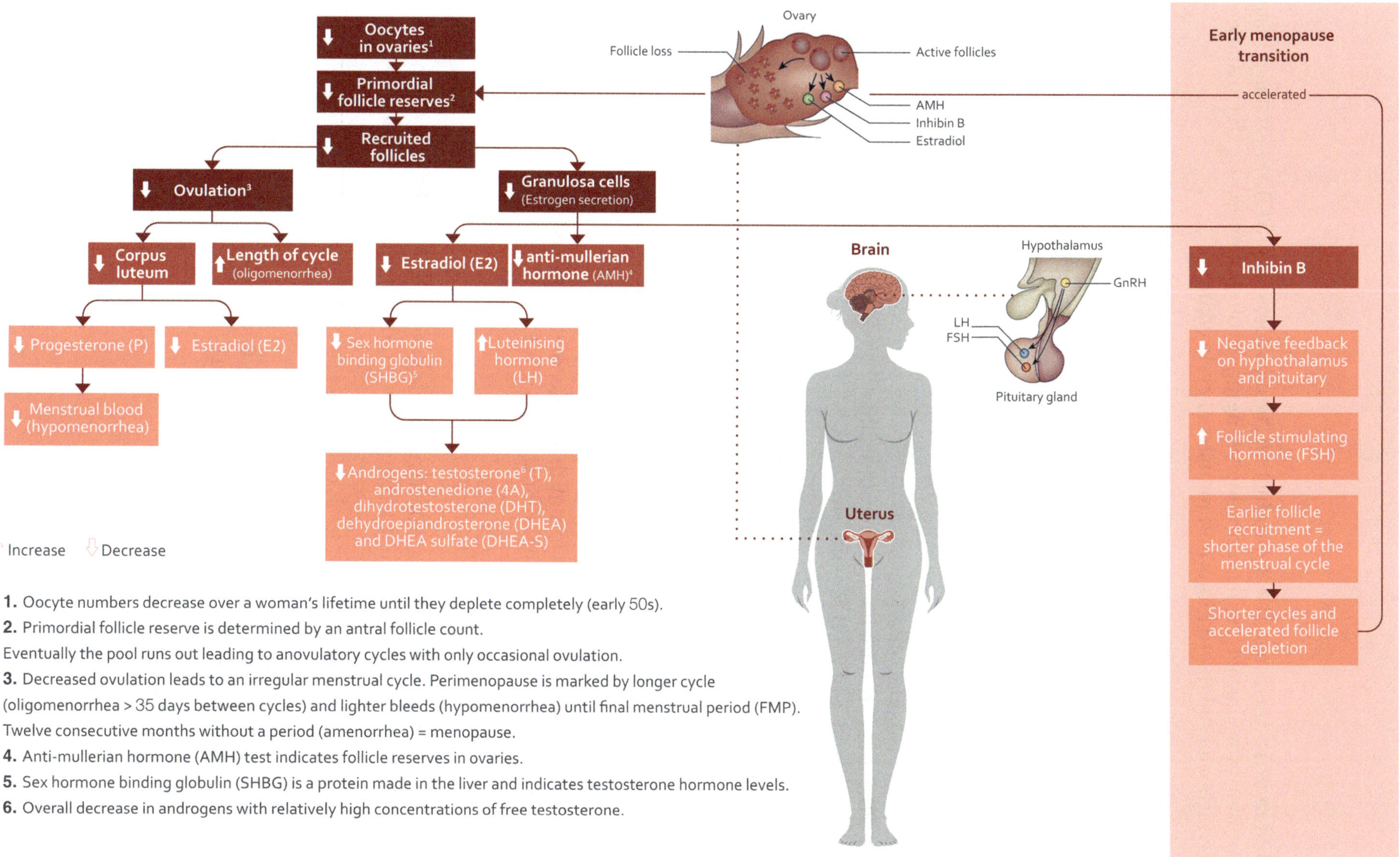

1. Oocyte numbers decrease over a woman's lifetime until they deplete completely (early 50s).

2. Primordial follicle reserve is determined by an antral follicle count.

Eventually the pool runs out leading to anovulatory cycles with only occasional ovulation.

3. Decreased ovulation leads to an irregular menstrual cycle. Perimenopause is marked by longer cycle (oligomenorrhea > 35 days between cycles) and lighter bleeds (hypomenorrhea) until final menstrual period (FMP).

Twelve consecutive months without a period (amenorrhea) = menopause.

4. Anti-mullerian hormone (AMH) test indicates follicle reserves in ovaries.

5. Sex hormone binding globulin (SHBG) is a protein made in the liver and indicates testosterone hormone levels.

6. Overall decrease in androgens with relatively high concentrations of free testosterone.

Figure 2.2e: The pathophysiology of menopause.

Summary

Throughout the menopausal transition, a woman's primary form of estrogen switches from estradiol to estrone. This shift is responsible for many of the physiological and psychological changes that occur during this period.

However, menopause also significantly impacts a range of other reproductive hormones and these can be used as markers to determine a woman's reproductive status and distinguish between the various stages of menopause.

References

Robinson. B., (2011). Understanding and Treating Menopause from a Western Medical Perspective. Treating Women Academy: Online Menopause Masterclass: Online Menopause Masterclass. https://www.treatingwomen.com/store/5tpUJ3Fk

Moon, J-Y., Choi, MH., Kim, J., (2016). Metabolic profiling of cholesterol and sex steroid hormones to monitor urological diseases, PMC US National Library of Medicine, National Institutes of Health, Endocrine-Related Cancer: Endocr Relat Cancer. 2016 Oct; 23(10): R455–R467. Published online 2016 Oct 1. doi: 10.1530/ERC-16-0285. https://www.ncbi.nlm.nih.gov/pmc/articles/PMC5064754

Mesen, TB., Young, SL., (2015). Progesterone and the luteal phase: a requisite to reproduction. National Library of Medicine, National Center for Biotechnology Information : HHS Public Access, Author Manuscript: Published online 2015 Jan 5. doi: 10.1016/j.cgc.2014.10.003. https://www.ncbi.nlm.nih.gov/pmc/articles/PMC4436586

Regidor, P-A., (2014). Progesterone in Peri- and Postmenopause: A Review, PMC US National Library of Medicine, National Institutes of Health, Geburtshilfe und Frauenheilkunde, Thieme: Geburtshilfe Frauenheilkd. 2014 Nov; 74(11): (pp 995–1002). doi: 10.1055/s-0034-1383297 https://www.ncbi.nlm.nih.gov/pmc/articles/PMC4245250

Nedresky, D., Singh, G., (2021). Physiology, Luteinizing Hormone, NCBI StatPearls [Internet]. https://www.ncbi.nlm.nih.gov/books/NBK539692

Orlowski, M., Sarao, MS., (2021). Physiology, Follicle Stimulating Hormone, NCBI, StatPearls [Internet]. https://www.ncbi.nlm.nih.gov/books/NBK535442

Gass, MLS., Rebar, RW., (2008). The Menopause, The Global Library of Women's Medicine's 10.3843/GLOWM.10079 https://www.glowm.com/section_view/heading/TheMenopause/item/79

Gruijters, MJG., Visser, JA., Durlinger, ALL., et al, (2003). Anti-Müllerian hormone and its role in ovarian function, NIH, National Library of Medicine, National Center for Biotechnology Information: Mol Cell Endocrinol 2003 Dec 15;211(1-2):(pp 85-90). doi: 10.1016/j.mce.2003.09.024. https://www.ncbi.nlm.nih.gov/pubmed/14656480

Chada, M., Prusa, R., Bronský, J., et al. (2003). Inhibin B, follicle stimulating hormone, luteinizing hormone, and estradiol and their relationship to the regulation of follicle development in girls during childhood and puberty, NIH, National Library of Medicine, National Center for Biotechnology Information: Physiol Res. 003;52(3):(pp 341-6). https://pubmed.ncbi.nlm.nih.gov/12790766/

2.3 Menopausal Hormone Therapy

The idea that a chemical communication system exists within the body originated in the mid-19th century, although the term 'hormone' was not used until 1905. Ernest Starling, a professor at University College London, first defined the word, which he derived from the Greek meaning "to arouse or excite."

In the 1920s, American scientists Edgar Allen and Edward Doisy began work on isolating and purifying estrogen. Meanwhile, in Germany, Adolph Butenandt was simultaneously carrying out the same work and rushed his manuscript to print, winning the Nobel Prize for his efforts. The first estrogen to be purified and crystallized was estrone, followed somewhat later by estradiol and estriol. Since then, the study of female endocrinology has led to significant medical advances, including hormonal contraception, artificial reproductive technology (ART), and menopausal hormone therapy (MHT), formerly known as hormone replacement therapy (HRT).

Interestingly, doctors had unknowingly been using hormone therapy for years before estrogen was identified. In the 1880s, Robert Bartley discovered that performing oophorectomies led to hot flashes and vaginal atrophy in his patients. Then, in 1897, Hubert Fosbery successfully used ovarian extracts to treat a patient with hot flashes.

Indeed, it seems that the medicinal use of endocrine gland extracts dates back even further than this. It is thought that Sun Si Miao used animal thyroid extracts to treat goitre as early as the 7th century. It is also reported that during the 11th century, the Chinese used concentrated urine extracts to treat hypogonadism and dysmenorrhea.

The history of MHT as we know it began in the 1940s. It was during this decade that Premarin was developed, a conjugated equine estrogen product derived from the urine of pregnant mares. At around the same time, the American Food and Drug Administration (FDA) approved diethylstilbestrol, a synthetic form of estrogen.

Between the 1940s and 1970s, the use of MHT increased exponentially. It was marketed as a solution to hot flashes and urogenital symptoms, and to prevent bone loss. However, during the 1970s, it became apparent that unopposed estrogen therapy increased the risk of endometrial cancer and its popularity waned. In the 1980s, it was discovered that combining estrogen with a progesterone reduced this risk significantly, precipitating a brief MHT revival lasting into the 1990s.

However, this revival did not last long as the large-scale Women's Health Initiative (WHI) study cast the shadow of doubt over MHT's safety once more. In 2002, it reported that the risks of MHT outweighed the benefits, citing an increased incidence of coronary heart disease and breast cancer in women with intact uteri. This created a sense of panic among doctors and patients alike, and the prescribing of MHT drastically declined.

The WHI has since been criticised for both its methodology and reporting. One of the study's major limitations was that most participants were asymptomatic and more than a decade past their final menstrual period. Therefore, the results hold little relevance for younger, symptomatic women.

Although the use of MHT remains controversial, it is now widely accepted that for many symptomatic women under the age of 60, or within 10 years of their final menstrual period, the benefits outweigh the risks.

MHT may also offer significant protection against bone loss and fractures, providing it is administered at the right time.

One of the main advantages of using MHT is symptom reduction, including:

- Vasomotor symptoms
- Sleep disorders
- Urogenital dryness and atrophy
- Musculoskeletal pain

The best time to begin MHT for osteopenia and osteoporosis prevention is before the age of 60, or within 10 years of the final period. Furthermore, it is generally recommended that women with premature ovarian insufficiency receive MHT until at least the age of natural menopause.

Safety

There are numerous guidelines regarding the safe use of MHT. Some of the many factors that prescribers must consider include:

- Non-hysterectomized women should receive combined MHT, including a progestogen to protect the endometrium. Estrogen monotherapy is suitable for hysterectomized women.
- Estrogen therapy can increase the risk of thrombosis when taken orally, although the risk is still low overall. Women with additional risk factors, such as smoking or obesity, should use transdermal MHT instead of oral medication.
- MHT is contraindicated in women with pre-existing breast cancer.
- Perimenopausal women should use oral hormonal contraception (if appropriate) until they reach menopausal age and then transition to MHT if necessary.

Types of MHT

Most people associate MHT with estrogens and progestogens. Estrogens include conjugated equine estrogen and estradiol. Meanwhile, progestogens can be natural micronized progesterone or synthetic progestins; norethisterone acetate, levonorgestrel, medroxyprogesterone, and dydrogesterone.

There may also be some advantages to replacing testosterone at an appropriate dosage. They include improving libido and arousal.

Furthermore, there are different ways to administer MHT, including oral tablets, transdermal patches, and gels. Each presents its own advantages and disadvantages.

For more information see Appendix 2, page 369 A Practitioner's Toolkit for Managing the Menopause.

Oral Estrogen

Advantages	Disadvantages
• Offers a convenient way to use MHT • Reliable absorption rates	• Increased risk of thrombosis • Increased risk of gallstones • Increases sex hormone-binding globulin (SHBG) levels and decreases free testosterone • Increases thyroid-binding globulin (TBG) levels. Women taking levothyroxine may need to adjust their dosage • Higher total dose than transdermal estradiol

Transdermal Estradiol (Patches or Gel)

Advantages	Disadvantages
• Increased convenience (once or twice weekly patch changes) • No changes in SHBG or TBG • Little increased risk of thrombosis • Lower total dose than oral estrogen	• Patches may cause discomfort and skin irritation • Gel may be difficult to apply • Less reliable absorption than oral estrogen • Compliance issues: patch changes may be forgotten, etc.

Progestogen

Advantages	Disadvantages
• Protects endometrium and is necessary for non-hysterectomized women • Available in a wide variety of preparations (oral tablets, creams, intrauterine devices) • Transdermal products may alleviate some symptoms with sufficient dosage	• Long-term benefits and safety of transdermal progestogen are unclear • Micronized progestin is considered safer than synthetic progestin in terms of breast cancer and cardiovascular disease risk

Side Effects of MHT

Aside from the potential risks mentioned above, MHT can cause several less serious side effects. Some common side effects of estrogen replacement therapy include:
Nausea | Headaches | Breast tenderness

It is, therefore, advisable for women to start MHT with the lowest dose possible and only increase it if necessary. These side effects are less likely to occur with transdermal preparations compared with oral tablets. The side effects of progestin therapy include:
Low mood | Irritability

Furthermore, the side effects of combined MHT include irregular and potentially heavy vaginal bleeding. Any unexpected bleeding should be investigated, especially if it persists for 3–6 months after initiating therapy. All women taking synthetic MHT should have a medical review every six months, regardless.

Finally, MHT can increase the risk of breast cancer and is unsuitable for women with or at high risk of the condition. See Chapter 2.7. Breast Health for further details.

Bioidentical Hormones

Bioidentical hormone therapy has become more popular in recent years. The term refers to a wide range of products with chemical structures identical to human hormones. They are natural or plant-derived and may be compounded, containing several different hormones.

Many plant-based products are manufactured using diosgenin, a steroidal sapogenin extracted from several species, including *Dioscorea* (yams) *Trigonella* (fenugreek), *Costus* (spiral flag), and *Smilax* (a large genus, including greenbriers, sarsaparilla, and Tu Fu Ling, among others). The compound is used as the basis for numerous pharmaceutical preparations, including sex hormones and corticosteroids. It has apparent anti-inflammatory, antioxidant, and neuroprotective properties and has been researched for a range of conditions. However, data from human clinical trials are lacking.

Many individuals perceive bioidentical hormone therapy as more natural and, therefore, safer than traditional MHT. However, there is currently insufficient evidence on its safety and long-term side effects. Moreover, while some products are licensed, many are not, meaning that their overall quality and potential to cause harm are unknown.

Other Pharmaceutical Treatments

Other medications that may help to relieve symptoms when used alongside, or instead of, MHT include:
Tibolone (not to be taken with other MHT) | Estrogen + selective estrogen receptor modulator (e.g. bazedoxifene) | Ospemifene | Selective serotonin reuptake inhibitors (SSRIs) | Clonidine Gabapentin | Stellate ganglion blockade

Summary

The decision of whether to take MHT or not is very personal. Your role as a clinician is to provide clear and up-to-date information to help patients decide for themselves which, if any, treatments may be useful. A referral to the patient's GP and gynecologist will allow them to discuss whether the benefits outweigh the risks and which options may be best suited to their individual needs.

References

Tata, JR., (2005). One hundred years of hormones, PMC US National Library of Medicine, National Institutes of Health, EMBO Reports. EMBO Rep. 2005 Jun; 6(6): (pp 490–496).doi:10.1038/sj.embor.7400444
https://www.ncbi.nlm.nih.gov/pmc/articles/PMC1369102/

Santen, RJ., Simpson, E., (2019). History of Estrogen: Its Purification, Structure, Synthesis, Biologic Actions, and Clinical Implications, Endocrinology, Volume 160, Issue 3, March 2019, (pp 605–625), doi.org/10.1210/en.2018-00529.
https://academic.oup.com/endo/article/160/3/605/5250672

Kohn, GE., Rodriguez, KM., Pastuszak. AW., (2020). The History of Estrogen Therapy, PMC US National Library of Medicine, National Institutes of Health: Sex Med Rev. 2019 Jul; 7(3):(pp 416–421). Published online 2019 May 27. doi: 10.1016/j.sxmr.2019.03.006.
https://www.ncbi.nlm.nih.gov/pmc/articles/PMC7334883/

Cagnacci, A., Venier, M., (2019). The Controversial History of Hormone Replacement Therapy, PMC US National Library of Medicine, National Institutes of Health: Medicina (Kaunas). 2019 Sep; 55(9): (pp 602). Published online 2019 Sep 18. doi: 10.3390/medicina55090602
https://www.ncbi.nlm.nih.gov/pmc/articles/PMC6780820/

Vinogradova, Y., Coupland, C., Hippisley-Cox, J., (2020). Use of hormone replacement therapy and risk of breast cancer: nested case-control studies using the QResearch and CPRD databases, The BMJ: BMJ 2020; (pp 371) doi: https://doi.org/10.1136/bmj.m3873 (Published 28 October 2020) Cite this as: BMJ 2020;371:m3873
https://www.bmj.com/content/371/bmj.m3873

Files, JA., Ko, MG., Pruthi, S., (2011). Bioidentical Hormone Therapy, PMC US National Library of Medicine, National Institutes of Health: Mayo Clinic Proceedings, Mayo Clin Proc. 2011 Jul; 86(7): (pp 673–680).
doi: 10.4065/mcp.2010.0714
https://www.ncbi.nlm.nih.gov/pmc/articles/PMC3127562/

Jesus, M., Martins, APJ., Gallardo, E,, et al. (2016). Diosgenin: Recent Highlights on Pharmacology and Analytical Methodology, PMC US National Library of Medicine, National Institutes of Health: Journal of Analytical Methods in Chemistry, J Anal Methods Chem. 2016; 2016: 4156293. Published online 2016 Dec 28. doi: 10.1155/2016/4156293
https://www.ncbi.nlm.nih.gov/pmc/articles/PMC5225340

2.4 Genetics and Epigenetics

In TCEAM genetics and epigenetics could be compared to pre-heavenly and post-heavenly jing.

Genetics is the study of heredity, a gene being a single inherited unit in a specific location on a chromosome. Each gene consists of nucleotide bases arranged in pairs in a linear fashion. Their functions include coding for a particular protein or protein segment which is responsible for a specific characteristic or physiological process.

Meanwhile, epigenetics is the study of how environmental and lifestyle factors influence gene function. While genetic changes are permanent, epigenetic changes are reversible and do not alter the DNA sequence. However, they can impact the way the DNA sequence is read and may be retained as an 'epigenetic memory' leading to heritable changes.

Genetics and epigenetics play an essential role in an individual's susceptibility to certain diseases. Furthermore, they can influence response to nutrients, medications, and drugs. Therefore, by understanding their unique genetic profile, patients can take a personalized approach to their own wellbeing, increasing the chances of remaining healthy during and after menopause.

Genetic testing is now available through a variety of organizations with sophisticated reporting of results which may provide useful insights into an individual's genetics. However, the results may be difficult to interpret and it is beyond most practitioners' scope of practice to do so. Therefore, it is advisable that patients consult a qualified geneticist in order to fully understand the implications of their results and how to modify their lifestyle accordingly.

Genetics

All humans share the same basic DNA sequence. It consists of 23 chromosomes, containing approximately three billion nucleotide base pairs. These base pairs consist of adenine and thymine, and guanine and cytosine.

The genetic differences that occur between individuals are the result of changes in these base pairs, commonly known as mutations. The most common genetic mutations are single nucleotide polymorphisms (SNPs – pronounced 'snips'). SNPs represent a mutation in a single nucleotide pair and each person's DNA contains 4-5 million. While SNPs do not cause diseases in themselves, they do represent a genetic predisposition to certain conditions as well as affecting a person's response to external factors, including nutrients, medications, and drugs.

Epigenetics

Epigenetics has been referred to as "the science of change." The term describes alterations in gene function that occur without changing the genetic sequence. These changes occur prenatally and throughout a person's entire lifespan, playing a crucial role in development and the aging process.

Epigenetic changes have been associated with many different diseases, including cognitive dysfunction, respiratory disease, cardiovascular disease, reproductive disorders, autoimmune disorders, psychiatric disorders, and almost all types of cancer.

Some of the factors that are thought to induce epigenetic changes include exposure to toxins (heavy metals, pesticides, tobacco smoke, diesel exhaust, polycyclic aromatic hydrocarbons (PAHs), etc.), hormones, radioactivity, viruses, bacteria, and basic nutrients.

There are many types of epigenetic changes, but the best known is DNA methylation.

DNA Methylation

DNA methylation involves the addition or removal of a methyl (CH_3) group, predominantly at cytosine nucleotide bases, and especially when two of these bases occur consecutively. DNA methylation has been observed in cancer and many other conditions.

Methylation is a process that controls gene expression, turning specific genes on and off, without altering the overall DNA sequence. It is a dynamic process although some patterns are retained, leading to heritable epigenetic changes.

Among its many functions, methylation regulates protein synthesis and hormone metabolism. It can be influenced by genetic SNPs and modifiable factors such as diet. Abnormal methylation can lead to chronic diseases including cancer, autoimmune disorders, metabolic syndrome, and neurological disorders. It has also been implicated in the aging process and appears to be one of many factors that influence the timing of menopause and longevity.

Researchers have proposed the existence of an 'epigenetic clock' based on an individual's levels of DNA methylation. It seems that this phenomenon may play a role both in determining the age of menopause and the rate of aging, in general. Furthermore, early menopause, surgical menopause, and longer time since menopause are all associated with accelerated epigenetic aging, suggesting that the relationship may be bidirectional.

Gene symbol	Variant(s)	Environmental exposure	Outcome and nature of interaction
Genes for skin pigmentation *(for example, MC1R)*	Variants for fair skin color	Sunlight or ultraviolet light B	Risk of skin cancer is higher in people with fair skin color that are exposed to higher amounts of sunlight
CCR5	Δ-32 deletion	HIV	Carriers of the receptor deletion have lower rates of HIV infection and disease progression
MTHFR	Ala222Val polymorphism	Folic acid intake	Homozygotes for the low activity Ala222Val variant are at different risk of colorectal cancer and adenomas if nutritional folate status is low
NAT2	Rapid versus slow acetylator SNPs	Heterocyclic amines in cooked meat	Red meat intake is more strongly associated with colorectal cancer among rapid acetylators
F5	Leiden prothrombotic variant	Hormone replacement	Venous thromboembolism risk is increased in factor V Leiden carriers who take exogenous steroid hormones
UGT1A6	Slow-metabolism SNPs	Aspirin	Increased benefit of prophylactic aspirin use in carriers of the slow metabolism variants
APOE	E4 allele	Cholesterol intake	Exaggerated changes in serum cholesterol in response to dietary cholesterol changes in APOE4 carriers
ADH1C	Y-2 alleles	Alcohol intake	Inverse association between ethanol intake and myocardial infarction; risk is stronger in carriers of slow-oxidizing Y-2 alleles
PPARG2	Pro12Ala	Dietary fat intake	Stronger relation between dietary fat intake and obesity in carriers of the Pro12Ala allele
HLA-DPB1	Glu69	Occupational beryllium	Exposed workers who are carriers of the Glu69 allele are more likely to develop chronic beryllium lung disease
TPMT	Ala154Thr and Tyr240Cys	Thiopurine drugs	Homozygotes for the low-activity alleles of TPMT are likely to experience severe toxicity when exposed to thiopurine drugs
ADRB2	Arg16Gly	Asthma drugs	Arg16Gly homozygotes have a greater response in the airway to albuterol

Figure 2.4a: Tables of SNPs and diseases.[8]

[8] Table Source: Craig, J. (2008) Complex diseases: Research and applications. Nature Education 1(1):184. Sourced July 2022. https://www.nature.com/scitable/topicpage/complex-diseases-research-and-applications-748

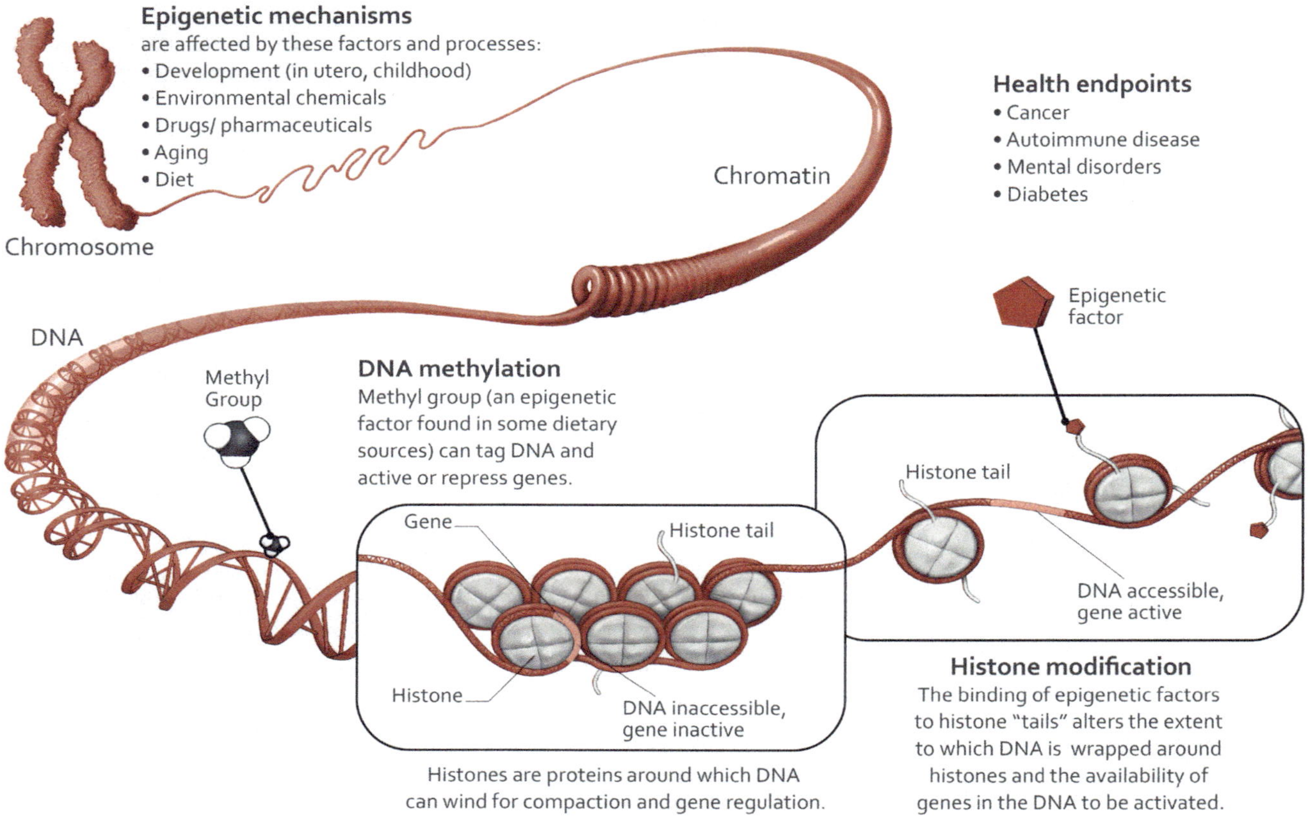

Figure 2.4b: A scientific illustration of how epigenetic mechanisms can affect health.[9]

Summary

Understanding one's genetic makeup can help individuals predict which chronic diseases they may be likely to develop and make appropriate lifestyle changes to reduce their risk of doing so.

By also taking into account the factors that can contribute to harmful epigenetic changes, individuals are empowered to take the necessary steps to maximize their chances of living a long and healthy life.

[9] Image source: National Institutes of Health, A Scientific Illustration of How Epigenetic Mechanisms Can Affect Health. Sourced July 2022. http://commonfund.nih.gov/epigenomics/figure.aspx

References

Journal of Human Genetics, (2007). SNPs in disease gene mapping, medicinal drug development and evolution: J Hum Genet 52, (pp 871–880) (2007).
https://doi.org/10.1007/s10038-007-0200-z. https://www.nature.com/articles/jhg2007117#Tab1

CDC, Centres for Disease Control and Prevention. (Sourced January 2021). What is Epigenetics?
https://www.cdc.gov/genomics/disease/epigenetics.htm

NIH, National Human Genome Research Institute. (Sourced January 2021). What is a genome?
https://www.genome.gov/human-genome-project/Completion-FAQ

NIH, National Library of Medicine, Medline Plus. (Sourced January 2021). What are single nucleotide polymorphisms (SNPs)?: Home > Genetics > Help Me Understand Genetics > Genomic Research > What are single nucleotide polymorphisms (SNPs)?
https://ghr.nlm.nih.gov/primer/genomicresearch/snp

Kim, M., Costello, J., (2017). DNA methylation: an epigenetic mark of cellular memory, EEM, Experimental & Molecular Medicine: Exp Mol Med 49, e322 (2017). https://doi.org/10.1038/emm.2017.10.
https://www.nature.com/articles/emm201710

Levine, ME., Lu, AT., Chen, BH., et al. (2016). Menopause accelerates biological aging, PHAS Proceedings of the National Academy of Sciences of the United States of America: PNAS August 16, 2016 113 (33) (pp 9327-9332); first published July 25, 2016 https://doi.org/10.1073/pnas.1604558113.
https://www.pnas.org/content/113/33/9327

Jin, BJ., Robertson, KD., (2011). Epigenetics: The Science of Change, PMC US National Library of Medicine, National Institutes of Health, ehp Environmental Health Perspectives: Environ Health Perspect. 2006 Mar; 114(3): A160–A167. doi: 10.1289/ehp.114-a160.
https://www.ncbi.nlm.nih.gov/pmc/articles/PMC1392256

Yoo, JW., Jones, PA., (2013). Cancer Genetics and Epigenetics: Two Sides of the Same Coin? PMC US National Library of Medicine, National Institutes of Health, HHS Public Access, Author Manuscript: Cancer Cell. Author manuscript; available in PMC 2013 Jul 10. Published in final edited form as: Cancer Cell. 2012 Jul 10; 22(1): (pp 9–20). doi: 10.1016/j.ccr.2012.06.008.
https://www.ncbi.nlm.nih.gov/pmc/articles/PMC3396881

Jin, B., Robertson, KD., (2011). DNA Methylation, Superior or Subordinate in the Epigenetic Hierarchy? PMC US National Library of Medicine, National Institutes of Health Genes & Cancer: Genes Cancer. 2011 Jun; 2(6): (pp 607–617). doi: 10.1177/1947601910393957.
https://www.ncbi.nlm.nih.gov/pmc/articles/PMC3174260

Lu, S., Niu, Z., Chen, Y., et al. (2018). Repetitive Element DNA Methylation is Associated with Menopausal Age. PMC US National Library of Medicine, National Institutes of Health, A&D Aging and Disease: Aging Dis. 2018 Jun; 9(3): (pp 435–443). Published online 2018 Jun 1. doi: 10.14336/AD.2017.0810.
https://www.ncbi.nlm.nih.gov/pmc/articles/PMC5988598

Bacon, ER., Mishra, A., Wang, Y., et al. (2020). Neuroendocrine Aging Precedes Perimenopause and is Regulated by DNA Methylation, PMC US National Library of Medicine, National Institutes of Health, HHS Public Access, Author Manuscript: Neurobiol Aging. Author manuscript; available in PMC 2020 Apr 2. Published in final edited form as: Neurobiol Aging. 2019 Feb; 74: (pp 213–224). Published online 2018 Oct 5. doi: 10.1016/j.neurobiolaging.2018.09.029.
https://www.ncbi.nlm.nih.gov/pmc/articles/PMC7117064

2.5 Medical and Surgical Menopause

Some women undergo premature or early menopause as a result of medical treatment or surgery. This is known as induced or iatrogenic menopause.

Although its underlying physiology differs from that of natural menopause, its clinical features are essentially the same. However, some symptoms, such as hot flashes, may be more severe in iatrogenic menopause compared to its natural equivalent. Furthermore, as with spontaneous premature ovarian insufficiency (POI), there may be an increased risk of post-menopausal diseases due to prolonged absence of estrogen.

Induced menopause can also have a significant psychological impact, including that of the primary illness, undergoing treatment, and menopause as a consequence. In some cases, psychological distress can be further amplified by infertility as a result of treatment. This may lead to feelings of remorse and grief if a woman has not previously conceived and wished to do so.

Medical menopause can be reversible but, in many cases, it is permanent. It is more likely to be reversible in women under 40 but still plays a major role in primary and secondary infertility.

Of course, all of these issues may become insignificant when dealing with a potentially terminal diagnosis such as cancer. Patients will likely require considerable emotional as well as physical support and it is essential to be sensitive yet realistic when discussing expected treatment outcomes.

Definitions

The distinction between surgical and medical menopause is an important one. The two terms can be defined as follows:

Medical Menopause
Menopause due to pharmaceutical drugs that cause POI, including the chemotherapy drugs cyclophosphamide, cisplatin, and doxorubicin.

Surgical Menopause
Menopause due to removal of the female reproductive organs and pelvic radiation therapy.

Surgical Menopause

There are several different procedures that may lead to surgical menopause, outlined below:

Procedure	Description	Reason
Oophorectomy	Removal of one (unilateral oophorectomy) or both (bilateral oophorectomy) ovaries	Ovarian, cervical, and endometrial (uterine) cancer Endometriosis BRCA gene mutations Benign tumors Cysts Ectopic pregnancy Pelvic inflammatory disease Tubo-ovarian abscess Torsion of the ovary Chronic pelvic pain
Radical (or total) hysterectomy	Removal of the uterus and ovaries	Uterine fibroids Uterine prolapse Cancer of the uterus, cervix, or ovaries Endometriosis Abnormal vaginal bleeding Chronic pelvic pain Adenomyosis
Abdominoperineal Resection (APR)	Removal of the lower colon and rectum, it can also include partial or total removal of the uterus and ovaries, as well as the rear wall of the vagina.	Colon cancer Rectal cancer
Total pelvic exenteration	Removal of pelvic organs including the bladder, urethra, and part of the rectum and reproductive organs: i.e., the uterus, cervix, ovaries, fallopian tubes, and vagina	Recurrent cervical cancer not responsive to surgery and radiation

Table 2.5: Surgical interventions that cause premature menopause.

Medical Menopause and Cancer

The ovarian reserve is highly sensitive to chemotherapy and radiation therapy, which induce cell death and atresia (breakdown) of developing follicles. These treatments also damage blood vessels and promote inflammation.

The most common reason for undergoing chemotherapy or radiotherapy is cancer. However, chemotherapy may also be used in the treatment of some autoimmune disorders and hematological disorders, such as sickle cell disease.

Systemic MHT should be avoided in women living with, or in remission from, estrogen receptor positive cancers, including breast cancer and some other estrogen-dependent cancers. These are cancers in which the affected cells have estrogen receptors and become active when the hormone binds to them. This can alter gene expression and stimulate the cancerous cells to grow.

Alternative, non-hormonal methods of managing menopausal symptoms include cognitive behavioral therapy, hypnotherapy, selective serotonin reuptake inhibitors (SSRIs), serotonin noradrenaline reuptake inhibitors (SNRIs), clonidine, and gabapentin. Data on the safety of vaginal estrogen in these patients is currently lacking.

It is also worth noting that hormonal cancer treatments such as aromatase inhibitors and tamoxifen can cause menopause-like symptoms.

Aromatase Inhibitors

Aromatase inhibitors, including anastrozole, letrozole, and exemestane work by blocking the activity of aromatase, an enzyme responsible for the conversion of androgens to estrogens via a process known as demethylation. This process occurs in the skin, adrenal glands, muscle, and adipose tissue and is the primary estrogen production pathway in post-menopausal women.
It appears that some breast cancer cells also display aromatase activity, likely fueling the growth of estrogen-sensitive tumors. Side effects include:

• Hot flashes • Weakness • Arthritis or arthralgia • Osteoporosis and increased risk of fractures • Bone pain • Vaginal dryness • Sexual dysfunction • Uterine atrophy • Thromboembolic disease • Hypertension • Hyperlipidemia • Cardiac and cerebrovascular events • Insomnia • Nausea

Tamoxifen

Tamoxifen acts as a selective estrogen receptor modulator. It has both agonistic and antagonistic effects in different parts of the body, making it a highly patient-specific treatment. In breast tissue, it competes with estrogen for binding sites and, thus, reduces its activity.
Side effects include:

• Hot flashes • Weakness • Arthritis or arthralgia • Irregular menstruation • Vaginal discharge • Mood changes • Peripheral odema • Lymphedema • Hypertension • Increased risk of pulmonary embolism and stroke in high-risk patients • Increased risk of uterine and endometrial cancer

Gender Affirming Hormone Therapy

A growing number of people have a gender identity that differs from that assigned to them at birth. Some of these individuals opt to take gender affirming hormone therapy (GAHT) or undergo gender affirming surgery.

Transmen (i.e., individuals assigned female sex at birth but identifying as male) may take testosterone in order to masculinize their features. This results in decreased levels of estrogen and progesterone.

Transwomen (i.e., individuals assigned male sex at birth but idetifying as female) may take estrogen and anti-androgens in order to feminize their features. Withdrawing estrogen therapy or reductions in dose may result in menopause-like symptoms, such as hot flashes.

Although GAHT tends to have an overall positive influence on mood and mental health, the long-term effects of this treatment and how it impacts menopause are currently underexplored.

Summary

Various medical and surgical interventions can result in premature or early menopause, known as induced or iatrogenic menopause.

The symptoms of iatrogenic menopause may be more severe than those of its natural equivalent. Furthermore, the risk of post-menopausal diseases is increased. Therefore, using MHT or oral hormonal contraceptives until the age of natural menopause may be beneficial where appropriate. The patient's consultant should discuss the options with them prior to surgery or the initiation of treatment.

References

Robinson. B., (2011). Understanding and Treating Menopause from a Western Medical Perspective. Treating Women Academy: Online Menopause Masterclass.
https://www.treatingwomen.com/store/5tpUJ3Fk

Spears, N., Lopes, F., Stefansdottir, A., et al, (2019). Ovarian damage from chemotherapy and current approaches to its protection, Oxford Academic, Human Reproduction Update, Volume 25, (Issue 6), November-December 2019, (pp 673–693), https://doi.org/10.1093/humupd/dmz027.
https://academic.oup.com/humupd/article/25/6/673/5585503

Okeke, TC., Anyaehie, UB., Ezenyeaku, CC., (2013). Premature Menopause, amhsr, Annals of Medical & Health Sciences Research: Ann Med Health Sci Res. 2013 Jan-Mar; 3(1): (pp 90–95). doi: 10.4103/2141-9248.109458.
https://www.ncbi.nlm.nih.gov/pmc/articles/PMC3634232

Szabo, RA., Marino, JL., Hickey, M., (2019), Managing menopausal symptoms after cancer, Taylor Francis Online, Climacteric, Volume 22, 2019 – (Issue 6): Life after cancer for women. (pp 572-578).
https://www.tandfonline.com/doi/abs/10.1080/13697137.2019.1646718

Peters, A., Tadi, P., (2021). Aromatase Inhibitors, NCBI, StatPearls [Internet]. Treasure Island (FL): StatPearls Publishing; 2021 Jan-.
https://www.ncbi.nlm.nih.gov/books/NBK557856

Farrar, ME., Jacobs, TF., (2021), Tamoxifen, NCBI StatPearls [Internet], Treasure Island (FL): StatPearls Publishing; 2021 Jan-.
https://www.ncbi.nlm.nih.gov/books/NBK532905

Mohamed, S., Hunter, MS., (2019). Transgender women's experiences and beliefs about hormone therapy through and beyond mid-age: An exploratory UK study, PMC US National Library of Medicine, National Institutes of Health, International Journal of Transgenderism, Taylor & Francis: Int J Transgend. 2019; 20(1): (pp 98–107). Published online 2018 Oct 23. doi: 10.1080/15532739.2018.1493626.
https://www.ncbi.nlm.nih.gov/pmc/articles/PMC6831003

Nguyen, HB., Chavez, AM., Lipner, E., et al. (2018). Gender-Affirming Hormone Use in Transgender Individuals: Impact on Behavioral Health and Cognition, PMC US National Library of Medicine, National Institutes of Health, HHS Public Access, Author manuscript: Curr Psychiatry Rep. Author manuscript; available in PMC 2019 Jan 31. Published in final edited form as: Curr Psychiatry Rep. 2018 Oct 11; 20(12): (pp 110). Published online 2018 Oct 11. doi: 10.1007/s11920-018-0973-0.
https://www.ncbi.nlm.nih.gov/pmc/articles/PMC6354936

Nguyen, HB., Loughead, J., Lipner, E., et al. (2018). What has sex got to do with it? The role of hormones in the transgender brain, NIH, National Library of Medicine, National Center for Biotechnology Information, Neuropsychopharmacology: 2019 Jan; 44(1): (pp 22–37). Published online 2018 Jul 5. doi: 10.1038/s41386-018-0140-7.
https://www.ncbi.nlm.nih.gov/pmc/articles/PMC6235900

2.6 Premature Ovarian Insufficiency

The terms premature menopause, premature ovarian insufficiency (POI), and premature ovarian failure (POF), are often used interchangeably. However, POI is now considered more accurate as there have been cases of intermittent ovarian function (oligomenorrhea) and even spontaneous pregnancy among women diagnosed with this condition.

POI can be subcategorized into primary and secondary amenorrhea. The former is defined by the absence of menarche, possibly with abnormal ovarian development. The latter is defined by the cessation of ovarian function and premature follicle depletion before age 40.

The condition is associated with an increased risk of postmenopausal diseases as well as having a severe psychological impact due to its effects on fertility and family planning.

Pathophysiology

POI can occur for a variety of reasons and, in many cases, the underlying cause is unknown. However, there are several factors that appear to contribute to the pathophysiology of POI as detailed below.

In many cases, POI is iatrogenic and occurs as a result of chemotherapy, radiation therapy, or pelvic surgery.

Risk Factors

Genetics
Genetic mutations are one of the most common causes of POI. These mutations may occur on the X-chromosome (as is common in cases of primary amenorrhea), autosomes, or other genes. Women with a family history of menstrual irregularities appear to be at increased risk of POI.

Early Puberty
Early puberty (menarche before 11 years old) increases the risk of early menopause by as much as 80%. This figure is further increased if the woman has no children.

Infections
Several infectious diseases can cause inflammation and damage the ovaries, potentially leading to POI. Some common examples include mumps, varicella, cytomegalovirus, tuberculosis, malaria, and shigella.

Autoimmune Disorders
POI often occurs alongside various autoimmune disorders. Lymphocytic oophoritis (autoimmune inflammation of developing follicles) was first described in association with Addison's disease. However, POI may also affect people with thyroid disorders (Graves' and Hashimoto's disease), parathyroid disorders, and type 1 diabetes.

Exposure to Environmental Toxins
Exposure to environmental toxins, including cigarette smoke, PAHs - found in industries that produce or use coal tar, coke, or bitumen /asphalt, industrial chemicals, and household products may result in follicle damage and degeneration, leading to POI.

Diagnosis and Treatment

Young women experiencing oligomenorrhea or amenorrhea should undergo testing to determine the underlying cause. A diagnosis of POI can be confirmed by low levels of estrogens and inhibins, coupled with elevated LH and FSH levels, ultrasound, and histological examination of laparoscopic biopsies. Other possible causes of oligomenorrhea and amenorrhea should also be excluded.

Patients will usually be advised to take MHT or oral hormonal contraceptives (OHC) until the age of natural menopause, which may offer some protection against osteoporosis and other conditions that affect post-menopausal women. However, these treatments are not suitable for all patients, including those with estrogen-sensitive conditions, such as breast cancer.

Summary

POI, or premature menopause, is associated with an increased risk of post-menopausal complications due to the prolonged absence of estrogen. It can also have a significant psychological impact due to the loss of fertility at an earlier age than expected.

Patients should work closely with their gynecologist to develop a suitable treatment plan, including MHT or OHC where appropriate. It may also be beneficial to receive psychological support in order to express and explore the challenging emotions that may arise as a result of this diagnosis.

References

Mishra, GD., Pandeya, N., Dobson, AJ., et al. (2017). Early menarche, nulliparity and the risk for premature and early natural menopause, Oxford Academic, Human Reproduction: Human Reproduction, Volume 32, Issue 3, March 2017, (pp 679–686),
https://doi.org/10.1093/humrep/dew350
https://academic.oup.com/humrep/article/32/3/679/2937790

Ebrahimi, M., Asbagh, FA., (2011). Pathogenesis and Causes of Premature Ovarian Failure: An Update, International Journal of Fertility & Sterility. Int J Fertil Steril. 2011 Jul-Sep; 5(2): (pp 54–65). Published online 2011 Sep 23.
https://www.ncbi.nlm.nih.gov/pmc/articles/PMC4059950

Wang, H., Chen, H., Qin, Y., et al (2015). Risks associated with premature ovarian failure in Han Chinese women, Elsevier: Reproductive BioMedicine Online (2015) 30, (pp 401–407).
https://www.rbmojournal.com/article/S1472-6483(15)00006-1/pdf

Beck-Peccoz, P., Persani, L., (2006). Premature ovarian failure, Orphanet Journal of Rare Diseases Article number: 9 (2006). https://ojrd.biomedcentral.com/articles/10.1186/1750-1172-1-9

Komorowska, B., (2016). Autoimmune premature ovarian failure, PMC US National Library of Medicine, National Institutes of Health, Menopause Review, Przeglad Menopauzalny: Prz Menopauzalny. 2016 Dec; 15(4): (pp 210–214). Published online 2017 Feb 8. doi: 10.5114/pm.2016.65666.
https://www.ncbi.nlm.nih.gov/pmc/articles/PMC5327623

NICE (2015) Premature menopause (premature ovarian insufficiency), NICE National Institute for Health and Care Excellence. NICE guideline {NG23} Published: 12 November 2015 Last updated: 05 December 2019.
https://www.nice.org.uk/guidance/ng23/ifp/chapter/Premature-menopause-premature-ovarian-insufficienc

2.7 Breast Health

No discussion on women's health would be complete without a mention of breast health. The breasts are highly sensitive to hormonal fluctuations and undergo significant changes between puberty and menopause, as well as throughout each menstrual cycle.

Therefore, the incidence and nature of breast disorders vary greatly at different life stages.

Breast Anatomy

The breasts comprise milk-producing glands called lobules, and ducts that carry milk to the nipple. These structures are surrounded by connective and fatty tissues, collectively known as stroma.

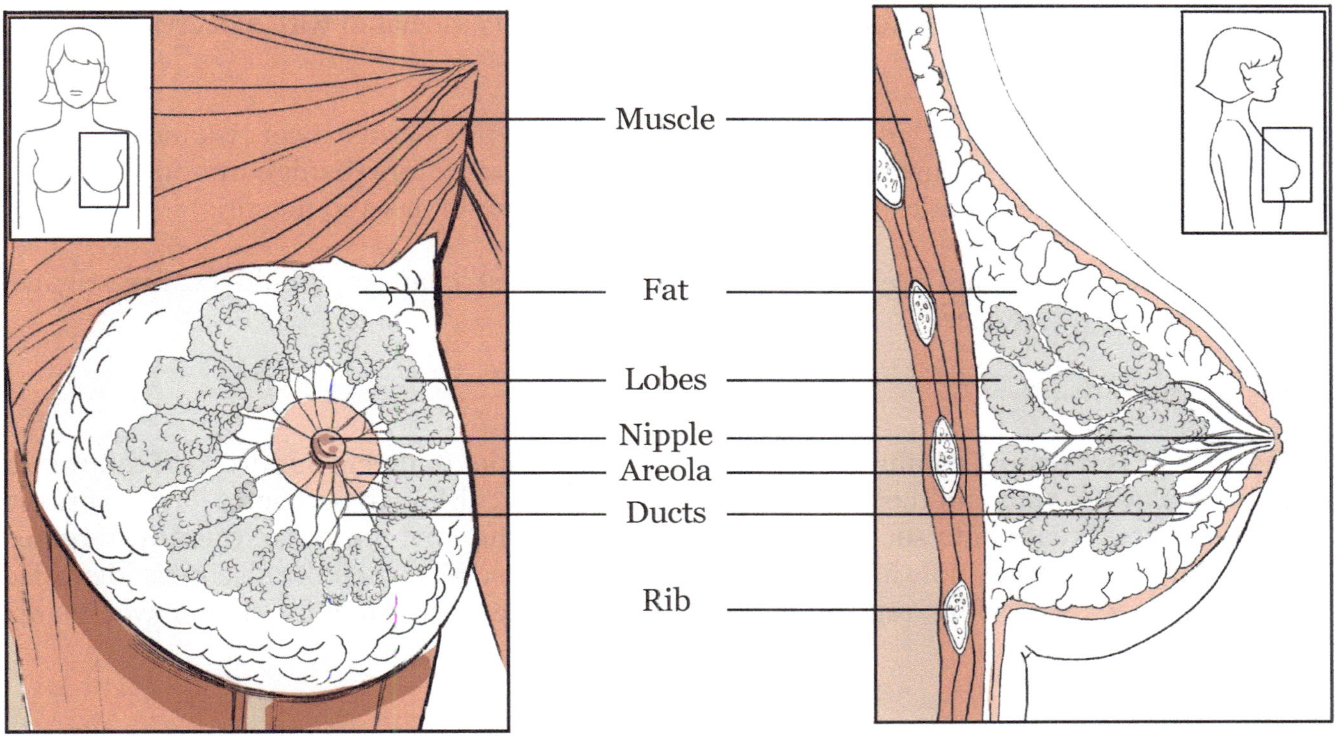

Figure 2.7a: Breast anatomy.

Ductal tissue development is initiated by increasing estrogen levels at puberty, while progesterone is responsible for ductal branching and lobulo-alveolar development. At maturity, these structures form a complex, branching network with 5-10 primary milk ducts, 20-40 segmental ducts, and 10-100 subsegmental ducts. Milk production is stimulated by the hormone prolactin, which is secreted by the pituitary gland during pregnancy and after birth.

Benign Breast Lesions

There can be substantial variations in breast composition between women. Some have a predominance of ducts, lobes, and stroma, whereas others have a predominance of fibrous tissues and cysts, known as fibrocystic changes. Fibrocystic changes can give the breasts an uneven and lumpy feel, which may cause some patients concern. However, these changes are extremely common, are not considered pathological, and do not increase the risk of breast cancer.

The breasts' composition changes with age as glandular tissue shrinks and is replaced by additional stroma and fatty tissue. Therefore, women may notice that their breasts become less firm and increasingly uneven following menopause. Again, this is not usually a cause for concern. In fact, the shrinkage of glandular tissue has been associated with a decreased risk of breast cancer.

Other benign breast lesions that are not associated with an increased cancer risk include:
• Periductal fibrosis • Hamartomas, lipomas, and phyllodes tumors (benign tumors)
• Neurofibromas • Traumatic lesions • Inflammation (granulomas and mastitis)

Although these conditions are not dangerous, any breast changes should be investigated promptly to rule out cancer.

Breast Cancer

Breast cancer is the most common form of cancer worldwide. It affects hundreds of thousands of individuals each year and the mortality rate is significant, although outcomes have improved in recent years. Treatments such as radiotherapy, chemotherapy, hormonal therapy, targeted therapy, and mastectomy now have a high success rate, especially when the disease is identified in its early stages. Therefore, regular self-checks and medical screening for eligible women are essential.

Pathophysiology

Breast cancer occurs due to DNA damage and genetic changes leading to abnormal cell growth. If the immune system is unable to control the growth of these cells, a tumor will develop and can metastasize if left untreated.

Breast cancer cells may be estrogen receptor-positive (ER+) or negative (ER-). ER+ cancer cells have estrogen receptors and are sensitive to the hormone's presence, further fueling their growth. ER+ cancers are most common in westernized countries, accounting for approximately 75% of cases.

Risk Factors

Gender

Female sex is the strongest risk factor for developing breast cancer, although it can also affect men.

Age

The risk of breast cancer increases with age and is most frequently diagnosed in the over 50s. While menopause is not a risk factor for breast cancer in itself, the incidence of the disease does increase markedly following menopause.

Genetics

Women with a family history of breast cancer have a higher risk of developing the disease, although most women with breast cancer do not have a known family history of it.

Mutations in the BRCA1, BRCA2, and PALB-2 genes increase the risk significantly, and risk reduction strategies, such as double mastectomy should be considered for these patients.

Breast Density

Having denser breast tissue (i.e., more glandular and less fatty tissue) increases the risk of breast cancer.

Breast Lesions

Some breast lesions in early life can increase the risk of going on to develop breast cancer. They include fibroadenomas, hyperplasia without atypia, papillomatosis, radial scars, blunt duct adenosis, and sclerosing adenosis.

Estrogen Exposure

Estrogen exposure is also a significant risk factor. Early menarche and late menopause can both prolong estrogen exposure and are considered risk factors, especially early menarche.

Estrogen-containing medicines, such as OHC and MHT can also increase the risk, as can nulliparity or late childbearing. Conversely, childbearing and breastfeeding are associated with a decreased risk of breast cancer.

Body Mass Index

Overweight and obese women tend to have enhanced estrogenic activity, thus increasing exposure to the hormone and their risk of breast cancer.

Lifestyle Factors

Smoking and excessive alcohol consumption can precipitate DNA changes and increase the risk of cancer in general.

Radiation

Exposure of the breasts or chest to radiation at an early age can increase the risk of breast cancer.

Breast Cancer and MHT

Much has been written about the correlation between MHT and breast cancer. Since estrogen exposure is a major risk factor, and MHT introduces exogenous estrogen to the body, it stands to reason that this treatment will have an impact.

There is strong evidence that MHT increases the risk of breast cancer, although numerous factors can influence the extent of the risk. The age of first use, duration of use, and type of MHT are the primary variables.

For example, older age at first use, longer duration of use, and combined MHT (estrogen + progestin) are associated with a greater risk of developing breast cancer. The type of progestin also appears to play a role, with norethisterone presenting the greatest risk and dydrogesterone presenting the lowest. The only form of MHT that does not appear to increase the risk of breast cancer at all is vaginal estrogen.

The risk decreases with time following the discontinuation of MHT, although it can remain elevated for up to 10 years, depending on the preparation. Therefore, MHT should be prescribed at the minimum effective dose and for the shortest duration possible, in order to minimize the risks.

Checking the Breasts

Historically, patients have been encouraged to check their breasts regularly and have any changes investigated as soon as possible. However, it has recently been suggested that this has limited value and does not appear to reduce the risk of breast cancer-specific or all-cause mortality in populations at average risk. As a result, the emphasis has shifted from recommending monthly self-examinations on a fixed schedule to promoting 'breast self-awareness', whereby all over-20s familiarize themselves with the normal appearance and feel of their breasts and report any changes.

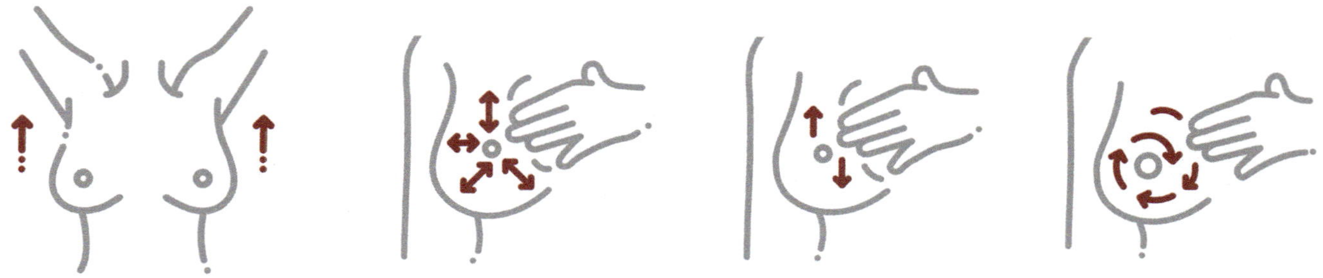

Figure 2.7b: Checking the breasts.

The most obvious sign of breast cancer is a lump in the breast or armpit. However, patients should also check for nipple retraction or discharge, dimpling, crusting, scaling, or flaking skin, swelling, and changes to the overall shape of the breast.

Summary

Understanding breast health is critical for patients and clinicians alike. Breast cancer affects thousands each year and has a significant mortality rate. Educating patients about the risk factors, signs, and symptoms of this disease, and encouraging them to perform regular self-checks and undergo screening where available can help to facilitate early diagnosis and treatment, delay disease progression, improve outcomes, and prevent unnecessary death.

References

Santen, RJ., (2018). Benign Breast Disease in Women, NCBI: Endotext [Internet]: Feingold KR, Anawalt B, Boyce A, et al., editors. South Dartmouth (MA): MDText.com, Inc.; 2000.
https://www.ncbi.nlm.nih.gov/books/NBK278994

World Health Organization. (2021). Breast Cancer,
https://www.who.int/news-room/fact-sheets/detail/breast-cancer

Dall, GV., Britt, KL., (2017). Estrogen Effects on the Mammary Gland in Early and Late Life and Breast Cancer Risk, Frontiers in Oncology: Front. Oncol., 26 May 2017 |
https://doi.org/10.3389/fonc.2017.00110
https://www.frontiersin.org/articles/10.3389/fonc.2017.00110/full

Surakasula, A., Nagarjunapu, GC., Raghavaiah, KV., (2014). A comparative study of pre- and post-menopausal breast cancer: Risk factors, presentation, characteristics and management, Journal of Research in Pharmacy Practice: J Res Pharm Pract. 2014 Jan-Mar 3(1): (pp 12–18). doi: 10.4103/2279-042X.132704
https://www.ncbi.nlm.nih.gov/pmc/articles/PMC4078652

Beral, V., Peto, R., Pirie, K., et al (2019). Type and timing of menopausal hormone therapy and breast cancer risk: individual participant meta-analysis of the worldwide epidemiological evidence, The Lancet: Volume 394, Issue 10204, (pp 1159-1168), September 28, 2019
https://www.thelancet.com/journals/lancet/article/PIIS0140-6736(19)31709-X/fulltext

Vinogradova, Y. (2020). Use of hormone replacement therapy and risk of breast cancer: nested case-control studies using the QResearch and CPRD databases, The BMJ: BMJ 2020; 371 doi:
https://doi.org/10.1136/bmj.m3873
(Published 28 October 2020) Cite this as: BMJ 2020;371:m3873.
https://www.bmj.com/content/371/bmj.m3873

Cameron, AM., (2020). Screening for Breast Cancer, Breast Self Examination, Science Direct, from Abeloff's Clinical Oncology, (6th edition).
https://www.sciencedirect.com/topics/medicine-and-dentistry/breast-self-examination

SECTION 3 - Menopause in Traditional Chinese and East Asian Medicine

«Wanting to illuminate bright virtue under heaven, the ancients first governed their states. Wanting to govern their states, they first put their families in order. Wanting to put their families in order, they first cultivated their body. Wanting to cultivate their body, they first rectified their heart. Wanting to rectify their heart, they first made their intentions sincere. Wanting to make their intentions sincere, they first extended their knowledge. The extension of knowledge lies in the investigation of things.»

Confucius, Great Learning (Da Xue), 5th Century BCE.

Source: Deadman, P., (2016). Live Well, Live Long: Teachings from the Chinese Nourishment of Life Tradition and Modern Research. The Journal of Chinese Medicine Ltd: Hove, England.

3.1 Traditional Chinese and East Asian Medicine Perspectives

Menopause is a natural phenomenon rather than a pathology. Therefore, every person experiences it differently, making it difficult to determine a one-size-fits-all approach to treatment. This is one of the major advantages of TCEAM, as these practices are far more flexible than allopathic medicine, allowing treatments to be tailored to meet the individual patient's needs. Even so, many practitioners tend to focus on treating one particular aspect of menopause - Kidney deficiency.

It is widely accepted that Kidney qi declines with age and that this can impact both Kidney yin and Kidney yang. However, the idea that declining Kidney qi equates to declining estrogen levels is a relatively modern one. It arose during the 1950s and 60s as Chinese doctors came under pressure to standardize their treatments and correlate TCEAM concepts with biomedical science.

Historically, there were no specific references to menopausal symptoms in Chinese medicine texts. This could possibly be due to the fact that East Asian women tend to experience fewer troublesome symptoms than their western counterparts and perhaps historically were not long-lived.

The first mention of menopause as a specific 'medical problem' did not occur until 1964. Prior to this, its symptoms were simply categorized according to their etiology and characteristics. Some common examples include visceral agitation (sometimes translated as hysteria), lily disease (*baihe bing*), metrorrhagia and metrostaxis, palpitations, and insomnia.

It is interesting to note that the primary focus was on emotional manifestations rather than physical symptoms like hot flashes.

Although the term *chaore*, meaning 'tidal heat effusion,' can be used to describe hot flashes, its historical use was far more general and did not relate specifically to menopause. Brian Grosam, PhD, LAc suggests that hot flashes are, in fact, 'bursts of qi' that occur as the body attempts to regain balance in a state of fluctuating yin and yang.

Another point of interest is that Japanese Kampo and traditional Korean and Taiwanese medicine approach menopause treatment very differently from Chinese traditions, despite having the same origins. For example, in Kampo there is no focus on Kidney deficiency. In fact, symptoms are more frequently seen as being a sign of excess than deficiency. It has been suggested that this healing system views menopausal symptoms as primarily the result of autonomic nervous system dysregulation rather than estrogen deficiency. Therefore, it is perhaps unsurprising that there is little overlap between the Kampo and Chinese formulas prescribed for menopausal women.

The Role of the Zang Organs

The link between the Kidneys and the reproductive hormones likely stems from the description of the seven and eight-year cycles of development described in Chapter 1 of the *Su Wen*. But other crucial features mentioned in this chapter, such as the role of the *renmai*, *chongmai*, and the *yangming*, are often overlooked.

Furthermore, the other *zang* organs, especially the Spleen, Liver, and Heart are also implicated in many pathologies that occur during and after menopause. Of course, all of these organs have a close relationship with the Kidneys, but it is essential that practitioners do not ignore the distinct role that each one of them plays.

"During their childhood, before they menstruate [and are fertile], women's [physiology] is subordinated to the lesser yin [i.e. the Kidneys]. When they menstruate [and are fertile] it is subordinated to the terminal yin [i.e. the Liver]. When menstruation [and fertility] ceases, it is subordinated to the greater yin [i.e. the Spleen]." [10]

This description suggests that many of the pathologies that occur in association with menopause are due to a decline in Spleen function. Indeed, many post-menopausal conditions involve pathogenic phlegm, the result of inadequate transformation and transportation of food essences. The problem is likely to be exacerbated further by the poor eating habits and unhealthy diets that are so commonplace in modern society.

It is also vital not to overlook the role of the Liver and Blood. Women lose a significant amount of Blood each month during menstruation, while pregnancy and childbirth deplete the Blood further. By the time a woman reaches middle age, her reserves will likely be greatly diminished. Since Blood is a yin substance, Blood deficiency can be considered a form of yin deficiency, potentially leading to empty heat and dryness. The Blood also houses the *shen*, meaning that Blood deficiency leads to *shen* disturbance and the emotional symptoms that are so common throughout the menopausal transition.

Finally, the Heart is often intricately involved in the development of menopausal symptoms. It has a close relationship with the Kidney, since the Kidney governs water (yin) and the Heart governs fire (yang). The Heart relies on Kidney yin to balance Heart yang and nourish Heart yin, while the Kidney relies on Heart yang to warm Kidney yang and generate Kidney yin. Disharmony between the Heart and Kidney is at the root of many menopausal symptoms.

[10] Wang Ketang, cited by Scheid, V., (2007). Traditional Chinese medicine—What are we investigating? The case of menopause., PMC US National Library of Medicine, National Institutes of Health, Complementary Therapies in Medicine : 2007, 10.10162/j.ctim.2005.12.002 https://www.ncbi.nlm.nih.gov/pmc/articles/PMC2233879

Etiological Factors

Menopause is not a disease and, therefore, cannot be considered as having an etiology in the ordinary sense of the word. However, there are several etiological factors that can contribute to the development of menopausal symptoms from a TCEAM perspective:

Emotional stress

Long-term worry, anger, fear, anxiety, sadness, shock, pensiveness, guilt, and shame can all weaken the Kidney, leading to yin deficiency. These issues are exacerbated by physical and mental overwork, which is so common in modern society.

A more detailed discussion of the specific stressors that may occur at this stage of life can be found in Chapter 5.2. Stress, Trauma and Stress Resistance.

Overwork

Working long hours without sufficient rest and long commutes to and from work can also tax the Kidney. Overwork is also often associated with irregular eating habits and emotional stress, which harm the Spleen and Liver, respectively.

Sexual Activity and Childbearing

Excessive sexual activity is often considered a cause of disease in TCEAM. Frequent orgasms, without sufficient recovery time, deplete Kidney yin and essence. Most practitioners see this phenomenon as more applicable to men who lose essence with every ejaculation. However, it can also affect women. Engaging in intercourse when intoxicated, tired, or otherwise unwell is particularly harmful.

Giving birth to too many children, too close together can also damage the uterus, leading to significant loss of Kidney yin and essence.

Smoking

In TCEAM terms, tobacco is considered a hot, pungent, drying, and toxic substance with no medicinal effect. Smoking injures both the Lungs and Kidneys, burning *jing* and leading to Kidney yin deficiency. It also damages the throat and Stomach, exhausts Blood, and injures *shen*.

Irregular diet

This includes irregular eating habits and overconsumption of sweet, greasy, and fried foods, bread, and dairy which lead to phlegm. Phlegm accumulation is one of the primary patterns underlying premature ovarian insufficiency and many post-menopausal conditions. Furthermore, overconsumption of caffeine and alcohol may lead to excess heat and aggravate vasomotor symptoms.

Summary

Hopefully, this preface highlights some of the complexities involved in the diagnosis and treatment of menopausal symptoms.

The following chapters are based on the teachings of highly experienced practitioners, including Giovanni Maciocia, Brian Grosam, Bob Flaws, Honora Lee Wolfe, Julian Scott, Rebecca Averne, and Anastacïa White. However, these treatment plans should be viewed as foundations to be built upon depending on each patient's unique presentation. There is no substitute for a practitioner's own observational and questioning skills when formulating an accurate diagnosis and treatment plan.

References

Grosam, B., (2021). Understanding and Treating Hot Flashes in Menopause with Chinese Medicine. Singing Dragon. London and Philadelphia.

Scheid, V., (2007). Traditional Chinese medicine—What are we investigating? The case of menopause., PMC US National Library of Medicine, National Institutes of Health, Complementary Therapies in Medicine : 2007, 10.10162/j.ctim.2005.12.002
https://www.ncbi.nlm.nih.gov/pmc/articles/PMC2233879 Cite: Wang Ketang.

Yu, Q., (2018). Traditional Chinese medicine: perspectives on and treatment of menopausal symptoms, Taylor & Francis Online: Climacteric, Volume 21, 2018 - Issue 2.
https://www.tandfonline.com/doi/full/10.1080/13697137.2018.1434983

Scheid, V., Tuffrey, V., Bovey, M., (2017), Chinese Herbal Medicine for Treating Menopausal Symptoms in London Women: Developing a Good Practice Protocol via the Factor Analysis of Prescribing Patterns in a Clinical Study, University of Westminster: WestminsterResearch: 10.1016/j.ctim.2017.03.008
https://core.ac.uk/outputs/161106244

Dharmananda, S. (Sourced January 2021). Towards a Spirit at Peace. Understanding the Treatment of Shen Disorders with Chinese Medicine, Chapter 6. ITM, Institute for Traditional Medicine.
http://www.itmonline.org/shen/

3.2 Jing (Essence) and Menopause

According to the *Su Wen* (Basic Questions) section of the Inner Canon of the Yellow Emperor (composed between 400 BCE and 260 CE), a woman's life can be divided into seven-year cycles which represent the unfolding of the 'Three Treasures' *jing*, *qi*, and *shen*.

The Three Treasures are three of the vital substances that are essential for sustaining human life. They can be defined as follows:

Jing (精): This vital substance is stored by the Kidney and maintains the body's physiological functions. It can be seen as a manifestation of Kidney yin. Also known as 'essence,' it can be further subdivided into pre-heavenly and post-heavenly *jing*.

Qi (气): Qi is most often translated as vital energy or life force. However, its Chinese character has a far broader range of interpretations, including gas, air, and breath. The meaning of the word can also change significantly when combined with other characters.

Shen (神): The term *shen* may be used to describe a supernatural being, immortal, or deity. In TCEAM terms, it is usually translated as the mind-spirit, which is housed within the Heart.

Seven-Year Cycles of Jing

The seven-year cycles discussed in the *Su Wen* relate primarily to *jing*. With a focus on the stages of reproductive development, the female cycle of *jing* theory ends at 49 years old. This is close to the age at which natural menopause occurs.

Cycle	Age in years	Su Wen Description
1	7	A girl's Kidney energy grows strong, the teeth change, and the hair grows longer and stronger.
2	14	The *renmai* (the sea of yin/essence) flows, and the qi and Blood in the *chongmai* (the sea of Blood) becomes prosperous. Menstruation (*tiangui*) arrives, and conception is possible.
3	21	Kidney energy is balanced, the adult teeth completely develop, and the body grows to full height.
4	28	The bones and muscles are strong, and the body is in optimal condition for reproduction.
5	35	Peak condition declines gradually. Energy in the *yangming* channel declines. The face starts withering, and the hair starts to lose lustre.
6	42	The three yang channels: *taiyang*, *yangming*, and *shaoyang*, begin to decline. The face wanes, and she starts to have white hair.
7	49+	The *renmai* and *chongmai* decline, menstruation dries up, and the physique declines. She is no longer able to conceive.

Table 3.2a: Seven-year cycles of jing.

Commentary

The first two seven-year periods are defined by an increase in Kidney qi, which allows for rapid growth and development. This includes the growth of hair and teeth in younger girls as well as the development of sexual characteristics at the onset of puberty.

The third and fourth seven-year periods are characterized by a surplus of Kidney qi, which levels out throughout a woman's 20s and early 30s. During this period, the wisdom teeth emerge and the bones and muscles reach their maximum strength.

From the fifth seven-year period onwards, a stage of gradual decline begins. First, the face begins to wrinkle and the hair thins and turns white. By the seventh seven-year period, a woman is no longer considered fertile.

Therefore, the general assumption is that puberty will occur at 14 years old (2 x 7 years) and menopause at 49 (7 x 7 years). Pregnancy and childbirth, on the other hand, could occur at any point in between, at multiple times, if at all.

Jing Deficiency: Premature Ovarian Insufficiency

Premature ovarian insufficiency (POI) can occur either due to Kidney yin or yang deficiency with or without Blood stasis, or qi and Blood deficiency with or without Blood stasis. The underlying pathology of these patterns is *jing* deficiency.

Jing deficiency may be constitutional and inherited from one's parents (pre-heavenly *jing* deficiency). In these cases, there may be a family history of premature or early menopause.

Alternatively, it may be the result of lifestyle factors (post-heavenly *jing* deficiency). For example, overwork, early or excessive sexual activity, drug and alcohol use, repeated ART cycles, recurrent miscarriages, chemotherapy or radiotherapy, surgery, and toxin exposure can deplete *jing*.

Finally, POI may also occur due to the accumulation and stagnation of phlegm.

A detailed description of these patterns and their associated symptoms can be found in Section 4 of this book.

> **Note:** Because of the repurposing of *jing* previously devoted to menstruation, many women find that they become forces to be reckoned with following menopause. The relative increase in Kidney yang allows them to act and communicate in a way that may not have been possible before, becoming more steadfast and vocal. It is perhaps no coincidence that some of the world's most powerful leaders have been post-menopausal women!

Childhood Illnesses Reoccurring in Menopause

According to pediatric acupuncturist Dr. Julian Scott, illnesses at different stages of childhood can reoccur in later life if left untreated. This makes menopausal women vulnerable to a resurgence of a previous illness or condition.

Childhood condition	Menopausal symptoms
Heat	Hot
Cold	Fibroids[11]
Damp	Sweating
Cranial compression	Migraines
Lingering pathogenic factors	Various
Damp-phlegm in Liver and Gallbladder	Hot flashes
Lingering pathogenic factor plus qi deficiency	Prolapse

Table 3.2b: Childhood conditions that can reoccur during menopause.

In the next section we discuss the two most problematic childhood conditions that may reoccur at menopause; lingering pathogenic factors, and damp-phlegm in the Liver and Gallbladder.

Lingering Pathogenic Factors

Lingering pathogenic factors (LPFs) arise from a childhood illness that was never fully cured or systemic damage due to childhood immunizations. LPFs sit in the channels, causing an echo of the original disease that comes and goes throughout a person's lifetime, usually during times of stress or when the immune system is compromized.

[11] The risk of fibroids actually decreases at menopause as they are related to estrogen (of course, this is complicated by MHT): Ulin, M., Ali, M., Chaudhry, ZT., (et al). (220). Uterine fibroids in menopause and perimenopause. NIH, National Library of Medicine, National Center for Biotechnology Information:
PMID: 31834160 PMCID: PMC6994343 DOI: 10.1097/GME.0000000000001438
https://pubmed.ncbi.nlm.nih.gov/31834160/

Thick Phlegm

One especially problematic consequence of LPFs is very thick phlegm which obscures the shen. Obscuring the shen causes a hazy connection to one's inner self, so "one cannot hear their inner voice pointing the way forward." This can cause one to move along the wrong path, pursue an unsuitable career, or stay in an unsatisfactory relationship, for example. The symptoms of thick phlegm can vary according to a person's age:

Age	Symptoms
2 years onwards	Symptoms of the original disease, skin problems, digestive problems
14–25 years	Glandular fever, self-harm
Fertile years	Chronic fatigue, depression, fibroids, food allergies
Menopause	Gallstones, migraine, panic attacks, mid-life crisis, divorce
Post-menopause	Arthritis, a wide range of issues

Table 3.2c: Age and varying symptoms of thick phlegm from LPFs.

Treatment for thick phlegm could include acupuncture at points including Baliao MHN-30, Ganshu BL-18, Pishu BL-20, Shenshu BL-23, Shenting DU-24.

It is also important to advise women to find a new outlet for creative energy. Failure to do this can cause palpitations, anxiety, and fatigue.

Damp Phlegm in the Liver and Gallbladder

Another potential problem is damp-phlegm in the Liver and Gallbladder:

Age	Symptoms
2 years onwards	Slight green vaginal discharge/excess smegma
14–25 years	Acne, greasy skin
Fertile years	PCOS, premature ejaculation, erectile dysfunction
Menopause	Hot flashes
Post-menopause	Hip degeneration

Table 3.2d: Age and varying symptoms of damp-phlegm in the Liver and Gallbladder from LPFs.

Treatment could include acupuncture at points including Ligou LIV-5, Ququan LIV-8, Zulinqi GB-41 (possibly combined with Waiguan SJ-5), Daimai GB-26.

Summary

According to the *Su Wen*, women move through seven-year cycles of *jing*, with menopause occurring at 7x7 years (49). *Jing* deficiency can underlie patterns of disharmony that lead to early cessation of menstruation, i.e., premature ovarian insufficiency.

During menopause, childhood illnesses may reappear, and this significant energetic change can present an opportunity to throw out these old diseases for good. However, treatment must begin years before menopause in order to be effective.

References

Larre, C., Translated from the French by Peter Firebrace (1987). The Way of Heaven: Neijing Suwen Chapters 1 & 2. Monkey Press 1994 : Cambridge, England.

Wu, Y., Leonard, C., Haeberle, M., (2019). Female Infertility & Reproductive Gynecology. A Comprehensive Clinical Manual of Integrated Chinese Medicine and Biomedicine. The Journal of Chinese Medicine Ltd: Hove, UK.

Health CMi, (2017) Acupuncture Premature Ovarian Failure Finding, Health CMi, Healthcare Medicine Institute. https://www.healthcmi.com/Acupuncture-Continuing-Education-News/1794-acupuncture-premature-ovarian-failure-finding

Health CMi (2018) Acupuncture Benefits Premature Ovarian Failure Patients, Health CMi, Healthcare Medicine Institute https://www.healthcmi.com/Acupuncture-Continuing-Education-News/1923-acupuncture-benefits-premature-ovarian-failure-patients

Scott, J., (2019). Gates of Life: Puberty and Menopause. Treating Women Academy: Online Menopause Masterclass. https://www.treatingwomen.com/store/5tpUJ3Fk

3.3 The Gates of Life

According to Dr. Shen, heralded as the greatest physician of Chinese medicine in the late 20th century, the 'Gates of Life' are significant physiological and psychological changes that every person undergoes throughout their lives. Women pass through more gates than men, since they experience more dramatic hormonal changes at various stages.

The Gates of Life Theory

The three main gates for women are puberty, pregnancy/childbirth, and menopause. There are also countless minor gates, including teething, first sex, leaving home, university, graduation, marriage, divorce, and retirement. Accidents and major illnesses could also be considered minor gates along with significant celestial influences such as the Saturn returns (29.5 and 56 years).

Of course, not every woman will experience all of these minor gates. Furthermore, some women do not pass through the major gate of pregnancy and childbirth either due to fertility issues, not finding a suitable partner, personal choice, or other circumstances.

However, the gates of puberty and menopause are certainties and these events present a great opportunity for change. They are times when pre-existing imbalances may either penetrate deeper or significantly improve, depending on one's attitude, lifestyle, and treatment.

Puberty

The average age of menarche in economically developed countries is 12–13 years old. This differs only slightly from the idea widely accepted by TCEAM practitioners that menarche occurs at 14 years old.

Early menarche is associated with an earlier menopause and, therefore, an increased risk of developing conditions such as cardiovascular diseases, diabetes, and osteoporosis later in life.

The risk of early menopause is amplified further for women who have an early menarche and do not have children.

Physiology

Puberty involves a series of hormonal changes in females. The first stage occurs between six and eight years old, as adrenal androgen production begins.

A few years later, disinhibition of the hypothalamic-pituitary-ovarian axis (HPOA) triggers the release of gonadotropin-releasing hormone (GnRH), which in turn stimulates the release of LH and FSH.

LH and FSH act upon gonadal cells to stimulate the release of estrogens and androgens. Specifically, LH stimulates the production of estrogen precursors. Meanwhile, FSH acts on ovarian follicles to convert these precursors into estrogen.

This process leads to the development of breasts, while the adrenal glands are responsible for the development of pubic hair.

TCEAM Viewpoint

In TCEAM terms, puberty coincides with a huge surge in Kidney qi. This results in *renmai* becoming fully functional, *chongmai* increasing in power, and the arrival of *tiangui* (menstrual Blood).

Risks and Opportunities

From around the age of nine, it is possible to see significant changes occurring in a female child. These changes follow the first surge of Kidney qi that occurs at age seven by approximately two years.

At this age, a child becomes increasingly aware of their own emotions, potentially leading to surliness and contradictory behavior. They also develop an increased ability to focus on tasks and activities.

Further changes happen at age 16, which some consider the age of 'emotional puberty.' At this age, there is an increased awareness of individuality and development of one's own ideas. Moodiness and defiance are common during these later stages of puberty.

Treating children with TCEAM at this age provides an opportunity to throw out old childhood diseases. One key strategy is clearing away dampness, which tends to accumulate earlier in life. Doing this can significantly improve digestive issues and skin problems such as eczema and acne.

However, during puberty, insulin sensitivity changes lead to an increased risk of developing diabetes. It is also a time when hay fever, migraines, and fatigue can emerge. In later puberty, there is a greater susceptibility to glandular diseases, such as mononucleosis.

Puberty presents a variety of consequences, behavior, opportunities, and dangers that if left untreated, may resurface in the menopausal years.

Age/ Energy Change	Physical Change	Mental/ Emotional Change	Consequences	Behavior	Common Illnesses	Opportunities	Dangers
2 y/old: First surge of Kidney yang	Teeth emerge	First assertion of individuality	Desire for world domination	'Terrible twos'	Fevers, febrile convulsions	Clear excess dampness	Asthma, epilepsy
9 y/old: Second (small) wave of Kidney yang	Self awareness	Awareness of emotions	Suppress emotions, ability to stay focused	Grumpiness, contradicting parents	Low blood sugar, diabetes, adult disease	Improve digestion	Hay fever, diabetes, migraines
16 y/old: Huge surge of Kidney yang	Ability to reproduce	Awareness of individuality	Own ideas	Maximum grumpiness	Diabetes, glandular problems	Throw out old illnesses	Glandular fever, chronic fatigue

Table 3.3: Developmental stages of puberty from a TCEAM perspective.[12]

[12] Table source: Scott, J., (2019). Gates of Life: Puberty and Menopause. Treating Women Academy: Online Menopause Masterclass. https://www.treatingwomen.com/store/5tpUJ3Fk

Pregnancy/Childbirth

In Dr. Shen's Gates of Life theory, pregnancy and childbirth are used synonymously. However, it is essential to recognize the differences between the two and how this might impact the journey through menopause.

Pregnancy

Parous
one or more live births.

Nulliparous
one or more pregnancies but no live births due to miscarriage, termination of pregnancy, or stillbirth.

Nulligravida
no pregnancies or live births.

Pregnancy can happen at any time between menarche and menopause. According to the World Health Organization (WHO) women of reproductive age refers to all women aged 15–49 years .[13]

For some women this particular gate may not happen at all, either due to personal choice or circumstance. This is significant, because whether a woman has children or not can impact how she experiences the menopause.

For example, a woman who does not have children by choice will likely have a more positive attitude towards the menopause than one whose choice has been removed. In the latter situation, menopause can represent an unwelcome sense of finality and even grief as the doors of fertility close. The summation being that women who have experienced infertility, miscarriages or undergone terminations may suffer from a greater sense of loss as they reach the end of their fertile years.

Examples include:

- **Primary or secondary infertility:** not being able to get pregnant despite having frequent, unprotected sex for at least one year.
- **Surgery:** removal of both ovaries (bilateral oophorectomy) or the uterus (hysterectomy).
- **Medications:** such as chemotherapy.
- **Psychosocial:** not finding a suitable partner, mental health challenges, financial instability, same-sex relationships, etc.

Whether menopause is medically induced or occurs naturally also plays a vital role. Women who experience surgical or medical menopause report greater levels of discomfort than those who reach their natural age of menopause.

---

[13] World Health Organization (2022). Critical considerations and actions for achieving universal access to sexual and reproductive health in the context of universal health coverage through a primary health care approach. WHO Geneva https://www.who.int/publications/i/item/9789240052659

Physiology

During early pregnancy, both progesterone and estrogen levels rise and help to maintain the pregnancy until the placenta takes over. A range of other hormones are also released during pregnancy, which all play a role in supporting the pregnancy, fetal development, and preparing the body for labor.

With regards to menopause, nulliparous women (which includes nulligravida) retain higher estrogen levels in comparison with those who do have children. Therefore, they may report fewer menopausal symptoms, including hot flashes and vaginal dryness. They also appear to be at a decreased risk of cognitive decline but an increased risk of breast cancer. Nulliparous women also have an increased risk of hip and spine, but not wrist, fractures. However, there is no apparent difference in bone mineral density between parous and nulliparous women.

Therefore, whether a woman has children or not will significantly influence her health during menopause and midlife, although both scenarios present distinct advantages and disadvantages.

TCEAM Viewpoint

During pregnancy, qi and Blood undergo significant changes. Blood increases along with a rise in Liver qi. Meanwhile, Kidney qi decreases and there is a propensity to develop excessive dampness or heat.

Childbirth

The fields of obstetrics and midwifery have advanced greatly in the past century, saving the lives of countless mothers and babies. However, these advances have also led to huge increases in the rates of interventions such as fetal monitoring, inductions, epidurals, ventouse suction cups, forceps, and cesarian sections. These interventions can be extremely traumatic for the women involved and this trauma can be challenging to deal with postnatally since much of her time will be taken up caring for her newborn.

Physiology

Childbirth involves a series of hormonal changes, which play crucial roles in facilitating labor. They include:

- An increase in estrogen levels, which primes the uterus for an efficient labor.
- Increases in oxytocin and prostaglandin activity, which contribute to cervical ripening.
- Increases in uterine oxytocin receptors also allow for effective contractions.
- Increased inflammation, which further activates the cervix and uterus.

Following childbirth, estrogen levels fall, and this reduction is maintained for approximately one year. Lactation has the effect of reducing estrogen levels further still.

Postpartum Depression (PPD)

Experts have proposed a link between PPD and perimenopausal depression for women aged 45-49. The risk of depression is already increased during perimenopause, and it appears that women with histories of hormone-related mood disorders (PPD, depression during pregnancy, or premenstrual syndrome) are at even higher risk. Research suggests that there may be a link between higher-than-average FSH levels and depressive episodes.

TCEAM Viewpoint

Childbirth can cause severe Blood deficiency, especially if traumatic. This can leave women susceptible to cold diseases and has led to the Chinese tradition of 'sitting the month.' The practice involves minimizing activity and accepting care and nourishment in the month following childbirth in order to replenish one's reserves.

Risks and Opportunities

Like puberty, pregnancy and childbirth present the opportunity for pre-existing conditions to either improve or worsen. For example, Blood loss during labor can leave a woman vulnerable to a whole range of physical and psychological issues later in life.

However, some women find that pregnancy and childbirth have a beneficial effect on their health. It may regulate their menstrual cycle if they previously suffered from painful or irregular periods. It can also have a significant impact on a woman's personality, making her more assertive and commanding.

Menopause

The average age of natural menopause in economically developed countries is 51, which is not too dissimilar to that age of 49 given by the *Su Wen*. This is particularly true given that many Asian cultures consider individuals to be aged one at birth.

Of course, menopause may occur much earlier, either due to genetic or environmental factors, premature ovarian insufficiency, or medically-induced menopause.

As discussed above, the age at which a woman passes through this gate can also be influenced by the previous two gates. Early menarche and not having children can both contribute to an earlier menopause.

Physiology

In the years leading up to menopause, a woman's ovarian function gradually declines. At birth, a woman has approximately 300,000 follicles, a figure which diminishes to approximately 25,000 by the age of 37. By menopause, there are very few to none remaining.

This reduction coincides with falling estrogen levels, specifically estradiol. Ovarian inhibin and AMH levels also decrease, with the latter being used as a measure of ovarian reserve. Meanwhile, FSH levels increase.

These hormonal changes cause a woman's menstrual cycle to become increasingly irregular and finally stop altogether. They may also be accompanied by various menopausal symptoms.

TCEAM Viewpoint

As *jing* steadily decreases, the balance between Kidney yin and Kidney yang changes. Kidney yin often enters a phase of relative deficiency, while Kidney yang becomes predominant. This switch can allow empty heat to flare up as well as other patterns of disharmony. A decline in the function of other *zang* organs with age and due to various lifestyle factors, coupled with Blood deficiency and the possible presence of pathogenic factors, contribute to the risk of menopausal symptoms.

Risks and Opportunities

Like all of the gates, menopause is a time when health may deteriorate or improve. Without the protective properties of estrogen, the risk of chronic diseases increases dramatically. This leaves women susceptible to weight gain, cardiovascular disease, diabetes, osteoporosis, and cognitive decline.

A Word About Contraception and Assisted Reproductive Therapy (ART)

Since hormonal contraception and ART both interfere with a woman's natural hormonal cycle, it is reasonable to assume that they might influence her experience of menopause. Unfortunately, there is currently little research on the subject.

There is some limited evidence that the use of high-dose oral contraceptives (as prescribed prior to 1972) could delay the onset of natural menopause. However, little information is available pertaining to the lower dose contraceptives that are used today.

In terms of ART, it is unclear whether the process influences the age of natural menopause. However, there is some evidence that poor responses to in-vitro fertilization (IVF), such as low oocyte retrieval, could be a useful predictor of early menopause.

From a TCEAM perspective, it is certainly feasible that the drugs used in IVF cycles could impact menopause in women who have taken them. For example, clomiphene citrate blocks estrogen receptors and is considered a hot, yang-stimulating drug. It has the side effects of consuming yin fluids, depleting Kidney yin and Liver Blood. Furthermore, aromatase inhibitors such as letrozole suppress estrogen production and are sometimes used to induce ovulation in ART cycles. This process stimulates Kidney yang and generates empty heat.

Overall, the act of recruiting multiple follicles during IVF draws on a woman's *jing*, meaning less Blood is formed to fill the *renmai* and *chongmai*. Not to mention the emotional toll of the experience, which adversely affects the Liver, leading to stagnation, and qi and Blood disorders.

Summary

The Gates of Life are among the myriad factors that can influence how a woman transitions through menopause. These include the major gates of puberty, pregnancy and childbirth and numerous other 'minor gates.'

For this reason, it is important to ask our menopausal patients in detail about their reproductive history* using the following checklist:

- ☐ Childhood illnesses
- ☐ Age of menarche
- ☐ Nature of PMS symptoms
- ☐ Experience of puberty
- ☐ Sexual activity
- ☐ Contraception
- ☐ Fertility issues
- ☐ Pregnancies
- ☐ Miscarriages
- ☐ Termination of pregnancies
- ☐ Childbirth
- ☐ Postpartum issues (mother)
- ☐ Postnatal issues (baby)
- ☐ Number of live births

It is also crucial to discuss their feelings surrounding these issues in order to get a clearer picture and provide an opportunity to heal past trauma that may not have been addressed at the time.

* Note: Sexual history, including sexual abuse are dealt with in Chapter 5.2. Stress, Trauma, and Stress Resistance.

References

Scott, J., (2019). Gates of Life: Puberty and Menopause. Treating Women Academy: Online Menopause Masterclass. https://www.treatingwomen.com/store/5tpUJ3Fk

Rowlands, IJ., Redshaw. M., (2012). Mode of birth and women's psychological and physical wellbeing in the postnatal period, BioMed Central : BMC Pregnancy Childbirth. 2012 Nov 28;12:138. doi: 10.1186/1471-2393-12-138. https://pubmed.ncbi.nlm.nih gov/23190575

Buckley, SJ., (2015). Executive Summary of Hormonal Physiology of Childbearing: Evidence and Implications for Women, Babies, and Maternity Care, The Journal of Perinatal Education: J Perinat Educ. 2015; 24(3): (pp 145–153). doi: 10.1891/1058-1243.24.3.145
https://www.ncbi.nlm.nih.gov/pmc/articles/PMC4720867

de Vries, E., den Tonkelaar, I., van Noord, PA., et al. (2001). Oral contraceptive use in relation to age at menopause in the DOM cohort, Human Reproduction: Hum Reprod. 2001 Aug;16(8): (pp 1657-62). doi: 10.1093/humrep/16.8.1657. https://pubmed.ncbi.nlm.nih.gov/11473959

de Boer, EJ., den Tonkelaar. I., te Veldel, ER., et al. (2003). Increased risk of early menopausal transition and natural menopause after poor response at first IVF treatment, Human Reproduction: Hum Reprod. 2003 Jul;18(7): (pp 1544-52). doi: 10.1093/humrep/deg278.
https://pubmed.ncbi.nlm.nih.gov/12832386

Dr. Shen - IN MEMORIAM Dr.. John Shen Alan Papier, Giovanni Maciocia, Peter Deadman & Leon Hammer, JCM 67, 2001.
https://www.jcm.co.uk/in-memoriam-Dr.-john-shen.html

Larre, C., Translated from the French by Peter Firebrace (1987). The Way of Heaven: Neijing Suwen Chapters 1 & 2. Monkey Press 1994 : Cambridge, England.

Betts, D., (2006). The Essential Guide to Acupuncture in Pregnancy & Childbirth. The Journal of Chinese Medicine Ltd. Sussex, England.

Jane, FM., Davis, SR., (2014). A Practitioner's Toolkit for Managing the Menopause, Taylor Francis online: Climacteric, Volume 17, 2014 - Issue 5. doi.org/10.3109/13697137.2014.929651.
https://www.tandfonline.com/doi/full/10.3109/13697137.2014.929651

Biro, FM., Pinney, SM., Huang, B., et al. (2014). Hormone Changes in Peripubertal Girls, PMC US National Library of Medicine, National Institutes of Health: The Journal of Clinical Endocrinology & Metabolism: J Clin Endocrinol Metab. 2014 Oct; 99(10): (pp 3829–3835). Published online 2014 Jul 16. doi: 10.1210/jc.2013-4528.
https://www.ncbi.nlm.nih.gov/pmc/articles/PMC4184081

Pierce, M., Hardy, R., (2012). Commentary: The decreasing age of puberty—as much a psychosocial as biological problem? PMC US National Library of Medicine, National Institutes of Health: International Journal of Epidemiology: Int J Epidemiol. 2012 Feb; 41(1): (pp 300–302). Published online 2012 Jan 13. doi: 10.1093/ije/dyr227
https://www.ncbi.nlm.nih.gov/pmc/articles/PMC3383190

Emmanuel, M., Bokor, BR., (2020). Tanner Stages, NCBI Resources, StatPearls [Internet]. Treasure Island (FL): StatPearls Publishing; 2022 Jan -
https://www.ncbi.nlm.nih.gov/books/NBK470280

References

Hoyt, LT., Falconi, A., (2015). Puberty and Perimenopause: Reproductive Transitions and their Implications for Women's Health, PMC US National Library of Medicine, National Institutes of Health: Social Science & Medicine: Soc Sci Med. 2015 May; 132: (pp 103–112). Published online 2015 Mar 14. doi: 10.1016/j.socscimed.2015.03.031
https://www.ncbi.nlm.nih.gov/pmc/articles/PMC4400253

Petrakis, NL., Wrensch, MR., Ernster, VL., et al. (1987). Influence of pregnancy and lactation on serum and breast fluid estrogen levels: implications for breast cancer risk, NIH, National Library of Medicine, National Center for Biotechnology Information: International Journal of Cancer: Int J Cancer. 1987 Nov 15;40(5):(pp 587-91). doi: 10.1002/ijc.2910400502.
https://www.ncbi.nlm.nih.gov/pubmed/3679587?dopt=Abstract

Kumar, P., Magon, N., (2012). Hormones in pregnancy, PMC US National Library of Medicine, National Institutes of Health: Nigerian Medical Journal: Niger Med J. 2012 Oct-Dec; 53(4): (pp 179–183).doi: 10.4103/0300-1652.107549.
https://www.ncbi.nlm.nih.gov/pmc/articles/PMC3640235

3.4 Body Type

Before even beginning the consultation to determine which patterns may be causing a patient's symptoms, it is possible to make assessments based on their body type and complexion. These observations can help the practitioner to form a hypothesis and guide their line of enquiry in order to confirm or deny it.

This technique is taught by Honora Lee Wolfe and Bob Flaws, and can significantly expedite the diagnostic process. That said, it is essential to note key information deliberately and methodologically. It is also crucial to understand how to interpret this information accurately. In general practice, other factors, including age and gender, can also assist a practitioner in forming their hypothesis. However, we already know that our menopausal patients are, generally speaking, women within the 45–60 age group. Based on this information, we can make the following assumptions:

- In women, the primary vital substance to consider is Blood, whereas in men, it is qi.
- Women tend toward Blood deficiency due to menstruation, gestation, and lactation.
- Women tend to experience yin deficiency and, often, Spleen deficiency.
- Spleen deficiency usually begins in the late 30s to 40s.
- By age 40, Kidney yin will have reduced by half.
- Spleen qi deficiency evolves into Kidney yang deficiency in the 50s to early 60s.
- Liver qi is responsible for how smoothly women transition through this change.
- The Liver controls free flow during this major transformation.
- If the free flow of qi is impaired, heat will arise.
- Heat causes dryness and a reduction of fluids.
- Rising heat impacts the Heart, Lungs, and sense organs.
- An unhappy Liver can also overact on earth via the *ke* (controlling) cycle, leading to dampness, phlegm, and reduced qi and Blood formation (see Chapter 3.6. Five Elements, Five Phase).
- Aging can lead to visceral dysfunction, phlegm, and Blood stasis and these patterns are common in elderly patients.

Body Types

In the 1940s, US-based psychologist William H. Sheldon developed a system of classification of human physical types (somatotypes) based on a person's degree of slenderness, angularity, and fragility. These are mesomorph, ectomorph, and endomorph. This differs slightly from the TCEAM view that there are four different body types: *shaoyang, shaoyin, taiyang,* and *taiyin*. This framework provides an overview of the state of a patient's qi, Blood, yin, yang, and likely pathogenic factors.

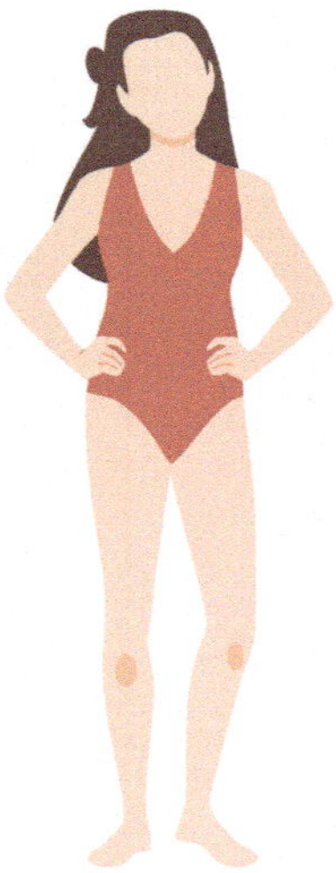

Shaoyang
Mesomorph

- Athletic, strong, and solid build
- Little body fat
- Neither overweight nor under-weight
- Can gain and lose weight relatively easily

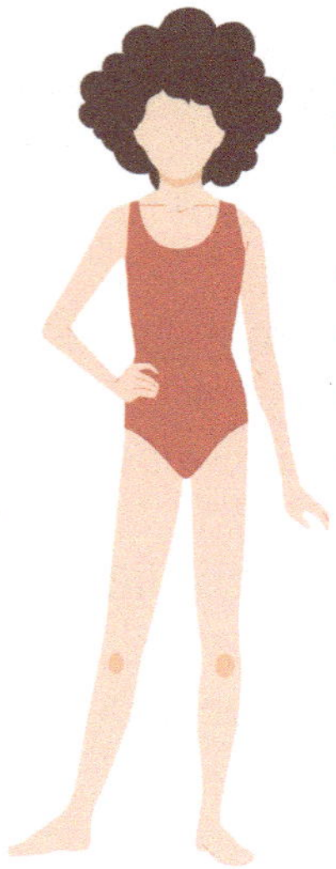

Shaoyin
Ectomorph

- Lean and may be underweight
- Little body fat or muscle
- Difficulty gaining weight
- May lack curves

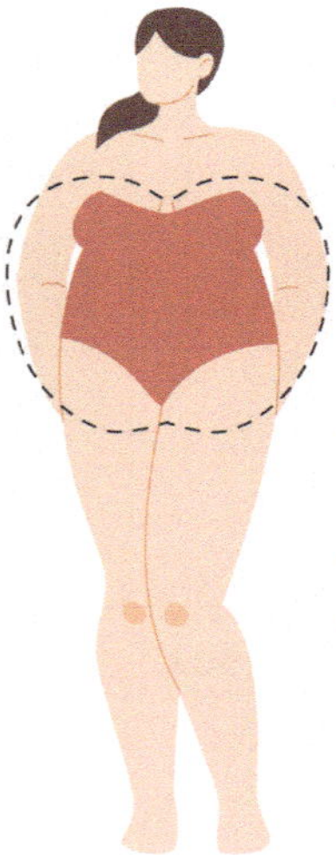

Taiyang
Apple-shaped endomorph

- Substantial body fat and muscle
- Gains weight easily, but not necessarily overweight
- Greater fat distribution in the upper body
- Larger breasts and abdomen
- Smaller hips and thighs

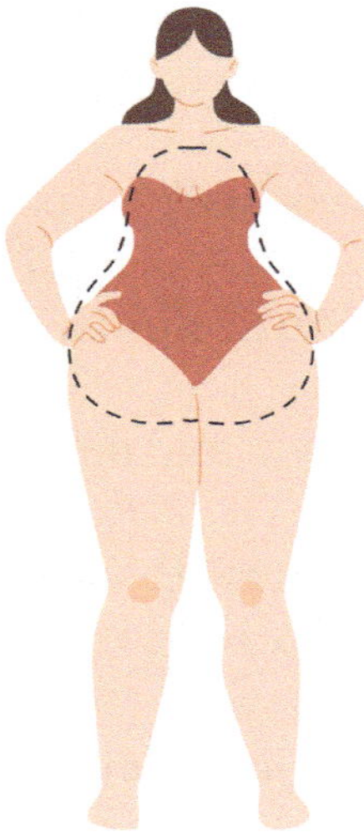

Taiyin
Pear-shaped endomorph

- Substantial body fat and no muscle
- Gains weight easily
- Greater fat distribution in the lower body
- Poor muscle tone
- Larger hips and thighs
- Smaller breasts and abdomen

Figure 3.4a: W.H. Sheldon's somatotypes; mesomorph, ectomorph, and endomorph and TCEAM differentiation.

Body Type	Significance	Treatment Focus	Acupuncture and other Modalities
Shaoyang	Yin and yang harmonize appropriately Qi and Blood flow freely	Often easiest to treat since yin, yang, qi, and Blood are relatively in balance. Aim to maintain this body type for as long as possible. Suggest focus on keeping Spleen strong and managing Liver qi. Exercise and a good diet can do most of the work for these women.	Hegu LI-4 Taichong LIV-3 (aid global qi flow) Zusanli ST-36 Zhongwan REN-12 Sanyinjiao SP-6 (strengthen Spleen)
Shaoyin	Insufficient Blood and yin	Gentle Blood nourishing and yin enriching with herbal medicine (caution with cloying herbs that are hard to digest). Short and shallow needle treatments. Moxa is usually applicable on the lower body unless there is upper-body injury. Focus on diet, moderate regular exercise, adequate sleep.	Taixi KID-3 or Fuliu KID-7 Sanyinjiao SP-6, Guanyuan REN-4 (nourish Blood and yin) Food, herbs, rest, stress control, and regular, gentle exercise are more important than acupuncture.
Taiyang	Exuberant yang with phlegm, dampness, and turbidity	Heat and dampness will be more prominent than in the first two body types. Acupuncture may benefit Liver qi, and herbs can help clear heat, but exercise will be the most important component in this body type.	Xingjian LIV-2 or Taichong LIV-3, angled toward LIV-2 (clear heat and eliminate dampness) A drop of blood from Zuqiaoyin GB-44 Ear apex Shangyang LI1 Avoid moxa No oil when massaging
Taiyin	Insufficient yang qi with phlegm, dampness, and turbidity	Dampness is the critical factor. Focus treatment on the Spleen. Digestion may not be good in these women, so herbs must be easily digestible if taken over long time periods. Dietary improvements are key. Exercise must be moderate and regular.	Zusanli ST-36 Yinlingquan SP-9 Yanglingquan GB-34 Zhangmen LIV-13 Moxa: - Zhongwan REN-12 - Qihai REN-6 - Guanyuan REN-4 - Pishu BL-20 - Zusanli ST-36 Note: Diet is more important than treatment.

Table 3.4a: Body types.

Symptom	Body Type	Treatment Principle	Acupuncture points
Hot flashes	Shaoyang	Control Liver/Spleen disharmony	Sanyinjiao SP-6 Yanglingquan GB-34 Taichong LIV-3 Zusanli ST-36 Hegu LI-4 even method
	Shaoyin	Nourish Blood and yin	Taixi KID-3 Taichong LIV-3 Sanyinjiao SP-6 Guanyuan REN-4
	Taiyang	Clear heat	Taixi KID-3 Zhaohai KID-6 Hegu LI-4 Quchi LI-11 Waiguan SJ-5 Neiguan P-6 Qihai REN-6
	Taiyin	Eliminate damp-heat	Yinlingquan SP-9 Zhongji REN-3 Zhigou SJ-6 Tianshu ST-25 Yanglingquan GB-34 Danzhong REN-17 Quchi LI-11 Ququan LIV-8
Dry skin and vagina	Worst in shaoyin	Nourish Blood and yin	Xuehai SP-10 Guanyuan REN-4 + Qugu REN-2 Taixi KID-3 Sanyinjiao SP-6 Ququan LIV-8
Fatigue	Worst in taiyin	Supplement Spleen Eliminate dampness	Guanyuan REN-4 + Zhongwan REN-12 + Danzhong REN-17 Taibai SP-3 Zusanli ST-36 Baihui DU-20 Yangchi SJ-4

Symptom	Body Type	Treatment Principle	Acupuncture points
Insomnia	Shaoyang	Calm Liver Reduce caffeine and alcohol	Qimen LIV-14 Ganshu BL-18 Sanyinjiao SP-6 Guanyuan REN-4 Neiguan P-6 Yintang EX-HN3
	Shaoyin	Nourish Blood and yin Herbs Stress management Improve diet Nutraceuticals	Taixi KID-3 Taichong LIV-3 Sanyinjiao SP-6 Guanyuan REN-4 Shenmen HT-7 Yintang EX-HN3
	Taiyang	Clear heat Supplement Spleen/Heart Avoid spicy and greasy/ meaty foods	Bleed Lidui ST-45 Zuqiaoyin GB-44 + ear apex if hypertension present Add points to anchor *mingmen* fire, such as: Guanyuan REN-4 or Qihai REN-6 Taixi KID-3 Sanyinjiao SP-6
	Taiyin	Eliminate damp-heat Strengthen Spleen	Yinlingquan SP-9 Zhongji REN-3 Zhigou SJ-6 Tianshu ST-25 Yanglingquan GB-34 Danzhong REN-17 Quchi LI-11 Ququan LIV-8 Add points to clear the mind, such as: Baihui DU-20 Shenting DU-24 Benshen GB-13

Table 3.4b: Body types and menopause symptoms.

Summary

When seeing a patient for the first time, noting their body type, along with their age, gender, and complexion (collectively known as the 'four firsts') can greatly assist in the diagnostic process. This information can be used to guide questioning, pulse and tongue expectations, etiology of the main complaint, and treatment planning.

This process, also known as hypothetico-deductive reasoning, must be done deliberately and requires accurate interpretation to be effective. However, when performed correctly, it can be an invaluable clinical tool.

References

Flaws, B., (2014). The Four Firsts of Diagnosis, online course. Blue Poppy Press ; Portland, Oregon, USA. https://bluepoppy.myabsorb.com

Wolfe, HL., (2019). The Four Firsts in Diagnosing Women. Treating Women Academy: Online Menopause Masterclass. https://www.treatingwomen.com/store/5tpUJ3Fk

Wolfe, HL., (1998). Managing Menopause Naturally with Chinese Medicine. Blue Poppy Press ; Portland, Oregon, USA.

3.5 Skin, Complexion, and Hair

There is an abundance of estrogen receptors located throughout the skin's dermis and epidermis. Therefore, menopause can have a significant effect on the skin. This includes normal, age-related changes, such as wrinkles and sagging, and more severe disorders of the skin, nails, and hair (dermatosis).

Estrogen receptors are most concentrated around the face, genitals, and lower limbs, meaning that these areas are more susceptible to changes in estrogen levels.

One of the most obvious examples is atrophic vulvovaginitis, which occurs due to a narrowing and shortening of the vagina, coupled with atrophy of the vaginal tissues. A full discussion of this condition can be found in Chapters 4.4 and 5.4. However, a broad range of other issues may also occur.

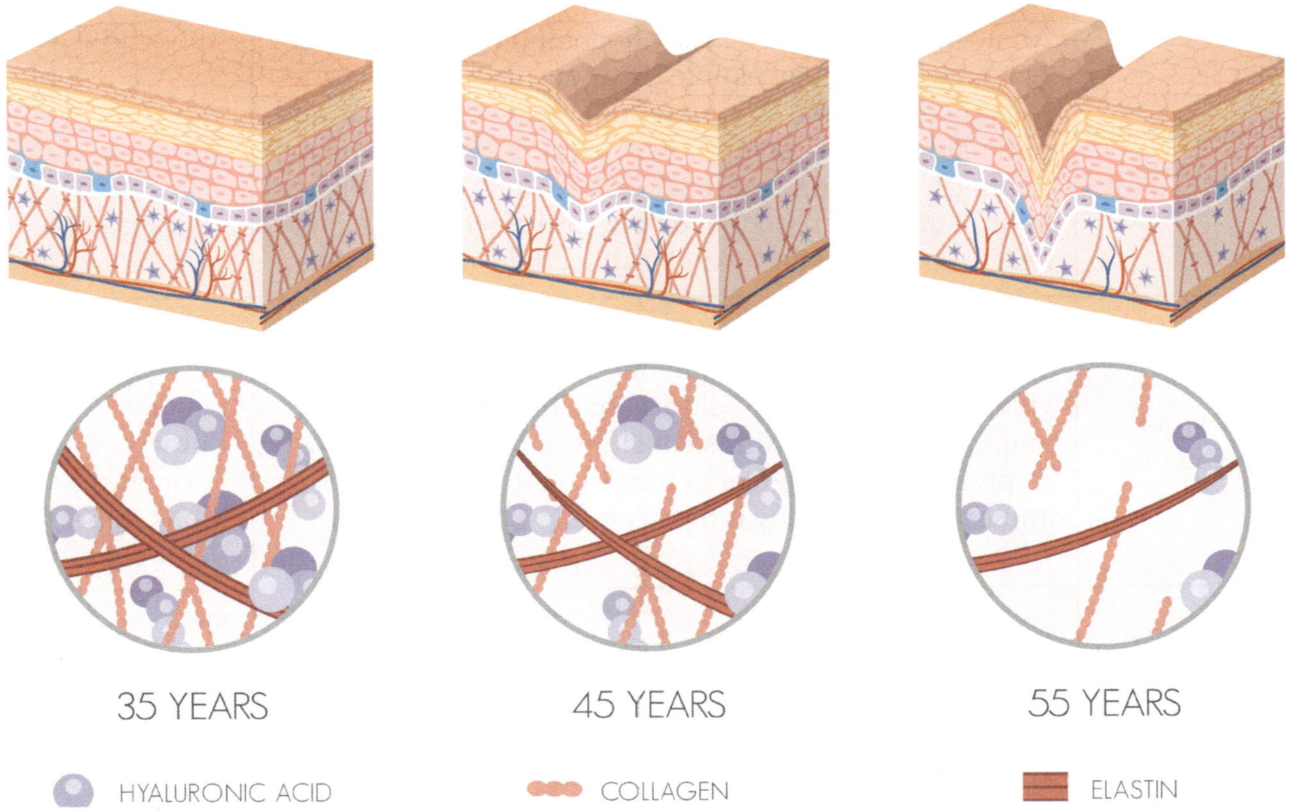

Figure 3.5a: Age-related changes to skin.

Skin Conditions

Menopausal dermatological issues may occur due to physiological, age-related, or hormonal changes. The latter includes both estrogen deficiency and hormone therapies. Some common examples are listed in table 3.5a.

Condition	Description	Affected area
Acne	Decreasing estrogen levels result in a relative excess of androgens, which can lead to the onset or recurrence of acne. Other possible triggers include cosmetics, diet, stress, lack of sleep, obesity, smoking, and UV radiation.	Mainly facial, less commonly affects the torso
Atrophic vulvovaginitis	Thinning of the vagina and vestibule, leading to symptoms such as dryness, burning, itching, tenderness, and painful intercourse. This may be accompanied by urogenital atrophy, with urinary urgency or frequency, incontinence, and painful or difficult urination.	Vagina Vulva Urogenital system
Vulvar lichen sclerosus	An atrophic disorder of the anogenital area, presenting as white, flat-topped papules forming plaques in a figure-of-eight formation and extending into the vulval and perianal regions. Symptoms include severe nocturnal itching, irritation, painful intercourse, difficult or painful urination, vaginal or urethral discharge, urinary or fecal incontinence, skin fissures, itchy or sore vulva.	Anogenital area
Dysesthetic vulvodynia	Widespread and spontaneous pain throughout the vulva, vestibule, labia, clitoris, perineum, mons pubis, and inner thighs. Pain is constant and related to touch or pressure, although activities like intercourse, cycling and horse riding may intensify it.	Vulva Vestibule Labia Clitoris Perineum Mons pubis Inner thighs
Menopausal flashing	Reddening of the skin in association with vasomotor symptoms.	Face Neck Upper chest
Keratoderma climactericum (Haxthausen's disease)	Thickened skin on the palms and soles. May be accompanied by redness and cracked skin, which can make walking painful. It is more common in obese or hypertensive patients.	Palms of hands Soles of feet, especially the heels
Vulvovaginal candidiasis	A common fungal infection of the vagina or vulva. Symptoms include itching, burning, and thick, white, curd-like discharge. Aggravated by hormone therapy, including oral hormonal contraceptives, steroid or antibiotic use, and diabetes.	Vagina Vulva

Condition	Description	Affected area
Pruritus (itching skin)	Dry skin can lead to itching, especially in the vulvar region.	Especially vulva and perianal region
Melasma (skin discoloration / pigment change)	Melanocytes (melanin producing cells) are highly sensitive to estrogen. Hyperpigmentation can occur as a side effect of oral hormonal contraceptives or estrogen-containing creams or ointments. Melasma can also occur for a variety of other reasons. It is exacerbated by sun exposure.	Genitals Mammary areola Abdomen Face
Sunburn	Sunburn and sun damage, in general, can contribute to premature aging. It also increases the risk of skin cancer, which often becomes evident during midlife.	Any areas overexposed to the sun
Delayed wound repair	Aging is associated with delayed healing, which may lead to chronic unhealed wounds and ulcers.	Any injured area
Bruises easily	As the skin becomes thinner during menopause, bruises may occur more easily.	Any injured area
Sensitivity and rashes (contact dermatitis)	Sensitivity and redness when exposed to irritating substances like itchy fabrics, perfumes, and dyes. May be accompanied by itching or soreness.	Any areas exposed to the irritant
Wrinkles	Aging is associated with a decrease in collagen synthesis and, therefore, skin elasticity. It also tends to decrease fibroblasts (collagen-producing cells), mast cells (immune cells located in the connective tissue), and blood vessels. These changes cause the skin to become thinner, drier, and more fragile. Skin aging can be accelerated by environmental factors, including smoking, alcohol consumption, poor nutrition, and UV light exposure.	The skin, especially in exposed areas such as the face

Table 3.5a: Dermatological conditions during menopause.

Facial Complexion

During and after menopause, the body produces less collagen, causing many changes to the skin. Skin elasticity reduces and a certain amount of fat may be lost from under the skin. In combination with hormonal changes, which result in dryness, this can lead to sagging, especially around the neck, jawline, and cheeks, as well as fine lines and wrinkles.

TCEAM Viewpoint

Clear and lustrous skin relies upon healthy Blood, qi, yin, and yang.

Blood provides nutrition, keeping the skin soft and moist. Deficiency can lead to general dryness and may also allow wind to arise, causing itching.

Qi enables the pores to open and close efficiently. Deficiency can cause difficulty in adapting to temperature changes, and spontaneous sweating.

Yin provides moisture, ensuring an abundance of thin fluids and preventing thick fluids from stagnating. Therefore, deficiency can lead to stagnation and empty heat.

Finally, yang generates warmth. Deficiency can lead to cold and clammy skin.

The impact of Blood, qi, yin, and yang on the skin is summarized in table 3.5 b below:

Skin Type	Reason
Thin, dry skin	Blood and yin deficiency
Thin, dry, itchy skin	Blood and yin deficiency with wind-heat
Thick, dry skin	Qi deficiency and damp stagnation
Thick, inflamed, itchy skin	Blood or damp stagnation with heat or wind
Thick, oily, raised skin	Excessive dampness

Table 3.5b: Skin conditions and associated TCEAM patterns.

Furthermore, all of the organs can directly or indirectly impact skin health. However, the Lungs have the greatest influence due to their role in dispersing qi and ascending and descending fluids. In menopausal patients, Kidney yin deficiency can lead to Lung yin deficiency, since the Lung is the mother of the Kidney according to five phase theory. The result of this is thin, dry skin with fine lines and wrinkles.

The Spleen also plays a vital role as it is responsible for extracting nutrition from food, which goes on to form qi and Blood. Therefore, Spleen qi deficiency can lead to general Blood and qi deficiency, both of which impact the skin. The Spleen also controls the raising of qi. If it fails to do this, the skin may become loose and saggy.

Complexion and Pathogenic Factors

A patient's complexion can indicate the presence of pathogenic factors as well as the state of the qi, Blood, and body fluids:

Complexion	Pathogenic Factor
Red	Heat (including deficiency heat, Stomach heat, Liver and Stomach heat, damp-heat)
Pale	Blood vacuity (including Heart, Kidney, or Spleen Blood vacuity)
Purple/sooty	Blood stasis
Oily	Dampness
Dry (skin or vagina)	Yin, Blood or body fluid insufficiency
Lustrous	Abundant qi and Blood
Liver lines (i.e. two vertical lines between the eyebrows)	Liver depression/qi stagnation

Table 3.5c: Skin complexion and associated TCEAM patterns.

Face Reading

Face reading is an ancient Chinese practice that has its roots in Daoism. It has now been adopted by TCEAM practitioners as a way to evaluate the state of a person's *jing* and qi.

The face is seen as an outward expression of the internal world. It is influenced by genetics and ethnicity, but also life experiences and emotions, which manifest on the face as a result of repetitive expressions. Different areas of the face relate to different organs and emotions, creating a visual map of a person's physical and psychological health.

Face reading can reveal a lot of information, although it is an art that takes many years and a great deal of experience to perfect. Some of the most common features and their correspondences are shown in the images below.

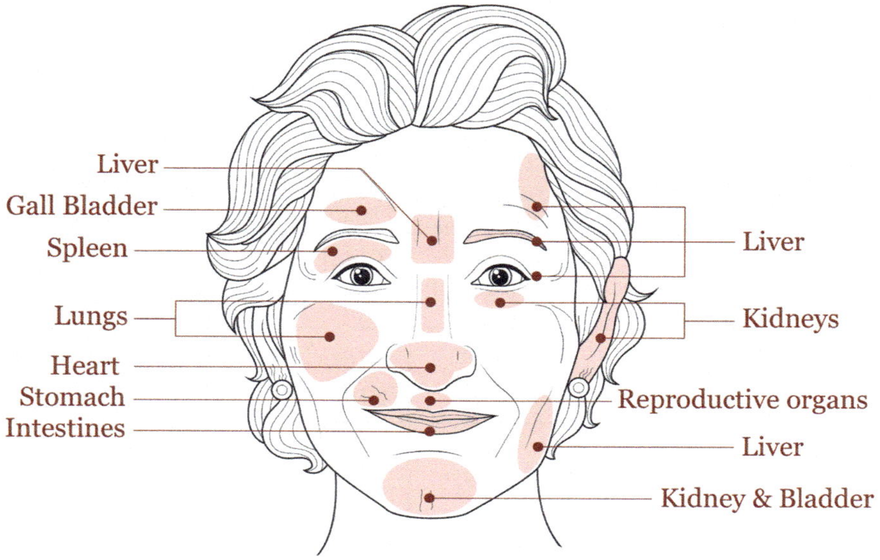

Figure 3.5b: Face map of organ correspondences.

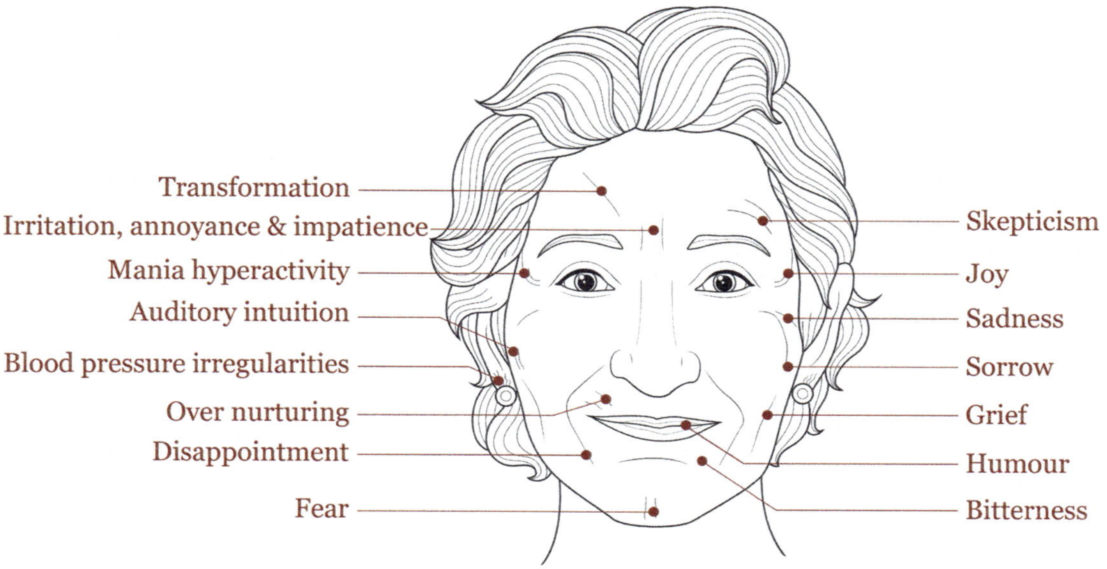

Figure 3.5c: Face map of emotional correspondences.

Hair

As with the skin, the hair becomes thinner and drier with age, as well as eventually losing its color. Meanwhile, hair in other regions, such as the face, may become thicker and more noticeable. In addition to these normal, age-related changes, more severe pathologies can occur:

Condition	Description	Affected area
Hirsutism	Excessive hair growth. Hirsutism may be genetic and results from increased testosterone. As progesterone levels decrease during the menopausal transition, the impact of androgens on hair follicles increases, altering the type of hair present. This symptom is often associated with polycystic ovary syndrome (PCOS).	Face Torso Arms Legs
Androgenetic alopecia	Hair loss due to a genetic sensitivity to dihydrotestosterone (DHT). Hair thinning during menopause gives the appearance of decreased hair coverage and may lead to severe emotional distress. Androgenic alopecia can be caused by various factors tied to the actions of hormones, including some ovarian cysts, taking high androgen index birth control pills, pregnancy, and menopause.	The top, front or temporal regions of the scalp. May resemble male pattern baldness

Table 3.5d: Hair conditions during menopause.

TCEAM Viewpoint

The hair's condition depends upon the Lungs and the Kidneys, specifically *jing*. The Lungs provide moisture and nourish the hair. Meanwhile, strong *jing* allows the hair to grow thick and maintain its color. Conversely, if *jing* becomes weakened or deficient, the hair will thin and gray.

The growth of facial hair is due to Blood in the *chongmai* no longer being directed downward to the uterus. Once menstruation ceases, it instead travels upward to nourish the face, resulting in hair growth.

Summary

Menopause causes numerous changes to the skin and hair. Many of these can be considered natural, although some are pathological. Either way, women may report feeling self-conscious about their changing appearance as they age and this may contribute to depression, anxiety, and loss of confidence.

Cosmetic acupuncture treatments can be effective in reducing the appearance of fine lines, wrinkles, and sagging skin. However, it may be more beneficial to a patient's overall health if they are able to come to terms with the idea of aging and reframe it as a positive experience.

As practitioners, we can reassure our patients that aging does not need to mean a loss of physical attractiveness. We might encourage them to focus on wearing clothing or hairstyles that make them feel good about themselves and to look toward older female role models for inspiration.

References

Nair, PA., (2014). Dermatosis associated with menopause, PMC US National Library of Medicine, National Institutes of Health, Journal of Mid-Life Health: J Midlife Health. 2014 Oct-Dec; 5(4): (pp 168–175). doi: 10.4103/0976-7800.145152
https://www.ncbi.nlm.nih.gov/pmc/articles/PMC4264279

Thornton, MJ., (2013). Estrogens and aging skin, PMC US National Library of Medicine, National Institutes of Health Dermato-Endocrinology: Dermatoendocrinol. 2013 Apr 1; 5(2): 264–270. Published online 2013 Apr 1. doi: 10.4161/derm.23872.
https://www.ncbi.nlm.nih.gov/pmc/articles/PMC3772914

Handel, AC., Miot, LDB., Miot, HA., (2014). Melasma: a clinical and epidemiological review, PMC US National Library of Medicine, National Institutes of Health, Anais Brasileiros de Dermatologia: An Bras Dermatol. 2014 Sep-Oct; 89(5): (pp 771–782). doi: 10.1590/abd1806-4841.20143063.
https://www.ncbi.nlm.nih.gov/pmc/articles/PMC4155956

Khunger, N., Mehrotra, K., (2019). Menopausal Acne – Challenges And Solutions, PMC US National Library of Medicine, National Institutes of Health, Dovepress, Iternational Journal of Women's Health: Int J Womens Health. 2019; 11: (pp 555–567). Published online 2019 Oct 29. doi: 10.2147/IJWH.S174292.
https://www.ncbi.nlm.nih.gov/pmc/articles/PMC6825478

Thambirajah, R., (2015). Cosmetic Acupuncture. Second edition. Singing Dragon. London, England.

Bridges, L., (2012). Face Reading in Chinese Medicine. Second edition. Elsevier: Amsterdam, Netherlands.

3.6 Five Elements, Five Phases

Five element (*wuxing* or five phase) theory is one of the fundamental concepts of Chinese and East Asian medicine. It describes the natural cycle of birth, maturation, and decline that governs the transition of the seasons and also human life.

Wuxing developed as a distinct philosophy during the Han dynasty (202 BCE to 220 CE). Prior to this, it functioned simply as a method of describing various natural processes. However, from the Han dynasty onward, it was extended to apply to various other phenomena, including esthetics, historical events, political and social structures, and more. It has now also become integral to many schools of acupuncture and TCEAM.

The Five Phases of Feminine Life

Although the elements/phases exist in a continuously flowing circuit, wood is generally taken as a starting point due to its association with the springtime and increasing yang. This also applies to the five phases of feminine life, which start with wood and end with water.

Anastacïa White, a TCEAM practitioner with over 30 years of experience, teaches that each of these phases is typically associated with certain characteristics and challenges. They can be viewed in the flowchart below.

Note that menopause begins after the earth phase and moves into the metal phase:

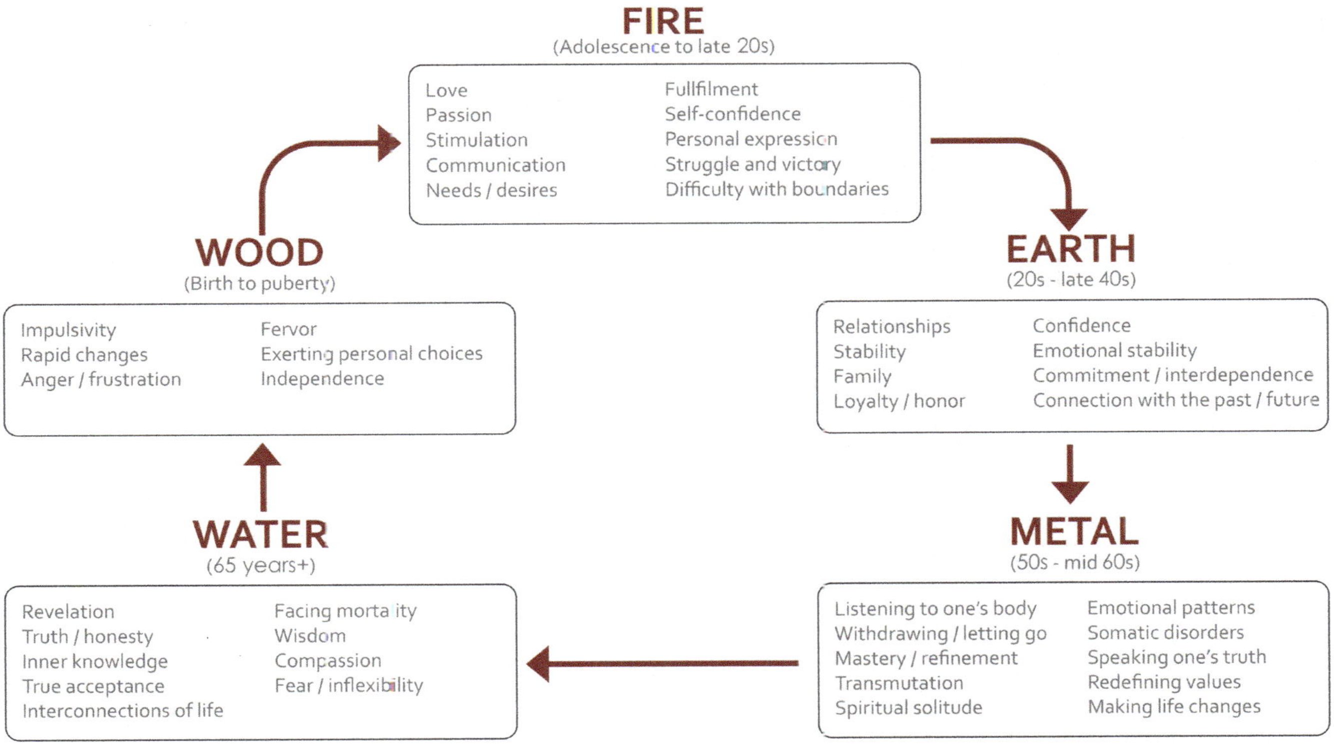

Figure 3.6a: Life cycle of the *wuxing* five phases or elements

Elemental Types and Imbalances

According to experienced five element practitioner Rebecca Avern, the way that a woman experiences menopause will depend upon the balance of the five elements within her body. In five element acupuncture, an elemental imbalance is seen as the root cause of menopausal symptoms (*ben*), whereas patterns of disharmony are considered the branches (*biao*).

Any of the elements can become imbalanced, although most women will tend towards imbalances in one particular element. By treating at this deep, constitutional level, acupuncturists can help women to flourish, thrive, and become empowered at every stage of their lives.

The primary methods of diagnosing elemental imbalances include observations of the patient's color, sound, odour, and emotion, in addition to routine questioning. Although this system may appear simple, five element diagnosis is highly nuanced and takes many years to perfect.

Element	Color	Sound	Odour	Emotion
Wood	Green	Shouting	Rancid	Anger
Fire	Red	Laughing	Scorched	Joy
Earth	Yellow	Singing	Fragrant	Sympathy/worry
Metal	White	Weeping	Rotten	Grief
Water	Blue	Groaning	Putrid	Fear

Table 3.6a: Primary methods of diagnosing elemental imbalances according to the Five Elements.

Each elemental type will have to deal with unique issues and symptoms and should, therefore, be treated accordingly. In five element acupuncture, there is a strong focus on the mind and spirit as well as physical symptoms. This allows for treatment of the whole person rather than just the presenting condition or issues.

Five Element Treatment and Protocols

Five element treatments tend to focus on the 'command points' of the relevant pair of channels. Command points include the *yuan* (source) points, *luo* (connecting) points, *xi*-cleft (accumulation) points, and elemental points. The elemental points have various functions depending upon the circumstances in which they are used.

It is customary to treat the yin and yang channels together, and practitioners will often only treat one pair at a time depending on which element they deem to be out of balance.

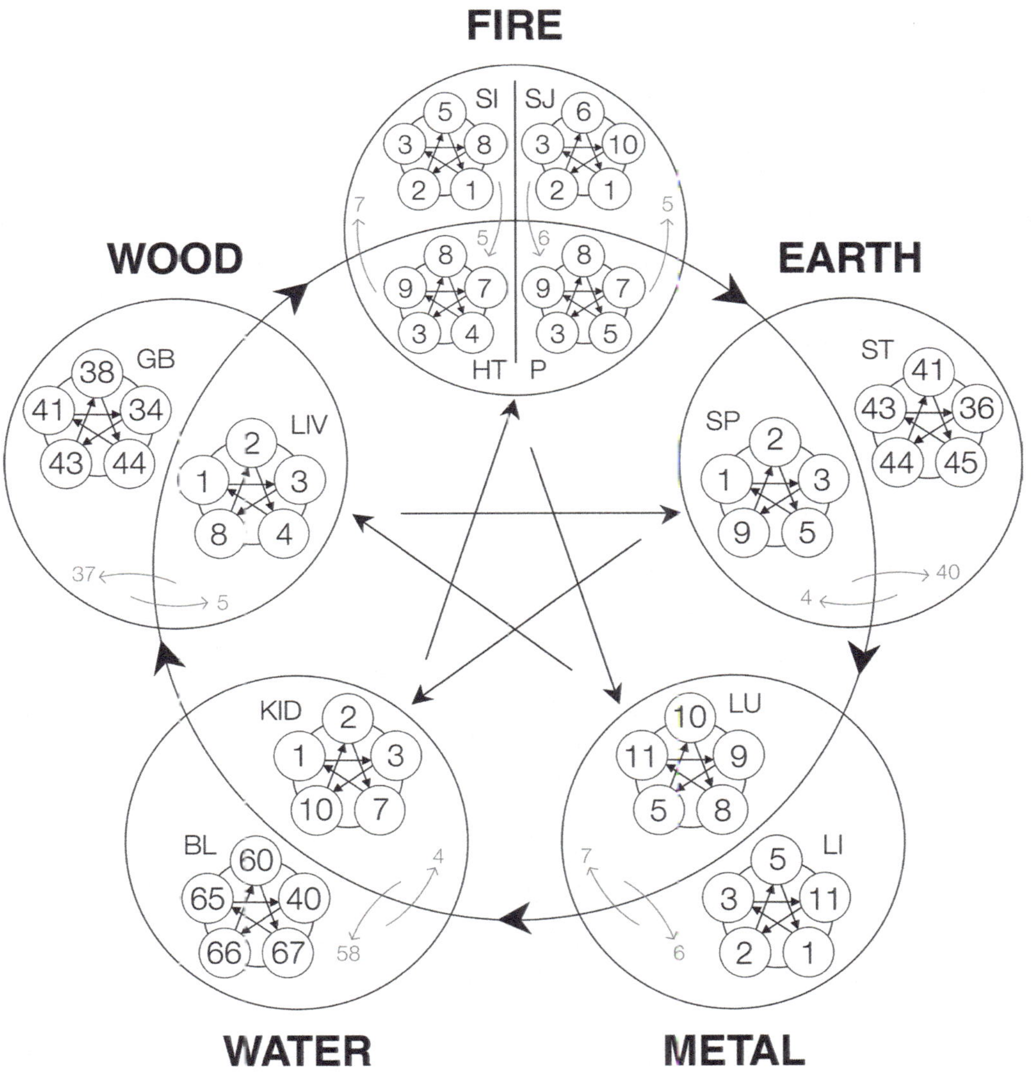

Organ	LU	LI	ST	SP	HT	SI	BL	KID	P	SJ	GB	LIV
Yuan Source	9	4	42	3	7	4	64	3	7	4	40	3
Xi Cleft	6	7	34	8	6	6	63	5	4	7	36	6

Figure 3.6b: Five element command points.

Below are some of the key issues faced by each elemental type as they progress through the menopausal transition. Symptoms, treatment principles, beneficial points, and dietary advice are also listed:

Wood

- Governs change
- Prevents getting 'stuck'
- Helps envisage the future
- Guides when to advance (Liver yang) and when to retreat (Liver yin)

Key Issues

- How to balance responsibility with freedom
- How to envision the next phase of life

Symptoms	Treatment	Points	Dietary Advice
Moodiness Irritability Intolerance Impatience Depression Changeability Headaches Declining vision Muscle stiffness/ pain/ spasms Irregular periods Heavy bleeding Hot flashes	Move qi/ Blood Nourish Liver Blood/yin Subdue Liver yang Clear Liver fire	Tianchong GB-9 (brings clarity and aids decision making) Benshen GB-13 Riyue GB-24 (recalibration of yin and yang) Guangming GB-37 (junction point) Zulinqi GB-41 Xingjian LIV-2 (frustration, agitation, hot flashes) Ligou LIV-5 (junction point) Ququan LIV-8 Qimen LIV-14	Avoid greasy/ fatty food Reduce heat-producing foods (red meat, alcohol, etc.) Reduce intake at each meal Move around after eating

Food

Leafy greens - cabbage, brassicas, dandelion leaf, kale, kohlrabi, parsley, spinach, etc.
Pulses and bean products - mung beans, aduki beans, black beans, kidney beans, haricot beans, etc.
Pungent foods - garlic, onions, radish, spring onion, mustard greens, watercress
Herbs and spices - aniseed, basil, caraway, cardamom, coriander, cumin, citrus peel, chive, fenugreek, turmeric
Sour foods - citrus zest, pickles, cider vinegar
Herbal teas - peppermint, chamomile, mint

Table 3.6b: Wood element treatment and protocols.

Fire
• Expression of individuality • Feeling loved and loveable • Connection with others • Inner calm and stability

Key Issues
• How to express one's authentic self at this stage of life • How to feel loved and connected

Symptoms	Treatment	Points	Dietary Advice
Insomnia (11pm-3am) Palpitations Forgetfulness Absent-mindedness Heavy bleeding Anxiety Agitation Panic attacks Depression	Nourish Blood/ yin Clear Heart-fire Resolve phlegm misting the mind Clear phlegm-fire harassing Heart	Jianshi P-5 (clears phlegm) Neiguan P-6 (opens the chest) Zhongchong P-9 Zhongzhu SJ-3 Tianyou SJ-16 (uplifts spirit) Jiquan HT-1 Shaohai HT-3 Yinxi HT-6 Shaofu HT-8 Houxi SI-3 Tianzong SI-11 (brings clarity)	Nourish Blood/yin Heating foods such as alliums in moderation Eat with others Make meals a joyful experience Beware of emotional eating due to loneliness, feeling unloved etc.

Food
Leafy greens - brassicas, dandelion leaf, kale, parsley, spinach, watercress **Vegetables** - avocado, beetroot, carrots **Pulses and seeds** - alfalfa, mung beans, aduki beans, sesame seeds, tahini **Fruit** - apricots, cherries, coconut products, dates, figs, goji berries **Grains** - wheat germ, oats, brown rice, corn, barley **Drinks** - green tea, chamomile, jasmine, mint

Table 3.6c: Fire element treatment and protocols.

<table>
<tr><th colspan="4">Earth</th></tr>
<tr><td colspan="4">• Balance of looking after self and others
• Changes in role as a mother (children growing up/sense of finality for women who did not have children)
• Feeling part of a community
• Governs thought and ideation (yi)
• Relationship with food</td></tr>
<tr><th colspan="4">Key Issues</th></tr>
<tr><td colspan="4">• How to meet one's own needs in the next phase of life
• Defining a new role once children have grown up/left home and finding other ways to feel needed</td></tr>
<tr><th>Symptoms</th><th>Treatment</th><th>Points</th><th>Dietary Advice</th></tr>
<tr><td>Digestive issues
Water retention
Weight gain
Muscle slackness
Fatigue
Worry
Feeling ungrounded
Feeling misunderstood
Feeling uncared for</td><td>Strengthen Spleen to hold Blood and raise qi

Resolve dampness</td><td>Renying ST-9 (reconnection with world and people)
Chengman ST-20
Qichong ST-30 (regulate chongmai)
Gongsun SP-4 (digestive issues)
Zhourong SP-20</td><td>Eat less

Avoid cold/damp-forming foods

Include foods to move qi (onions, garlic, spices etc.)

Make eating a communal experience

Regain enjoyment of cooking for one's self</td></tr>
<tr><th colspan="4">Food</th></tr>
<tr><td colspan="4">Root vegetables - carrots, celeriac, parsnips, pumpkin, squash, sweet potato
Fruit - small amounts of cooked fruits (esp. apples, blackberries, cherries, peaches)
Meat and fish - small amounts of chicken, chicken liver, herring, mackerel, tuna
Aromatic herbs and alliums - aniseed, basil, caraway, cardamom, clove, coriander, fennel, fenugreek, ginger, nutmeg, oregano, rosemary, thyme
Moderate amounts of beans and pulses
Grains - rye, buckwheat, basmati rice, toasted oats
Drinks - green tea, jasmine tea</td></tr>
</table>

Table 3.6d: Earth element treatment and protocols.

Metal
• Connection with that which is of value • Relationship with sadness/grief • Ability to let go of what no longer serves and take in the new

Key Issues
• How to create meaning in the next phase of life • Finding a source of self-esteem

Symptoms	Treatment	Points	Dietary Advice
Sadness Grief Feeling undervalued	Nourish and warm Lung qi Nourish Lung yin Resolve phlegm	Zhongfu LU-1 (reconnect with heavenly qi, aid digestion through connection with the Spleen) Tianfu LU-3 Chize LU-5 (resolve phlegm) Tianding LI-17 Futu LI-18	Good quality foods - metal constitutional types care about quality, easily feel 'polluted'

Food
To tonify qi - rice, carrots, sweet potato, cabbage and other brassicas, licorice, shiitake and reishi mushrooms **A little honey, barley malt, molasses** **Small amounts of pungent foods** - onions, garlic, leek, spring onion, horseradish, fresh ginger **To nourish Lung yin** - apples, apricots, figs, pears, honey, barley malt, rice syrup, almonds, avocados, barley, pine nuts, seaweed, sesame seeds, eggs

Table 3.6e: Metal element treatment and protocols.

Water			
• Underpins changeover of cycles • Houses willpower (*zhi*) to determine drive and libido • Ability to feel safe and trusting • Influences relationship with the future			
Key Issues			
• How to approach the next phase of life with serenity and courage			
Symptoms	**Treatment**	**Points**	**Dietary Advice**
Irregular periods Insomnia (4–5am) Lethargy Feeling cold Hot flashes Water retention Low libido Anxiety Depression Panic attacks Spiritual malaise	Nourish Kidney yin/yang Nourish Kidney *jing* Clear empty heat	Jingming BL-1 (allows a clear view of future) Tianzhu BL-10 (overcoming fear of future) Kunlun BL-60 Yongquan KID-1 Bulang KID-22 (overcoming fear of entering next stage of life)	Nourish *jing* Reduce cold and damp-forming foods Reduce heat-producing foods Be still and do not engage in other activities when eating
Food			
Nuts and seeds - especially walnuts, chestnuts, pistachios **Animal products** - anchovy, beef, chicken, kidney, lamb, liver, lobster, mussels **All fruit and vegetables**, especially alfalfa, artichoke, asparagus, tomato, turnip, yam **All pulses** **All nuts and seeds** **Royal jelly, bee pollen**			

Table 3.6f: Water element treatment and protocols.

Five Element Acupuncture Treatment Approaches

In addition to treatment according to each of the elemental types, there are also various protocols that are used within a five element acupuncture framework, especially within the early stages of treatment. These include the following:

Aggressive Energy

Aggressive energy (AE) treatments usually take place during the first five element acupuncture session, unless internal or external dragons are present (see below). AE is described as a form of pathological qi that travels through the yin organs via the *ke* (controlling) cycle. Therefore, it should be cleared before carrying out treatments that transfer qi from one channel to another.

AE treatments are sometimes referred to as a 'draining' treatment, and some practitioners liken them to a form of detox. These treatments also have a diagnostic role as they assist in the identification of potentially afflicted organs.

Although they are routinely conducted during the first session, AE treatments can be repeated later and are especially useful for people taking or coming off medication, including MHT. In these cases, they function to clear blocked qi and yang.

> *Protocol*
>
> AE treatments are usually conducted with the patient in a seated position. It is preferable to seat them on a stool or sideways on a chair, leaning forward over the treatment couch to prevent fainting. It is also possible to conduct an AE treatment with the patient lying face down, providing a face cradle is used to keep the head and neck straight.
>
> The treatment itself involves very superficial needling, without manipulation, of the yin back-shu points in the following order:
>
> 1. Feishu BL-13
> 2. Jueyinshu BL-14
> 3. Ganshu BL-18
> 4. Pishu BL-20
> 5. Shenshu BL-23
> 6. Xinshu BL-15 (some practitioners omit this point unless AE shows on Jueyinshu)
>
> If there is any AE in a particular organ, erythema (redness) will appear around the corresponding needle. However, some patients with sensitive skin will develop erythema regardless of the presence of AE. Therefore, it is necessary to place 'check' needles at adjacent non-acupoints for comparison. Usually, one check needle per segment of the back (upper, middle, and lower) is sufficient.
>
> If AE is present, the needles are retained until it clears, usually 20–30 minutes, although it may take longer. If there is no indication of AE after 5–10 minutes, the needles can be removed.
>
> Once the needles have been removed, the treatment is completed by needling the source points of the patient's primarily imbalanced element. The needle technique for this is gentle reinforcing without retention.

Internal and External Dragons

The internal and external dragons (IDs and EDs) are a form of deep energetic block and, if present, must be cleared before treatment can proceed. As the names suggest, IDs tend to stem from internal sources, such as long-term emotional issues, whereas EDs tend to stem from external sources. Examples include abusive relationships, traumatic experiences, or drug dependence.

Diagnosing IDs and EDs can be challenging. Common signs include patients who seem disconnected, 'spaced out,' or unable to maintain eye contact. The patient may also provide clues by using phrases such as "not feeling myself." Some practitioners also describe a 'masked' quality on the pulse.

IDs and EDs can occur together or in isolation. Determining which is present will ultimately depend upon the patient's individual case history. As the two are difficult to differentiate clinically, many practitioners choose to treat both blocks, starting with IDs and then progressing to EDs.[14]

> *Internal Dragons Protocol*
> With the patient lying on their back, the following points are needled in order:
>
> 1. Master point of Jiuwei REN-15 (just below REN-15, located by palpation)
> 2. Tianshu ST-25
> 3. Futu ST-32
> 4. Jiexi ST-41
>
> Needles are inserted perpendicularly, right to left, and turned a fraction anti-clockwise on insertion. Once all of the needles have been inserted and manipulated, it is necessary to turn them further to complete a 180-degree anti-clockwise turn.
>
> Patients should then be allowed to relax with needles in situ for at least 20 minutes or until a satisfactory pulse change occurs. Needles are removed in the same order as they were inserted.
>
> The treatment is completed by needling Shenmen HT-7 using a gentle reinforcing technique without retention.
>
> *External Dragons Protocol*
> With the patient lying on their front, the following points are needled in order:
>
> 1. Baihui DU-20
> 2. Dazhu BL-11
> 3. Shenshu BL-23
> 4. Pucan BL-61
>
> Needles are inserted and manipulated in the same fashion as for IDs.

---

[14] It is possible to conduct IDs and EDs treatments in the same session if the patient is constitutionally strong enough. However, many practitioners prefer to conduct them in consecutive sessions, followed by AE.

Husband-Wife Imbalance

Husband-wife (HW) imbalances are rare but serious energetic blocks that occur due to the separation of yin and yang. The primary sign of a HW imbalance is a pulse that is weaker on the left-hand side (the husband) than the right (the wife). It suggests a decrease in organ function and may precede the onset of serious disease.

These patients may be in a situation where they feel trapped but unable to act as that would destroy their personal identity. Therefore, it is common for those with HW imbalances to present with psychological symptoms or mood disorders. In menopausal women, this may manifest as a tortured state of indecision about the future. However, the key to diagnosis is the pulse and without this feature, a HW imbalance is unlikely to be the cause.

> *Protocol 1*
> The following points are needled in order, using a gentle reinforcing technique without retention:
>
> 1. Zhiyin BL-67
> 2. Fuliu KID-7
> 3. Taixi KID-3
> 4. Zhongfeng LIV-4
> 5. Wangu SI-4
> 6. Shenmen HT-7
>
> If the above fails to clear the block, a second protocol may be attempted (see below).

> *Protocol 2*
> The following points are needled in order, using a reducing technique:
>
> 1. Chize LU-5
> 2. Erjian LI-2
> 3. Taibai SP-3
> 4. Chongyang ST-42
> 5. Daling P-7
> 6. Yangchi SJ-4

Since the above protocols involve transferring qi from one channel to another, it is essential to perform an AE drain before conducting them. Therefore, the order of the first 3–4 treatments is as follows:

1. Internal Dragons (if present)
2. External Dragons (if present)
3. Aggressive Energy
4. Husband-Wife (if present)

Five Element Spirit Points

When treating menopause with TCEAM, there is a tendency to focus on underlying patterns of disharmony. However, it is also beneficial to help reframe menopause as a positive experience by attending to the patient's emotional and spiritual needs. Perhaps one of the most effective ways to do this is by adopting a five element approach to treatment.

While many five element practitioners have a strict approach whereby they treat only the constitutional element, there are some points that may benefit all menopausal patients.

Due to earth and metal's associations with the shift from the fertile years to menopause, points on these channels may be particularly appropriate. It may be especially helpful to select points according to their impact on the psyche, or what we might refer to as the 'spirit of the points.'

Some excellent examples include:

Point	Function
Renying ST-9	Supports new experiences and perspectives, engenders conscious change
Quepen ST-12	Facilitates the receiving and retention of nourishment, attenuates sense of loss
Liangmen ST-21	Integrates the body, mind, and spirit during periods of transition
Taiyi ST-23	Promotes harmony, integration, and a sense of wholeness
Tianshu ST-25	Provides stability during periods of transition (consider combining with Daheng SP-15)
Fenglong ST-40	Promotes a sense of harvest and abundance (consider combining with Gongsun SP-4)
Gongsun SP-4	Brings about a sense of harvest while looking toward the future
Diji SP-8	Promotes adaptability and creative transformation
Daheng SP-15	Promotes flexibility without weakness
Fuai SP-16	Counters feelings of sadness, especially those relating to the end of motherhood or fertility
Zhongfu LU-1	Engenders a sense of connection and security
Tianfu LU-3	Promotes balance between healthy boundaries and appropriate connection
Kongzui LU-6	Counters feelings of emptiness and depletion
Lieque LU-7	Facilitates the healthy expression of grief and sadness
Taiyuan LU-9	Counters depression and feelings of deprivation
Tianding LI-17	Promotes clarity of mind and spirit
Futu LI-18	Supports the ability to let go of the old and accept the new

Table 3.6h: Five Element Spirit Points.

Summary

The five elements/five phases can be used to describe the different stages that a woman passes through during her lifetime, with menopause occuring at the end of the earth phase and moving into metal.

The five elements can also provide a treatment framework that aims to rectify deep imbalances (the root - *ben*), thus alleviating multiple symptoms (the branches - *biao*) simultaneously. Five element acupuncture may be used as a standalone technique or combined with other methods, such as the eight principles.

Moreover, in five-element traditions, there is a strong focus on the 'spirits of points,' and how they can impact psychological wellbeing. Points on the earth and metal channels may be particularly helpful for menopausal patients, although there are many other powerful examples and points should always be selected on a case-by-case basis.

References

White, A., (2019). Chinese Herbal Medicines and Constitutional Types. Treating Women Academy: Online Menopause Masterclass.
https://www.treatingwomen.com/store/5tpUJ3Fk

Littlejohn, R., Wuxing (Wu-hsing). IEP., Internet Encyclopedia of Philosophy: (Sourced January 2021).
https://iep.utm.edu/wuxing

Avern, R., (2019). Midlife and Menopause - Five Element Perspective. Treating Women Academy: Online Menopause Masterclass.
https://www.treatingwomen.com/store/5tpUJ3Fk

Jarrett, L., (2006). The Clinical Practice of Chinese Medicine. Spirit Path Press. Stockbridge, Massachusetts.

Hatton, C.L., (2004). Acupuncture Point Compendium. Second Edition. College of Traditional Acupuncture: Royal Leamington Spa

SECTION 4 - Symptoms and Treatment

4.1 Vasomotor Symptoms

The vasomotor system includes the nerves and the structures from which they arise (e.g., the medulla oblongata or spinal cord) that regulate blood flow to specific organs or body parts by controlling the blood vessels' internal diameter.

Vasomotor symptoms (VMS) are synonymous with menopause, including hot flashes and night sweats. They affect the majority of individuals to some extent during the climacteric period. Vasomotor symptoms can be defined as periodic episodes of intense heat accompanied by sweating or flashing.

They usually affect the head, neck, chest, and upper back, lasting 3–10 minutes, and may occur multiple times each day. In some cases, vasomotor symptoms may be accompanied by feelings of anxiety and palpitations.

The severity of vasomotor symptoms usually peaks between late perimenopause and early post-menopause. However, they may occur much earlier, even before the onset of menstrual irregularities, and persist into a person's 60s or 70s. For this reason, it is essential that practitioners learn how to treat hot flashes and night sweats to alleviate their patients' suffering.

Pathophysiology

As women approach menopause, their 'thermoregulatory zone' narrows, meaning the range within which normal body temperature is maintained reduces. Thus, even small fluctuations in the external temperature can trigger a homeostatic response, including peripheral vasodilation and perspiration.

The exact physiological mechanism underlying vasomotor symptoms is unclear. However, they appear to be the result of multiple central and peripheral systems interacting abnormally due to fluctuating estrogen and FSH levels. The fact that estrogen replacement therapy reduces vasomotor symptoms suggests that reduced estrogen levels are a critical factor.

The serotonergic, noradrenergic, autonomic, and vascular systems may all play a role in the development of vasomotor symptoms. There is also some inconsistent evidence suggesting the involvement of the endogenous opioid system. One theory suggests that decreased estrogen levels increase noradrenaline release, upregulating hypothalamic serotonin receptors, which play a role in temperature control.

Risk Factors

Although vasomotor symptoms are extremely common, the following risk factors can predict more severe, more frequent, and longer-lasting problems:

Ethnicity

According to the large-scale Study of Women's Health Across the Nation (SWAN) study, the ethnic group most likely to be severely affected by vasomotor symptoms is African-Americans. The least likely groups to suffer are Chinese and Japanese women, while Caucasian and Hispanic women report similar rates of vasomotor symptoms.

The reason for these differences is unclear. In the past, it has been suggested that East Asian women suffer fewer vasomotor symptoms due to a higher soy intake. However, this does not appear to be the case. Other possible explanations are cultural differences in the way menopause is interpreted, experienced, and reported to health professionals, particularly in cultures where doctors are mostly male.

Obesity

Women with a higher body mass index, especially those carrying excess abdominal fat, have a higher risk of experiencing severe vasomotor symptoms. This could be due to increased endocrine dysregulation or the additional insulation of adipose tissue. However, the precise reasoning is not fully understood.

Smoking

Both active and passive smoking may increase the risk of severe vasomotor symptoms. Many of the chemicals in cigarette smoke have anti-estrogenic properties.

Negative Mood

Women who suffer from anxiety or depression tend to experience more severe vasomotor symptoms. There also appears to be a connection with childhood abuse or neglect and lower socioeconomic status (see Chapter 5.2 Stress, Trauma, and Stress Resistance).

Diet and Exercise

The direct link between diet, physical activity, and vasomotor symptoms has not been confirmed. However, eating a balanced, calorie-controlled diet and engaging in regular physical activity can contribute to a healthy body mass index, which in turn could reduce the risk of vasomotor symptoms.

TCEAM Viewpoint

Traditionally, VMS (and menopause in general) have been associated with Kidney deficiency, especially Kidney yin deficiency. In reality, the etiology of this symptom is usually far more complex.

While Kidney deficiency is common among older patients, either Kidney yin or Kidney yang deficiency may predominate. However, it is rare to see one without at least some degree of the other. Furthermore, other *zangfu* are frequently involved, as are qi and Blood deficiency or stasis.

In TCEAM terms, VMS may be seen as a form of tidal heat effusion, or *chaore*. There are several different patterns of disharmony that may underlie tidal heat effusion, which we will discuss below. These may occur in combination with a variety of other underlying patterns.

Pattern Differentiation

1. Predominance of Kidney yin deficiency
2. Predominance of Kidney yang deficiency
3. Kidney and Liver yin deficiency with Liver yang rising
4. Kidney and Heart not harmonized
5. Yin and Blood deficiency
6. Spleen and Stomach qi deficiency
7. *Yangming* repletion
8. Summer-heat invasion
9. Blood stasis

Rebellious Qi in the Penetrating Vessel (*Chongmai*)

Around menopause, the qi of the *chongmai* can become destabilized, causing symptoms such as hot flashes and anxiety. This is not a clinical pattern in itself, but may occur alongside other patterns, including cold, heat, stagnation, and phlegm. See Table 4.1a: Rebellious Qi in the Penetrating Vessel (*Chongmai*) on page 112.

Rebellious Qi in the Penetrating Vessel (*Chongmai*)			
The *chongmai* has two branches originating from Yinhui REN-1. One branch descends to the feet while the other ascends to the face. Around the time of menopause, qi in the *chongmai* may become destabilized causing it to rebel upward and fail to descend. This can occur as a result of various excess or deficiency factors, including heat, cold, stagnation, etc.			
Clinical Manifestations			
Feelings of heat in face, cold feet, headache, feeling of a lump in the throat, breast distension/pain, flutter in the chest or above the stomach, palpitations, slight breathlessness, sighing, chest tightness/oppression, abdominal fullness/distension/pain, irregular/painful/heavy periods, hypogastric fullness/distension/pain. To make a diagnosis, at least three symptoms must be present at different physical levels (i.e. hot face, cold feet, and abdominal symptoms), in combination with anxiety.			
Tongue	**Pulse**	**Treatment Principle**	**Points**
Variable, depending on coexisting excess and deficiency patterns	Firm and beating straight up and down in all three positions, from *chi* to *cun*, being most pronounced in the middle (*guan*) position However, the precise quality will vary depending on coexisting excess and deficiency patterns, meaning that patients may present with a wide variety of pulses	Harmonize the *chongmai*, subdue rebellious qi	Juque REN-14 Zhangmen LIV-13 Zhongji REN-3 Qichong ST-30 Youmen KID-21 Dahe KID-12 Qixue KID-13 Gongsun SP-4 Neiguan P-6 Taichong LIV-3
Prescription			
For cold: Wu Zhu Yu Tang For heat stagnation: Zuo Jin Wan For phlegm: Wen Dan Tang For food stagnation: Bao He Wan			

Table 4.1a: Rebellious qi in the penetrating vessel (*chongmai*).

1. Predominance of Kidney Yin Deficiency			
Deficient Kidney yin fails to subdue fire and leads to empty heat rising.			
Clinical Manifestations			
Night sweats, sensations of heat, dry mouth and throat at night, hot flashes, cold feet, frequent-pale urination, dizziness, vertigo, tinnitus, poor memory, hearing problems, lower backache, aching bones, tiredness, lassitude, depression, slight anxiety.			
Tongue	**Pulse**	**Treatment Principle**	**Points ***
Normal color without coating or rootless coating Red in severe cases	Floating-empty or weak on both Kidney positions	Nourish Kidney yin	Shenshu BL-23 Guanyuan REN-4 Taixi KID-3 Zhaohai KID-6 Sanyinjiao SP-6
Prescriptions			
Zhi Bai Di Huang Wan Zuo Gui Wan			

* For VMS, add: Baihui DU-20 | Shenmen HT-7 | Hegu LI-4 | Taichong LIV-3

Table 4.1b: Predominance of Kidney yin deficiency.

2. Predominance of Kidney Yang Deficiency

Yang becomes deficient and is unable to transform yin. This results in empty heat due to the ministerial fire flowing upwards along with excess yin. Patients with this pattern often present with a noticeable pale tongue, yet with other heat symptoms.

Clinical Manifestations

Hot flashes, hot sensation in the face, night sweats, lower backache, feeling cold, cold knees, back and feet, weak legs, bright white complexion, low libido, tiredness, lassitude, clear urination, nocturia, apathy, odema in legs, loose stools, depression.

Tongue	Pulse	Treatment Principle	Points *
Pale	Deep-weak	Tonify Kidney yang	Mingmen DU-4 Shenshu BL-23 Guanyuan REN-4 Taixi KID-3 Zusanli ST-36

Prescriptions

Jin Gui Shen Qi Wan
You Gui Wan

* For VMS, add: Baihui DU-20 | Shenmen HT-7 | Hegu LI-4

Table 4.1c: Predominance of Kidney yang deficiency

Acupuncture Points for Combined Kidney Yin and Kidney Yang Deficiency

Mingmen DU-4
Shenshu BL-23
Guanyuan REN-4
Taixi KID-3

Zhishi BL-52
Yongquan KID 1
Zhaohai KID-6
Sanyinjiao SP-6

For VMS symptoms add:
Baihui DU-20
Shenmen HT-7
Hegu LI-4
Zusanli ST-36
Qihai REN-6

3. Kidney and Liver Yin Deficiency with Liver Yang Rising			
Liver yin and Liver Blood rely on Kidney yin and Kidney essence for nourishment (water generating wood). Therefore, when Kidney yin becomes deficient, Liver yin will often follow suit. Deficient Liver yin allows Liver yang to rise upward, creating sensations of heat and other symptoms, such as irritability and headaches.			
Clinical Manifestations			
Hot flashes, night sweats, dizziness, tinnitus, blurred vision, dry eyes, dry skin, aching joints, sore back, irritability, headaches.			
Tongue	**Pulse**	**Treatment Principle**	**Points ***
Red without coating	Floating-empty, wiry on Liver position	Nourish Kidney and Liver yin, subdue Liver yang, calm the mind, settle the *hun*	Taichong LIV-3 Xingjian LIV-2 Xiaxi GB-43 Ganshu BL-18 Shenshu BL-23 Taixi KID-3 Sanyinjiao SP-6
Prescription			
Tian Ma Gou Teng Yin			

* For VMS, add: Baihui DU-20 | Shenmen HT-7 | Hegu LI-4 | Yinlingquan SP-9

Table 4.1d: Kidney and Liver yin deficiency with Liver yang rising.

4. Kidney and Heart Not Harmonized			
This pattern is a water-fire imbalance. It occurs due to a lack of Kidney yin (water), which fails to restrict Heart yang (fire), allowing it to flare upwards and cause hot flashes.			
Clinical Manifestations			
Hot flashes, palpitations, insomnia, mental restlessness, poor memory and night sweats, blurred vision, dizziness, tinnitus, anxiety, backache, malar flush, feeling of heat in the evening, dry mouth and throat, dry stools.			
Tongue	**Pulse**	**Treatment Principle**	**Points ***
Red without coating, redder tip	Rapid-fine, floating-empty, or weak-deep on both *chi* (proximal) positions, overflowing on both *cun* (distal) positions	Nourish Kidney yin, calm *shen*, clear empty heat	Xinshu BL-15 Shenshu BL-23 Taixi KID-3 Yongquan KID 1 Shenmen HT-7 Laogong P-8 Daling P-7 Sanyinjiao SP-6
Prescriptions			
Tian Wang Bu Xin Dan Huang Lian E Jiao Zi Huang Tang			

* For VMS, add: Baihui DU-20 | Shenmen HT-7 | Hegu LI-4 | Taichong LIV-3 | Juque REN-14 | Shenting DU-24

Table 4.1e. Kidney and Heart not harmonized.

5. Yin and Blood Deficiency			
Yin and Blood deficiency is one of the primary patterns underlying *chaore* in menopausal patients. Yin and Blood often become deficient due to decades of menstruation. This may be exacerbated by issues such as poor diet and impaired Stomach and Spleen function, Liver deficiency (the Liver stores Blood), and Heart deficiency (the Heart rules Blood). As the source of Blood, the Kidney is also often involved.			
Clinical Manifestations			
Intermittent waves of low-grade heat, heat in the palms and soles, heart vexation, palpitations, insomnia, night sweats. These symptoms are generally worse in the afternoon and evening or at night.			
Tongue	**Pulse**	**Treatment Principle**	**Points**
Red with scant coating	Fine and rapid	Nourish yin and Blood, clear heat	Rangu KID-2 Zhaohai KID-6 Sanyinjiao SP-6 Shaofu HT-8 Shenmen HT-7 Yuji LU-10 Dazhui DU-14 Jianshi P-5
Prescription			
Qing Gu San			

Table 4.1f. Yin and Blood deficiency.

6. Spleen and Stomach Qi Deficiency			
The most common cause of Spleen and Stomach deficiency is inappropriate diet and eating habits, including excessive consumption of unhealthy foods, overeating, undereating, etc. It may also occur as a result of chronic illness and often accompanies Kidney yin and yang deficiency.			
Clinical Manifestations			
Hot flashes that are worse in the morning, fatigue, weakness of the limbs, spontaneous sweating, pale complexion.			
Tongue	**Pulse**	**Treatment Principle**	**Points**
Pale	Weak	Tonify Spleen and Stomach qi, clear heat	Pishu BL-20 Weishu BL-21 Qihai REN-6 Zhongwan REN-12 Zusanli ST-36 Dazhui DU-14
Prescription			
Bu Zhong Yi Qi Tang			

Table 4.1g: Spleen and Stomach qi deficiency.

7. *Yangming* Repletion			
This is an excess pattern affecting the Stomach and Large Intestine and causing heat effusion as a result of stagnation in the digestive tract. It may occur in conjunction with Spleen qi deficiency and food stagnation. Stagnation causes heat to build up and then release at regular intervals throughout the day. The patient often presents with a history of constipation or difficult bowel movements, which must be addressed to treat the heat effusion successfully.			
Clinical Manifestations			
Hot flashes that become more severe between 3pm and 5pm, profuse sweating of the hands and feet, abdominal pain and distension, constipation, vexation, agitation.			
Tongue	**Pulse**	**Treatment Principle**	**Points**
Dry and yellow coating	Deep and forceful	Clear stagnation and heat in the *yangming* channels	Neiting ST-44 Hegu LI-4 Quchi LI-11 Pianli LI-6 Zusanli ST-36 Dachangshu BL-25 Dazhui DU-14 Jianshi P-5
Prescription			
Da Cheng Qi Tang			

Table 4.1h: *Yangming* repletion.

8. Summer-Heat Invasion			
In this pattern, sometimes known as damp-evil obstruction, hot and humid weather act as an external pathogenic factor, penetrating the body and impairing Spleen and Stomach qi. This leads to heat effusion that eases gradually as the weather cools. This pattern can also occur due to consuming contaminated food or water, or a diet that is too rich for the patient's constitution. While not necessarily a primary cause of hot flashes in menopausal patients, it may worsen pre-existing patterns and increase symptom severity.			
Clinical Manifestations			
Hot flashes, low-grade fever, thirst, poor appetite, vexation, agitation, fatigue, weakness, diarrhea.			
Tongue	**Pulse**	**Treatment Principle**	**Points**
Red with a greasy coating	Fine and rapid	Clear heat and dampness, support the Spleen and Stomach	Neiguan P-6 Hegu LI-4 Zusanli ST-36 Dazhui DU-14 Qihai REN-6 Pishu BL-20
Prescription			
Qing Shu Yi Qi Tang			

Table 4.1i: Summer-heat invasion.

9. Blood Stasis			
Blood stasis may occur as a result of long-standing qi stagnation or deficiency, and Blood deficiency impairing circulation and generating heat. It frequently occurs in combination with one of the above patterns.			
Clinical Manifestations			
Hot flashes that are worse in the afternoon, mental restlessness, very irregular periods preceding menopause, dark-clotted blood, insomnia, high blood pressure, abdominal pain, dry mouth, musculoskeletal pain.			
Tongue	**Pulse**	**Treatment Principle**	**Points**
Purplish or bluish, possibly with macules	Rough and fine	Invigorate Blood, eliminate stasis, move qi, eliminate stagnation	Geshu BL-17 Zhongji REN-3 Diji SP-8 Xuehai SP-10 Hegu LI-4 Taichong LIV-3 Baihui DU-20 Shenmen HT-7
Prescription			
For Blood stasis in the lower abdomen, affecting the menstrual cycle: Shao Fu Zhu Yu Tang For a milder formula: Tao Hong Si Wu Tang For deficiency cold of the *chongmai* and *renmai* with Blood stasis: Wen Jing Tang			

Table 4.1j: Blood stasis.

Patient Advice

> Reduce caffeine and alcohol consumption.
> Do not smoke.
> Keep rooms cool and use a desk, floor, or handheld fan if necessary.
> Sip cool water as needed throughout the day.
> Keep a spritzer bottle filled with water handy to spray the face as a hot flash comes on.
> Wear loose layers of clothing that can be easily removed.
> Wear natural fabrics, such as cotton, linen, or hemp.
> Layer sheets on the bed rather than a thick duvet so they can be easily removed if necessary.
> Bathe or shower in lukewarm, rather than hot, water.
> Some medication can cause hot flashes as a side effect - discuss this possibility with a doctor.

References

Thurston, RC., Joffe, H., (2011). Vasomotor symptoms and menopause: findings from the Study of Women's Health across the Nation. Obstetrics & Gynecology Clinics of North America,38(3): (pp.489-501).

NIH, National Library of Medicine, National Center for Biotechnology Information: Obstet Gynecol Clin North Am. 2011 Sep;38(3):489-501. doi: 10.1016/j.ogc.2011.05.006.
https://pubmed.ncbi.nlm.nih.gov/21961716/

Bolca, S., Bracke, M., Depypere, H., (2012). Soy consumption during menopause. Facts Views & Visions in ObGyn, 4(1): (pp.30-37). Facts Views Vis Obgyn v.4(1); 2012 PMC3991438.
https://www.ncbi.nlm.nih.gov/pmc/articles/PMC3991438/

Grosam, B., (2021). Understanding and Treating Hot Flashes in Menopause with Chinese Medicine. Singing Dragon. London and Philadelphia.

Maciocia, G. (1989). The Foundations of Chinese Medicine. First edition. Churchill Livingston Elsevier, London, UK.

Wolfe, HL., (1998). Managing Menopause Naturally with Chinese Medicine. Blue Poppy Press. Inc. Boulder, Colorado. USA

4.2 Mood Disorders

Mood is a concept that is subjective and difficult to define. It is less specific than emotions or thoughts and can be described as an ongoing state of mind that tends to be categorized as positive or negative.

Although one's mood has a significant influence over both psychological and physical health, our understanding of its neurological mechanisms is limited. It seems that numerous brain regions are involved, especially the hippocampus and amygdala. It also relies upon the release and binding of various neurotransmitters and activity in the hypothalamic-pituitary-adrenal axis. Furthermore, there is now mounting evidence that the gastrointestinal system, including the gut microbiota, plays a role.

It has been suggested that fluctuating moods are the result of our brains attempting to achieve a state of balance via allostasis, the process of maintaining homeostasis by anticipating change. Therefore, prediction errors may lead to alterations in mood depending on the desirability of the outcome, and negative moods have been linked with feelings of uncertainty and perceived lack of control.

Many different factors can impact mood, including genetics, epigenetics, life experiences, and exposure to stressors. Healthy individuals tend to experience moderate mood changes that are appropriate to the events affecting them on a daily basis.

However, mood disorders can lead to a narrowed spectrum of thoughts and emotions with a tendency to ruminate on negative themes. In some cases, they can cause rapid and extreme mood swings that are distressing to the individual and those around them. Therefore, it is essential that mood disorders are diagnosed and treated in a timely manner to attenuate their detrimental effects and reduce harm.

Mood and Menopause

Women are more likely to suffer from mood disorders, including depression and anxiety, as they transition through menopause. In addition to these common issues, perimenopausal and menopausal women may be more likely to experience other mood disorders for the first time or see an increase in pre-existing symptoms.

For example, the highest incidence of schizophrenia is during early adulthood. However, a second peak may occur in women aged 45–50 years. This second peak is not observed in men.

For women with bipolar disorder, the rate of depressive episodes may increase during the menopausal transition. There is also some inconclusive evidence that cycling between depressive and manic states may occur more rapidly.

During the menopausal years, panic disorder may occur for the first time, or pre-existing symptoms may worsen. The incidence of panic attacks may also increase.

A similar situation can be observed for obsessive-compulsive disorder, with menopause potentially triggering new cases, relapses, and changes in pre-existing symptoms.

However, the most thoroughly-researched mood disorders in relation to menopause remain depression and anxiety.

In terms of treatment, estrogen replacement therapy alone has not proven consistently effective. However, it may offer some value alongside a selective-serotonin reuptake inhibitor (SSRI) antidepressant in women who do not respond to SSRIs alone.

Depression

The term 'depression' covers a broad spectrum of mood disorders, ranging from mild and intermittent low mood to major depressive disorder. Symptoms include:

- Persistent low mood
- Irritability and tension
- Nervousness
- Tearfulness
- Feeling hopeless or helpless
- Low self-esteem
- Loss of motivation
- Loss of pleasure or enjoyment
- Difficulty making decisions
- Suicidal ideation or self-harm

Pathophysiology

Hormonal changes appear to contribute to the pathophysiology of depression during menopause. Women are twice as likely to suffer from depression than men at any stage in life, with this disparity evident from puberty. Depressive symptoms can fluctuate with hormonal changes, for example, premenstrual dysphoric disorder and postpartum depression.

Changing estrogen levels directly impact neurotransmitters, namely serotonin and norepinephrine, both of which are implicated in depressive disorders. Estrogen also reduces monoamine oxidase activity, delaying the metabolism of these chemicals.

Various psychosocial factors can also contribute to depressive symptoms during the menopausal transition. They include:

- Lack of social support
- Stressful life events such as divorce
- Unemployment or employment changes
- Financial stress
- Poor overall health
- Lack of a partner or relationship dissatisfaction
- Unsatisfactory sexual relationships
- Negative attitude towards aging and menopause
- A sense of finality regarding fertility
- Changes in one's role as a mother
- Aging and increasingly dependent parents
- Illness or death of a partner
- Feelings of self-doubt and loss of confidence
- Feelings of unattractiveness due to societal views of aging, weight gain or loss, changing body image

Risk Factors

In addition to the above, several risk factors can predict the likelihood of developing depression during the menopausal period:

Vasomotor Symptoms

Women who suffer from severe vasomotor symptoms are more likely to suffer from depression during menopause.

Ethnicity

According to the SWAN study, Caucasian, African-American, and Hispanic women have an increased risk of depressive symptoms during menopause compared to Chinese and Japanese women.

Smoking

Being a current smoker increases the risk of depression during the menopausal transition.

Body Mass Index

Having a higher body mass index is another predictor of depression during menopause.

Socioeconomic Factors

Women with less than a college education are more likely to suffer from depression. These women are also more likely to have other risk factors, including smoking, increased body weight, and employment/financial difficulties.

History of Depression

Menopausal mood disorders appear to have an association with a past history of depressive disorders treated with antidepressants, major depressive disorder, and oral contraceptive-induced dysphoria. This suggests that some psychiatrically vulnerable women may also have an increased sensitivity to reproductive hormones.

TCEAM Viewpoint

Mood disorders can arise as a result of an imbalance in any of the yin organs. For more information, see Chapter 3.6, Five Elements, Five Phases.

Pattern Differentiation

1. Liver qi stagnation
2. Predominance of Kidney yin deficiency
3. Predominance of Kidney yang deficiency
4. Phlegm

1. Liver Qi Stagnation			
Four distinct pathological factors contribute to the development of this pattern: **I.** Over three decades of a monthly menstrual cycle lead to qi and Blood deficiency. **II.** Qi and Blood deficiency increase the likelihood of Liver qi stagnation, especially combined with the additional lifestyle stressors associated with menopause. **III.** Liver qi stagnates along the channel, giving rise to localized symptoms in the upper and middle *jiao*, along with menstrual issues. **IV.** Stagnation generates heat. Liver fire harasses the Heart, causing emotional issues and insomnia.			
Clinical Manifestations			
Hypochondriac pain and distension, sighing, hiccups, nausea, vomiting, epigastric pain or pulsation, poor appetite, acid reflux, belching, difficulty swallowing, churning sensation in the stomach, abdominal distension, borborygmi, diarrhea, depression, mood swings, irritability, irregular or painful periods, premenstrual breast distension, premenstrual syndrome.			
Tongue	**Pulse**	**Treatment Principle**	**Points***
Normal body color	Wiry, especially on the left side	Disperse Liver and regulate qi	Ganshu BL-18 Neiguan P-6 Taichong LIV-3 Sanyinjiao SP-6 Zhangmen LIV-13 Zusanli ST-36 Xingjian LIV-2 Zhigou SJ-6 Yanglingquan GB-34
Prescription			
For stagnation without heat: Xiao Yao San For stagnation with heat: Jia Wei Xiao Yao San, Yue Ju Wan For stronger Liver qi stagnation: Chai Hu Shu Gan San			

* Additional points:
Taixi KID-3 Water nourishes wood
Hegu LI-4 Regulate qi and calm *shen*
Baihui DU-20 to Shenting DU-24 and Shenmen HT-7 to calm *shen*

Table 4.2a: Liver qi stagnation.

2. Predominance of Kidney Yin Deficiency			
As Kidney water declines throughout the menopausal transition, it becomes less able to quell Heart fire. This leads to *shen* disturbances, including anxiety, insomnia, and hot flashes. Eventually, the Heart qi becomes taxed and weakens, leading to fatigue and qi stagnation.			
Clinical Manifestations			
Night sweats, sensations of heat, dry mouth and throat at night, hot flashes, cold feet, frequent-pale urination, dizziness, vertigo, tinnitus, poor memory, hearing problems, lower backache, aching bones, tiredness, lassitude, depression, slight anxiety.			
Tongue	**Pulse**	**Treatment Principle**	**Points***
Normal color without coating or with rootless coating. Red in severe cases	Floating-empty or weak on both Kidney positions	Nourish Kidney yin	Shenshu BL-23 Guanyuan REN-4 Taixi KID-3 Zhaohai KID-6 Sanyinjiao SP-6
Prescription			
Liu Wei Di Huang Wan For signs of empty heat: Zhi Bai Di Huang Wan For true Kidney yin deficiency (at the *jing* level): Zuo Gui Wan			

* For mood disorders, add: Taichong LIV-3 | Shenmen HT-7 | Hegu LI-4 | Baihui DU-20

Table 4.2b: Predominance of Kidney yin deficiency.

3. Predominance of Kidney Yang Deficiency			
Declining Kidney yang fails to generate yin and activate qi, allowing stagnation and, thus, depression to occur. Kidney yang deficiency can cause fatigue, low libido, and apathy, all of which are frequently associated with depression.			
Clinical Manifestations			
Hot flashes, hot sensation in the face, night sweats, lower backache, feeling cold, cold knees, back, and feet, weak legs, bright white complexion, low libido, tiredness, lassitude, clear urination, nocturia, apathy, odema in the legs, loose stools, depression.			
Tongue	**Pulse**	**Treatment Principle**	**Points**
Pale	Deep-weak	Tonify Kidney yang	Mingmen DU-4 Taibai SP-3 Shenshu BL-23 Guanyuan REN-4 Taixi KID-3 Zusanli ST-36 Taichong LIV-3 Hegu LI-4 Baihui DU-20 Shenmen HT-7 Neiguan P-6
Prescription			
Jin Gui Shen Qi Wan You Gui Wan			

Table 4.2c: Predominance of Kidney yang deficiency.

4. Phlegm			
Phlegm may accumulate due to insufficient Stomach and Spleen activity and failure to transform food essences efficiently. Accumulated phlegm leads to qi stagnation and Blood stasis, which eventually consume qi and *jing*. According to many sources, phlegm obstructs the Heart orifices or combines with fire to 'harass the Heart,' leading to depression, restlessness, and agitation. In these cases, the symptoms tend to be more severe, including intractable depression and extreme anxiety or mania, in which the patient is not grounded.			
Clinical Manifestations			
Obesity, chest oppression, sputum in the chest, feeling of fullness in the epigastrium, feeling of breast distension, irritability, belching, nausea, lack of appetite, moodiness, depression.			
Tongue	**Pulse**	**Treatment Principle**	**Points**
Slightly red sides, sticky coating	Slippery	Move qi, resolve phlegm, pacify the Liver, eliminate stagnation, free the connecting channels	Zhongwan REN-12 Zusanli ST-36 Hegu LI-4 Fenglong ST-40 Yinlingquan SP-9 Tianshu ST-25 Qihai REN-6 Pishu BL-20 Taichong LIV-3 Neiguan P-6 Baihui DU-20
Prescription			
Er Chen Tang For stagnation generating phlegm (i.e. Liver overacting on Spleen): Yue Ju Wan			

Table 4.2d: Phlegm.

Anxiety

Anxiety is more difficult to define than depression as it can include a variety of distinct disorders, including generalized anxiety disorder, social anxiety disorder, phobias, and panic disorder. However, generally speaking, the symptoms of anxiety include:

- Irritability and tension
- Nervousness
- Restlessness
- Unexplained fear
- Racing or pounding heart
- Dry mouth
- Dizziness
- Tiredness
- Nausea
- Headaches
- Insomnia *
- Sweating
- Shortness of breath

> *** Insomnia**
>
> Brian Grosam clinical observation:
> "Interestingly, menopause transition (MT) anxiety, insomnia, and hot flashes all respond to acupuncture at the same equal rate in clinic whereas MT depression responds faster than MT anxiety."

Pathophysiology

The exact pathophysiology of anxiety during menopause is unclear. However, many of the factors that contribute to depression may also lead to anxiety.

One of the most significant predictors for anxiety during menopause is vasomotor symptoms, suggesting there may be a relationship between these two disorders.

Risk Factors

The risk factors for anxiety during menopause are similar to those of depression. They include ethnicity, socioeconomic, and health-related factors.

Interestingly, women with low anxiety levels prior to menopause are more likely to see increased anxiety symptoms during the climacteric period. No additional increases have been noted in women with previously high anxiety levels. Symptoms appear to decrease in both groups once the menopausal transition is complete.

Pattern Differentiation

1. Predominance of Kidney yin deficiency
2. Kidney and Liver yin deficiency with Liver yang rising
3. Kidney and Heart not harmonized

1. Predominance of Kidney Yin Deficiency			
Deficient yin leads to empty heat rising, restlessness, and anxiety.			
Clinical Manifestations			
Night sweats, sensations of heat, dry mouth and throat at night, hot flashes, cold feet, frequent-pale urination, dizziness, vertigo, tinnitus, poor memory, hearing problems, lower backache, aching bones, tiredness, lassitude, depression, slight anxiety.			
Tongue	**Pulse**	**Treatment Principle**	**Points***
Normal color without coating or rootless coating. Red in severe cases	Floating-empty or weak on both Kidney positions	Nourish Kidney yin	Shenshu BL-23 Guanyuan REN-4 Taixi KID-3 Zhaohai - KID-6 Sanyinjiao SP-6
Prescription			
Liu Wei Di Huang Wan For signs of empty heat: Zhi Bai Di Huang Wan For true Kidney yin deficiency (at the *jing* level): Zuo Gui Wan			

* For mood disorders, add: Taichong LIV-3 | Shenmen HT-7 | Hegu LI-4 | Baihui DU-20

Table 4.2e: Predominance of Kidney yin deficiency.

2. Kidney and Liver Yin Deficiency with Liver Yang Rising			
Liver yin and Liver Blood rely on Kidney yin and Kidney *jing* for nourishment (water generating wood). Therefore, when Kidney yin becomes deficient, Liver yin will often follow. A deficiency in Liver yin allows Liver yang to rise upward, creating sensations of heat and other symptoms, such as anxiety, irritability, and headaches.			
Clinical Manifestations			
Hot flashes, night sweats, dizziness, tinnitus, blurred vision, dry eyes, dry skin, aching joints, sore back, irritability, headaches.			
Tongue	**Pulse**	**Treatment Principle**	**Points***
Red without coating	Floating-empty, wiry on middle left (Liver) position	Nourish Kidney and Liver yin, subdue Liver-yang, calm the mind, settle the *hun*	Taichong LIV-3 Xingjian LIV-2 Yanglingquan GB-34 Xiaxi GB-43 Ganshu BL-18 Shenshu BL-23 Taixi KID-3 Sanyinjiao SP-6
Prescription			
Tian Ma Gou Teng Yin			

Table 4.22: Kidney and Liver yin deficiency with Liver yang rising.

3. Kidney and Heart Not Harmonized

Deficient Kidney yin (water) fails to restrict Heart yang (fire), leading to empty heat, *shen* disturbances, restlessness, anxiety, and insomnia.

Clinical Manifestations

Hot flashes, palpitations, insomnia, mental restlessness, poor memory and night sweats, blurred vision, dizziness, tinnitus, anxiety, backache, malar flush, feeling of heat in the evening, dry mouth and throat, dry stools.

Tongue	Pulse	Treatment Principle	Points*
Red without coating, redder tip	Rapid-fine, floating-empty, or weak-deep on both *chi* (proximal) positions, overflowing on both *cun* (distal) positions	Nourish Kidney yin, calm *shen*, clear empty heat	Xinshu BL-15 Shenshu BL-23 Taixi KID-3 Yongquan KID 1 Shenmen HT-7 Laogong P-8 Daling P-7 Sanyinjiao SP-6

Prescription

Tian Wang Bu Xin Dan
Gan Mai Da Zao Tang

Table 4.2g: Kidney and Heart not harmonized.

Patient Advice

The first-line treatment for mood disorders generally involves a combination of antidepressants and psychotherapy or behavioral therapy. While these treatments must be prescribed by an appropriately trained professional, there are also some lifestyle modifications that may prove helpful:

> Managing one's time effectively, prioritizing tasks, and taking regular breaks.
> Doing one thing at a time. Multitasking is no longer considered beneficial.
> Being assertive and saying no to tasks that are unmanageable or undesirable.
> Asking for help or delegating tasks when necessary.
> Regularly practicing relaxation techniques (meditation, breathing exercises, yoga, tai chi, etc.).
> Practicing mindfulness - the non-judgemental noticing of one's thoughts and feelings in the present moment.
> Engaging in sufficient physical activity.
> Spending time in nature and getting enough daylight each day.
> Eating a balanced and nourishing diet with a focus on B vitamins, vitamin C, vitamin D, healthy fats, and protein intake.
> Limiting alcohol and caffeine intake and the use of recreational drugs.
> Practicing good sleep hygiene.
> Connecting with friends and family to create a strong support network.
> Spending time with people who generate feelings of positivity.
> Joining a support group in person or online.
> Practicing kindness, compassion, and gratitude - towards others and oneself.
> Avoiding negative self-talk and challenging negative self-beliefs.
> Trying a new hobby or learning a new skill.
> Taking time out for enjoyment and self-care activities.

References

Clark, JE., Watson, S., Friston, KJ., (2018), What is mood? A computational perspective, PMC US National Library of Medicine, National Institutes of Health: Psychological Medicine: Psychol Med. 2018 Oct; 48(14): (pp 2277–2284). Published online 2018 Feb 26. doi: 10.1017/S0033291718000430.
https://www.ncbi.nlm.nih.gov/pmc/articles/PMC6340107

Clapp, M., Aurora, N., Herrera, L., et al. (2017) Gut microbiota's effect on mental health: The gut-brain axis, NIH, National Library of Medicine, National Center for Biotechnology Information: Clinic and Practice: Clin Pract. 2017 Sep 15; 7(4): 987. Published online 2017 Sep 15. doi: 10.4081/cp.2017.987 PMCID: PMC5641835PMID: 29071061.
https://www.ncbi.nlm.nih.gov/pmc/articles/PMC5641835

Carabotti, M, Scirocco, A, Maselli, MA, Severi, C. , (2015). The gut-brain axis: interactions between enteric microbiota, central and enteric nervous systems, NIH, National Library of Medicine, National Center for Biotechnology Information:Annals of Gastroenterology: Apr-Jun; 28(2): (pp 203–209. PMCID: PMC4367209PMID: 25830558.
https://www.ncbi.nlm.nih.gov/pmc/articles/PMC4367209

Bar, M., (2010). A cognitive neuroscience hypothesis of mood and depression, PMC US National Library of Medicine, National Institutes of Health: Trends Cogn Sci. Author manuscript; available in PMC 2010 Nov 1. Published in final edited form as: Trends Cogn Sci. 2009 Nov; 13(11): (pp 456–463). Published online 2009 Oct 12.
doi: 10.1016/j.tics.2009.08.009.
https://www.ncbi.nlm.nih.gov/pmc/articles/PMC2767460

Parry, BL., (2008). Perimenopausal Depression, The American Journal of Psychiatry: Published Online:1 Jan 2008
https://doi.org/10.1176/appi.ajp.2007.07071152
https://ajp.psychiatryonline.org/doi/10.1176/appi.ajp.2007.07071152

Stewart, DE., Boydell, KM., (1993): Psychologic distress during menopause: associations across the reproductive life cycle, International Journal of Psychiatry in Medicine (IJPM): Int J Psychiatry Med; 23: (pp 157–162) doi: 10.2190/026V-69M0-C0FF-7V7Y. https://pubmed.ncbi.nlm.nih.gov/8359998

Bromberger, JT., Kravitz, HM., (2011). Mood and Menopause: Findings from the Study of Women's Health Across the Nation (SWAN) over ten years, PMC US National Library of Medicine, National Institutes of Health: Obstet Gynecol Clin North Am. Author manuscript; available in PMC 2012 Sep 1. Published in final edited form as: Obstet Gynecol Clin North Am. 2011 Sep; 38(3): (pp 609–625). doi: 10.1016/j.ogc.2011.05.011
https://www.ncbi.nlm.nih.gov/pmc/articles/PMC3197240

Maciocia, G. (1989). The Foundations of Chinese Medicine. First edition. Churchill Livingston Elsevier, London, UK.

Wolfe, HL., (1998). Managing Menopause Naturally with Chinese Medicine. Blue Poppy Press. Inc. Boulder, Colorado. USA.

4.3 Insomnia and Sleep Disorders

Sleep is essential for good health and it is recommended that adults get at least seven hours of sleep each night. Lack of sleep can cause tiredness the following day, which reduces concentration and increases the risk of accidents. It can also affect mood, appetite, and immunity. Long-term sleep deprivation is also linked with weight gain and a number of chronic conditions, including high blood pressure, cardiovascular disease, and diabetes.

Unfortunately, sleep disorders are common among perimenopausal and postmenopausal women. Symptoms include:

- Difficulty falling asleep
- Difficulty maintaining sleep
- Waking routinely during the night or early in the morning
- Subjective lack of restorative sleep
- Daytime functional impairment

Pathophysiology

Fluctuating Hormone Levels

Reductions in both estrogen and progesterone may contribute to poor sleep. Progesterone, in particular, appears to have sedative and anxiolytic effects, potentially making it a key factor in menopausal sleep disorders.

Circadian Rhythm Disruptions

The human circadian rhythm is controlled by two hormones, cortisol and melatonin. Cortisol levels peak in the early morning and promote feelings of wakefulness and alertness. Meanwhile, melatonin induces sleepiness. It is produced by the pineal gland in response to darkness.

Increased age is associated with reduced melatonin levels in both males and females. However, these reductions are especially pronounced in post-menopausal women. Therefore, this could be a primary cause of poor sleep in older women.

Increased cortisol levels may also contribute to poor sleep. In addition to being a key component of the circadian clock, this hormone is released in response to physical and emotional stress. Therefore, women with high stress levels may be at even greater risk of sleep disorders during and after menopause.

Risk Factors

Numerous other factors can contribute to sleep disorders during and after menopause. They include:

Vasomotor Symptoms

Vasomotor symptoms may occur during the night and impair sleep quality and quantity. Night sweats may be particularly problematic as they can result in soaked bedclothes, making it harder to fall back to sleep.

Mood Disorders

Mood disorders, such as anxiety and depression are more prevalent during and after menopause. Both of these conditions can contribute to reduced sleep quality and duration.

Comorbidities

As women grow older, they are at increased risk of comorbidities that could impede their ability to sleep. Conditions such as chronic pain, fibromyalgia, and restless leg syndrome may all occur during midlife and could have a negative impact.

Furthermore, women tend to gain weight after menopause, which may contribute to obstructive sleep apnea. Another contributing factor to post-menopausal sleep apnea is decreased progesterone levels, as this hormone influences pharyngeal dilator muscle activity.

TCEAM Viewpoint

Pattern Differentiation

1. Kidney and Heart not harmonized
2. Liver Blood and Kidney yin deficiency
3. Heart Blood and Spleen qi deficiency
4. Heart yin and Blood deficiency
5. Phlegm-Fire harassing the heart
6. Blood stasis

1. Kidney and Heart Not Harmonized			
This pattern is a water-fire imbalance. It occurs due to a lack of Kidney yin (water), which fails to restrict Heart yang (fire), allowing it to flare upwards and cause hot flashes. When empty heat flares upward, it causes restlessness, insomnia (characterized by waking multiple times during the night), and other Heart-related symptoms, such as palpitations.			
Clinical Manifestations			
Hot flashes, palpitations, insomnia, frequent dreams, mental restlessness, poor memory and night sweats, blurred vision, dizziness, tinnitus, anxiety, backache, malar flush, feeling hot in the evening, dry mouth and throat, dry stools.			
Tongue	**Pulse**	**Treatment Principle**	**Points**
Red without coating, redder tip	Rapid-fine, floating-empty, or weak-deep on both *chi* (proximal) positions, overflowing on both *cun* (distal) positions	Nourish Kidney yin, calm *shen*, clear empty heat	Xinshu BL-15 Shenshu BL-23 Taixi KID-3 Yongquan KID-1 Shenmen HT-7 Laogong P-8 Daling P-7 Sanyinjiao SP-6 Taichong LIV-3 Juque REN-14 Shenting DU-24
Prescription			
Gan Mai Da Zao Tang Tian Wang Bu Xin Dan			

Table 4.3a: Kidney and Heart not harmonized.

2. Liver Blood and Kidney Yin Deficiency			
During the menopausal transition, Liver Blood often becomes deficient due to decades of regular menstrual bleeding. This, in turn, affects Liver yin and Kidney yin. Furthermore, Kidney yin is the basis of Liver yin and, thus, Liver Blood. Therefore, deficient Kidney yin can lead to deficient Liver Blood and its associated symptoms. Blood anchors the *shen* and Blood deficiency can lead to *shen* disturbance and poor sleep. A lack of yin also allows yang to flare upwards, leading to restlessness, hot flashes, night sweats, dizziness, etc.			
Clinical Manifestations			
Insomnia or dream-disturbed sleep, hot flashes and sweating (especially in the upper body), headaches, blurred vision, spots in front of the eyes, dizziness, vertigo, tinnitus, weak or sore lower back or legs, constipation, thirst, dry mouth.			
Tongue	**Pulse**	**Treatment Principle**	**Points***
Red with little to no coating or dry, scanty, yellow coating	Fine, bowstring and rapid	Nourish Kidney and Liver yin (thereby nourishing Liver Blood)	Guanyuan REN-4 Ganshu BL-18 Shenshu BL-23 Zusanli ST-36 Taixi KID-3 Zhaohai KID-6 Taichong LIV-3 Sanyinjiao SP-6
Prescription			
Liu Wei Di Huang Wan For Liver Blood deficiency affecting the Heart: Suan Zao Ren Tang			

* For any point prescription for insomnia, add:
Shenmen HT-7 | Baihui DU-20 | Shenting DU-24 | Hegu LI-4

Table 4.3b: Liver Blood and Kidney yin deficiency.

3. Heart Blood and Spleen Qi Deficiency			
Blood formation relies upon healthy Spleen function, since the Spleen is responsible for the transformation and transportation of food essences, which form the basis of Blood and qi. Therefore, deficient Spleen qi will eventually lead to deficient Heart Blood and affect its ability to house the *shen*. This pattern may be the result of inappropriate diet and eating habits or excessive worry and overthinking.			
Clinical Manifestations			
Insomnia and/or excessive dreaming, anxiety, emotional instability, poor memory, pale or sallow complexion, fatigue, itchy skin.			
Tongue	**Pulse**	**Treatment Principle**	**Points**
Pale and swollen with teeth marks	Fine and weak or empty	Tonify the Spleen and Heart, nourish the Blood, calm the *shen*	Xinshu BL-15 Pishu BL-20 Qihai REN-6 Shenmen HT-7 Zusanli ST-36 Xuehai SP-10 Sanyinjiao SP-6 Taixi KID-3 Taichong LIV-3 Hegu LI-4 Baihui DU-20 to Shenting DU-24
Prescription			
Gui Pi Tang			

Table 4.3c: Heart Blood and Spleen qi deficiency.

4. Heart Yin and Blood Deficiency			
Kidney yin is the foundation of Heart yin. Therefore, Kidney yin deficiency can lead to Heart yin deficiency, which usually coexists with Heart Blood deficiency (since Heart yin also encompasses Blood). In this state, the Heart is unable to house the *shen*, leading to symptoms of restlessness, insomnia, and dream-disturbed sleep.			
Clinical Manifestations			
Mental restlessness, insomnia, dream-disturbed sleep, poor memory, anxiety, startling easily, palpitations or racing heart, heat in palms, soles, and chest, low-grade fever (especially in the afternoon/evening), night sweats, dry mouth. Note: If Heart Blood deficiency predominates, the patient will have difficulty falling asleep but will sleep well once they do. If Heart yin deficiency predominates, they will have difficulty falling and staying asleep.			
Tongue	**Pulse**	**Treatment Principle**	**Points**
Pale if Heart Blood deficiency predominates, red if Heart yin deficiency predominates	Fine and weak if Heart Blood deficiency predominates, fine and rapid if Heart yin deficiency predominates	Tonify the Heart and Kidneys, nourish the Blood, calm the *shen*	Xinshu BL-15 Geshu BL-17 Juque REN-14 Sanyinjiao SP-6 Qihai REN-6 Shenmen HT-7 Neiguan P-6 Taixi KID-3 Baihui DU-20 Shenting DU-24 Taichong LIV-3
Prescription			
Si Wu Tang Gan Mai Da Zao Tang			

Table 4.3d: Heart yin and Blood deficiency.

5. Phlegm-Fire Harassing the Heart

A combination of Liver qi stagnation and Kidney yang deficiency contributes to an overall decline in Spleen function over time. If the Spleen is unable to properly transform fluids from food, they accumulate as dampness, which may combine with heat and eventually congeal into phlegm.

Phlegm can accumulate in the vessels and block the free flow of qi, leading to further stagnation. It can also 'obstruct the orifices' causing severe mental and emotional symptoms, including insomnia. Although it is rooted in deficiency, this is an excess pattern.

Clinical Manifestations

Mental restlessness, insomnia, dream-disturbed sleep, a sensation of stuffiness in the chest, depression, anxiety, startling easily, extreme emotional reactions (uncontrolled laughter or crying, shouting, physical aggression, etc.), confusion, palpitations, excessive mucus production, bitter taste in the mouth, the sensation of a lump in the throat, nausea, vomiting, obesity.

Tongue	Pulse	Treatment Principle	Points*
Red with sticky, yellow coating, midline crack containing yellow prickles	Full- rapid-slippery, rapid-overflowing slippery, or rapid-full-wiry	Clear Heart-fire, eliminate phlegm, calm the *shen*	Xinshu BL-15 Shenmen HT-7 Neiguan P-6 Yongquan KID-1 Shaofu HT-8 Sanyinjiao SP-6 Fenglong ST-40 Chize LU-5 Neiting ST-44 Yinlingquan SP-9 Taixi KID-3 Taichong LIV-3 Zhangmen LIV-13 Zhongji REN-3 Laogong P-8 Shenting DU-24 Yintang EX-HN3

Prescription

For phlegm fire: Wen Dan Tang
For severe phlegm fire: Sheng Tie Luo Yin
For predominant Liver fire: Long Dan Xie Gan Tang

* Moxa is contraindicated

Table 4.3e: Phlegm-fire harassing the Heart.

<table>
<tr><th colspan="4">6. Blood stasis</th></tr>
<tr><td colspan="4">Occurs in combination with one of the above patterns.</td></tr>
<tr><th colspan="4">Clinical Manifestations</th></tr>
<tr><td colspan="4">Hot flashes, mental restlessness, very irregular periods preceding menopause, dark-clotted blood, insomnia, high blood pressure, abdominal pain.</td></tr>
<tr><th>Tongue</th><th>Pulse</th><th>Treatment Principle</th><th>Points*</th></tr>
<tr><td>Purple</td><td>Wiry or choppy</td><td>Invigorate Blood, eliminate stasis, calm the shen, open the mind's orifices, move qi, eliminate stagnation</td><td>Geshu BL-17
Zhongji REN-3
Diji SP-8
Xuehai SP-10
Hegu LI-4
Taichong LIV-3</td></tr>
<tr><th colspan="4">Prescription</th></tr>
<tr><td colspan="4">Xue Fu Zhu Yu Tang
For stasis with Blood deficiency: Tao Hong Si Wu Tang</td></tr>
</table>

* For insomnia, add: Baihui DU-20 to Shenting DU-24 | Shenmen HT-7 | Taixi KID-3 | Neiguan P-6

Table 4.3f: Blood stasis.

Patient Advice

> Maintain a regular sleep routine, going to bed and waking at the same time each day.
> Dim the lights and reduce screen time in the evening to aid melatonin production.
> Reserve the bedroom for sleep and sexual activity.
> Keep the bedroom cool and dark.
> Invest in a comfortable mattress and bedding.
> Exercise sufficiently during the day and engage in calming activities before bed (reading, meditation, yin yoga, etc.).
> Do not eat large meals late in the evening.
> Avoid stimulants and alcohol.
> Replace caffeinated beverages with herbal teas or water.
> Short-term melatonin supplementation may be beneficial in some cases.

References

Lee, J., Han, Y., Cho, HH., et al. (2019). Sleep Disorders and Menopause, PMC US National Library of Medicine, National Institutes of Health: JMM, Journal of Menopausal Medicine, J Menopausal Med. 2019 Aug; 25(2): (pp 83–87). Published online 2019 Aug 5. doi: 10.6118/jmm.19192
https://www.ncbi.nlm.nih.gov/pmc/articles/PMC6718648

Maciocia, G., (2015). The Foundations of Chinese Medicine. 3rd Edition. Elsevier : Amsterdam, Netherlands.

Wolfe, HL., (1998). Managing Menopause Naturally with Chinese Medicine. Blue Poppy Press. Inc. Boulder, Colorado. USA.

4.4 Urogenital Symptoms

The urogenital system can be defined as the internal and external organs responsible for reproduction and the excretion of urine, including the vulva, vagina, urethra, and other associated structures. (See Chapter 2.1. Female Anatomy and Physiology).

A large proportion of women suffer from urogenital dryness and atrophy during and after menopause. However, many do not report their symptoms or seek treatment, making it difficult to know the exact figures.

This particular problem has a progressive course and tends to worsen throughout and following the menopausal period.

Associated symptoms include:

- Vaginal and vulvar burning or itching
- Painful urination
- Painful intercourse
- Reduced sexual satisfaction
- Spotting during or after intercourse
- Reduced libido
- Urinary frequency, urgency, or stress incontinence
- Pelvic organ prolapse

Vulvodynia

Vulvodynia is a chronic form of vulvar pain that may occur before, during, or after menopause. It is classified as generalized pain (involving all or much of the area between the mons pubis and anus), occuring in the absence of relevant clinical findings or identified neurological disorders.

Symptoms include vulvar burning, stinging, itching, or aching, and pain when inserting tampons or during intercourse. In general, there is little variation in these symptoms between pre and post-menopausal individuals, although there may be a higher incidence of vaginal burning following menopause.

Pathophysiology

There are many different factors that contribute to urogenital dryness and atrophy. However, the root cause of all of them is diminished estrogen levels.

Estrogen is responsible for the health of the vaginal mucosa. It ensures that the area receives sufficient blood flow and regulates its secretory function to provide lubrication. It also plays a role in the proliferation of the vagina's endothelial layer and smooth muscle, supporting collagen production and tissue folding.

Therefore, when estrogen levels decline, blood flow to the vagina reduces, secretions decrease, and the mucosa begins to thin. This increases the risk of trauma, inflammation, and pain.

Another effect of decreasing estrogen is an altered vaginal microbiota. Prior to menopause, the vagina is home to a large population of *Lactobacillus* bacteria, which produce lactic acid and keep the area at an optimal pH.

As estrogen levels fall, this population can reduce, causing a rise in vaginal pH. This not only contributes to vaginal atrophy but also increases the risk of infections such as candidiasis.

Risk Factors

The primary risk factors for urogenital dryness and atrophy are advanced age and menopausal stage. Women who undergo induced menopause are also more likely to suffer.

Other, lesser, associated factors include ethnicity and anxiety. The correlation with anxiety is reduced for women who remain sexually active.

TCEAM Viewpoint

Urogenital symptoms can be subdivided into urinary problems and vaginal dryness and atrophy. Although there may be some overlap in symptoms, the underlying TCEAM patterns may differ.

Pattern Differentiation

1. Kidney yin deficiency
2. Kidney qi not firm
3. Kidney and Liver yin deficiency
4. Blood deficiency
5. Body fluid deficiency

1. Kidney Yin Deficiency			
Deficiency of Kidney yin and *jing* leads to depletion of body fluids. The problem is exacerbated by the loss of fluids during night sweats or as a result of empty heat.			
Clinical Manifestations			
Night sweats, sensations of heat, dry mouth and throat at night, hot flashes, cold feet, frequent-pale urination, dizziness, vertigo, tinnitus, poor memory, hearing problems, lower backache, aching bones, tiredness, lassitude, depression, slight anxiety.			
Tongue	**Pulse**	**Treatment Principle**	**Points***
Normal color without coating, or rootless coating (red in severe cases)	Floating-empty or weak on both Kidney positions	Nourish Kidney yin	Shenshu BL-23 Guanyuan REN-4 Taixi KID-3 Zhaohai KID-6 Sanyinjiao SP-6 Local points for urogenital symptoms: Qihai REN-6 Guilai ST-29 Qixue KID-13
Prescription			
Liu Wei Di Huang Wan Zhi Bai Di Huang Wan Zuo Gui Wan			

* General additions: Baihui DU-20 | Shenmen HT-7 | Hegu LI-4 | Fuliu KID-7 | Taichong LIV-3

Table 4.4a: Kidney yin deficiency.

2. Kidney Qi Not Firm *(Also known as lower original qi not firm)*			
This is, in essence, a form of Kidney yang deficiency and weakness of ministerial fire. Kidney qi and original qi decline and cannot provide enough qi for the Bladder to function efficiently. The lower orifice of the urethra may also become weakened, resulting in urinary leakage or incontinence. Furthermore, deficient Kidney yang fails to nourish the Spleen, affecting its holding function. Therefore, vaginal discharge (this may present as a thin mucus) and prolapse may occur. This pattern is more likely to occur in women who have had many childbirths close together.			
Clinical Manifestations			
Sore or weak back, frequent clear abundant urination, weak urination flow, dribbling after urination, urinary incontinence, enuresis, nocturia, uterine prolapse, leucorrhea.			
Tongue	**Pulse**	**Treatment Principle**	**Points**
Pale	Deep-weak, especially the *chi* (proximal) positions	Reinforce Kidney qi	Guanyuan REN-4 Shenshu BL-23 Zhishi BL-52 Taixi KID-3 Fuliu KID-7 Mingmen DU-4 Sanyinjiao SP-6 Zusanli ST-36 Baihui DU-20
Prescription			
Jin Suo Gu Jing Wan			

Table 4.4b: Kidney qi not firm.

3. Kidney and Liver Yin Deficiency			
The Kidneys and Liver rule the genitals. When Kidney and Liver yin become deficient, body fluids in the genitals decline, leading to dryness. If there is also heat in the Liver channel, there may be vaginal itching and inflammation.			
Clinical Manifestations			
Hot flashes, night sweats, dizziness, tinnitus, blurred vision, dry eyes, dry skin, aching joints, sore back, irritability, headaches.			
Tongue	**Pulse**	**Treatment Principle**	**Points***
Red without coating	Floating-empty, wiry on Liver position	Nourish Kidney and Liver yin, subdue Liver yang, calm the *shen*, settle the *hun*	Shenshu BL-23 Ganshu BL-18 Guanyuan REN-4 Taixi KID-3 Zhaohai KID-6 Sanyinjiao SP-6 Zusanli ST-36 Taichong LIV-3 Local points for urogenital symptoms: Qihai REN-6 Guilai ST-29 Qixue KID-13
Prescription			
Liu Wei Di Huang Wan Zhi Bai Di Huang Wan			

* General additions: Baihui DU-20 | Shenmen HT-7 | Hegu LI-4

Table 4.4c: Kidney and Liver yin deficiency.

4. Blood Deficiency			
Blood deficiency usually arises from nutritional deficiency or weakness of the Stomach and Spleen. It can also occur due to extreme blood loss, for example, heavy menstruation or traumatic childbirth. Most menopausal patients will have some degree of Blood deficiency due to years of regular menstruation. Since Blood is yin and has moistening properties, Blood deficiency can result in dryness throughout the body, including vaginal dryness.			
Clinical Manifestations			
Dull complexion, pale lips, dizziness, poor memory, insomnia, palpitations, numbness, blurred vision, dry hair, skin, and nails.			
Tongue	**Pulse**	**Treatment Principle**	**Points***
Pale, slightly dry	Choppy or fine	Tonify the Spleen, nourish Blood	Guanyuan REN-4 Qihai REN-6 Geshu BL-17 Ganshu BL-18 Pishu BL-20 Shenshu BL-23 Zusanli ST-36 Taixi KID-3 Taichong LIV-3 Sanyinjiao SP-6 + Local points
Prescription**			
Ba Zhen Tang			

* Bleeding treatment is contraindicated.
** Dietary advice is also key.

Table 4.4d: Blood deficiency.

5. Body Fluid Deficiency			
Body fluid deficiency is, in essence, a form of yin deficiency. Body fluids are responsible for moistening the body's tissues, including the skin and muscles. They have a close relationship with qi, which is responsible for circulating them around the body. Furthermore, qi deficiency can lead to loss of body fluids via sweating. Body fluids are also somewhat interchangeable with Blood as both are yin substances. Blood deficiency can result in insufficient body fluids, and body fluid deficiency can cause the Blood to become thick and prone to clotting.			
Clinical Manifestations			
Dry skin, lips, and mucous membranes, dry cough, dry mouth at night, scanty urination, dry stools.			
Tongue	**Pulse**	**Treatment Principle**	**Points**
Dry, possibly with cracks	Deficient and thin, possibly hollow if *jing*, Blood, and body fluids are completely exhausted. Also possibly rapid in cases of deficiency heat	Nourish body fluids	Guanyuan REN-4 Qihai REN-6 Zusanli ST-36 Sanyinjiao SP-6 Taixi KID-3 Taichong LIV-3 Lieque LU-7 Baihui DU-20 Feishu BL-13 Pishu BL-20 Weishu BL-21 Shenshu BL-23
Prescription			
Zeng Ye Tang For dryness only in the lower jiao: You Gui Wan For signs of Lung dryness: Sha Shen Mai Men Dong Tang			

Table 4.4e: Body fluid deficiency.

Patient Advice

> Apply a vaginal moisturizer as required, but only use products specially formulated for vaginal use.
> To continue with Pap smears or similar procedures, it is usually advised that women apply estrogen cream a few weeks prior to the procedure to moisturize the vagina and lessen the experience of pain from dryness and atrophy.
> Use mild, unperfumed soaps and washes to prevent irritation.
> Wear underwear and clothing made from natural fibers to reduce the risk of yeast infections.
> Stay well hydrated to reduce urinary-tract irritation and infections.
> Apply a gentle, water-based lubricant to the vagina and penis before intercourse.
> Spend sufficient time on foreplay to increase arousal.
> Practise pelvic floor exercises such as Kegel exercises daily (see below).

How To Do Kegel Exercises

Kegel exercises involve tightening and relaxing muscles that control urine flow, the pelvic floor muscles (see figure 2.1c, page 20). To identify the pelvic floor muscles, stop urinating mid-stream. This causes the muscles of the bladder, vagina, and anus to tighten. The thighs, abdomen, and buttocks should remain relaxed. Once the correct muscles have been identified, Kegel exercises may be performed sitting or lying down. However, it is important to perform them with an empty bladder.

1. Empty the bladder
2. Mentally pull the internal pelvic floor muscles upwards toward the diaphragm
3. Tighten the pelvic floor muscles in three phases:
    a. *Phase 1. Lift and tighten*
    b. *Phase 2. Tighten deeper*
    c. *Phase 3. Tighten deeper again*
4. Engage the abdominal muscles along with pelvic floor muscles and hold for 3 - 5 seconds
5. Relax the muscles for 3-5 seconds
6. Perform 10 repetitions, three times a day (morning, afternoon, and night)

References

Phillips, NA., Brown, C., Foster, D., et al. (2016). Presenting Symptoms Among Premenopausal And Postmenopausal Women With Vulvodynia: A Case Series: NIH, National Library of Medicine, National Center for Biotechnology Information: Journal List > HHS Author Manuscripts > PMC4666723.
https://www.ncbi.nlm.nih.gov/pmc/articles/PMC4666723

Maciocia. G. (1989). The Foundations of Chinese Medicine. First edition. Churchill Livingston Elsevier, London, UK.

Chen, R., Song, D., Zhang. W., et al. (2018). Randomized, Double-Blind, Placebo-Controlled Study of Modified Erzhi Granules in the Treatment of Menopause-Related Vulvovaginal Atrophy, PMC US National Library of Medicine, National Institutes of Health, Hindawi: Evid Based Complement Alternat Med. 2018; 2018: 6452709. Published online 2018 Oct 14. doi:10.1155/2018/6452709.
https://www.ncbi.nlm.nih.gov/pmc/articles/PMC6204235

Shen Nong.com. (Sourced January 2021). Urinary and Vaginal Changes during Menopause.
http://www.shen-nong.com/eng/exam/specialties_menopause_urinary.html

4.5 Uterine Bleeding

Excessive or prolonged uterine bleeding is known as menometrorrhagia. It has numerous possible causes and may occur at irregular and/or frequent intervals, affecting almost a quarter of women aged 40-50.

Some women experience abnormal uterine bleeding following menopause, i.e. bleeding 12 months after the last menstrual period. It can be the result of vaginal dryness, polyps (noncancerous growths), or other changes in the reproductive system. It is also a red flag symptom for cancer and should be investigated by the patient's primary care doctor or gynecologist.

Uterine bleeding can be subclassified into two types depending on whether or not the woman is taking MHT:

- **Postmenopausal bleeding:**
  Uterine bleeding more than one year after the final menstrual period.
- **Breakthrough bleeding:**
  Unscheduled uterine bleeding in postmenopausal women taking MHT.

Pathophysiology

The most common cause of postmenopausal uterine bleeding is endometrial atrophy. It may also be the result of endometrial polyps or endometrial cancer. Non-uterine sources of bleeding include cervical or vaginal lesions, or bleeding from the urinary or gastrointestinal systems.

Risk Factors

The primary risk factors for postmenopausal uterine bleeding are obesity, diabetes, and hypertension. Other risk factors include:

- Advanced age
- Early menarche
- Late menopause
- Tamoxifen treatment
- Unopposed estrogen therapy
- Hereditary non-polyposis colorectal cancer

TCEAM Viewpoint

In TCEAM terms, any abnormal or excessive bleeding is the result of either heat, Spleen qi deficiency, or Blood stasis. Uterine bleeding in postmenopausal women is most often due to a combination of these patterns.

Pattern Differentiation

1. Blood heat
2. Spleen qi deficiency
3. Blood stasis

Note: In the case of bleeding, it is important to staunch the bleeding, treat the root cause, and correct the depletion caused by abnormal bleeding.

1. Blood Heat			
Common menopausal patterns such as qi stagnation and yin deficiency generate heat, which causes the Blood to become reckless and overflow.			
Clinical Manifestations			
I. General: Feeling hot, skin disease with red eruptions, dry mouth, and bleeding. **II.** Heart Blood heat: Anxiety, mood disorders, and mouth ulcers. **III.** Liver Blood heat: Skin diseases with itching, heat, and redness. **IV.** Blood heat in uterus and *chongmai*: Heavy menstrual or vaginal bleeding with fresh red or dark blood.			
Tongue	**Pulse**	**Treatment Principle**	**Points***
Red with yellow coating	Rapid and full	Disperse heat, cool Blood, stop bleeding	Geshu BL-17 Dazhui DU-14 Shenshu BL-23 Yinbai SP-1 Xuehai SP-10 Quchi LI-11 Taichong LIV-3 Dadun LIV-1 Rangu KID-2 Shuiquan KID-5 Neiguan P-6 Shenmen HT-7
Prescription			
For full heat: Qing Jing San For deficiency heat: Gu Jing Wan			

* Local abdominal points: Zhongji REN-3 | Dahe KID-12

Table 4.5a: Blood heat.

<table>
<tr><th colspan="4">2. Spleen Qi Deficiency</th></tr>
<tr><td colspan="4">Spleen qi is responsible for holding the Blood inside the vessels. Therefore, when it becomes deficient, Blood may leak out causing abnormal bleeding.</td></tr>
<tr><th colspan="4">Clinical Manifestations</th></tr>
<tr><td colspan="4">Lack of appetite, abdominal distension after eating, loose stools, fatigue, sallow complexion, weak limbs.</td></tr>
<tr><th>Tongue</th><th>Pulse</th><th>Treatment Principle</th><th>Points*</th></tr>
<tr><td>Pale or normal colored, possibly swollen with transverse cracks</td><td>Weak, soft, empty</td><td>Tonify Spleen qi, stop bleeding, nourish Blood and yin if depleted</td><td>Baihui DU-20
Zhongwan REN-12
Pishu BL-20
Shenshu BL-23
Zusanli ST-36
Sanyinjiao SP-6
Yinbai SP-1
Taichong LIV-3
Taixi KID-3
Shenmen HT-7</td></tr>
<tr><th colspan="4">Prescription</th></tr>
<tr><td colspan="4">Bu Zhong Yi Qi Tang with Dang Gui Bu Xue Tang
Gui Pi Tang</td></tr>
</table>

* Local abdominal points: Guanyuan REN-4 | Qihai REN-6 | Qixue KID-13

Table 4.5b: Spleen qi deficiency.

3. Blood Stasis			
When Blood stagnates, it blocks the vessels, forcing Blood to flow outside of its proper pathways and leading to abnormal bleeding.			
Clinical Manifestations			
Dark complexion, purple lips, purple nails, boring-fixed-stabbing pain, unmovable abdominal masses, bleeding with dark blood and clots.			
Tongue	**Pulse**	**Treatment Principle**	**Points***
Purple	Wiry, firm, or choppy	Invigorate Blood and dispel stasis, arrest bleeding and nourish Blood, yin, and qi if required	Geshu BL-17 Ganshu BL-18 Shenshu BL-23 Sanyinjiao SP-6 Diji SP-8 Taichong LIV-3 Dadun LIV-1 Rangu KID-2 Shuiquan KID-5 Neiguan P-6 Shenmen HT-7
Prescription			
For deficiency stasis: Tao Hong Si Wu Tang For excess stasis: Shao Fu Zhu Yu Tang For cold stasis: Wen Jing Tang			

* Local abdominal points: Zhongji REN-3 | Siman KID-14 | Qichong ST-30 | Chongmen SP-12

Table 4.5c: Blood stasis.

A Word on Feminine Hygiene Products

The term 'feminine hygiene products' refers to items such as tampons, sanitary pads, menstrual cups, sea sponges, and others designed to collect menstrual blood. Feminine hygiene products also include products meant to cleanse the vulva or vagina, such as douches, feminine wipes, and soap.

Product	Pros	Cons
Tampons	Widely available. More discreet than sanitary pads.	Some tampons are manufactured using harmful materials, including dioxin and pesticide residues. These are readily absorbed by the vaginal mucosa. May cause toxic shock syndrome. Many TCEAM practitioners consider tampons obstructive and a cause of stagnation.
Sanitary pads	Widely available. Not inserted into the vagina.	May contain chemicals that irritate the vulva or increase the risk of infections. Heavy flow may cause leakage. Most sanitary pads use plastic that requires as long as 800 years to decompose.
Reusable sanitary pad	Cloth pads can be washed and reused, reducing wastage. Not inserted into the vagina.	Heavy flow may cause leakage. Must be washed and dried hygienically. Must be stored carefully to prevent contamination.
Menstrual cup	No adverse effects on vaginal microbiota. Can last up to 10 years, decreasing waste. Many menstrual cup users report increased satisfaction compared with other products.	May be difficult to insert without experience. May leak if placed incorrectly or not changed before full. May present difficulty with emptying and cleaning the cup in public toilets. May cause toxic shock syndrome in rare cases.
Sea sponge	A natural alternative to synthetic tampons.	May contain contaminants, including sand, grit, bacteria, yeast, or mold. Although little evidence is available, sea sponges can be presumed to present the same risks as tampons regarding toxic shock syndrome, etc.

Table 4.5d: Feminine hygiene products.

Summary

Uterine bleeding can occur for a variety of reasons, many of which are benign. However, **this symptom should always be considered a red flag and referred to a medical doctor for further investigation.**

References

Donnez, J., (2012). Menometrorrhagia during the premenopause: an overview, NIH, National Library of Medicine, National Center for Biotechnology Information: Gynecol Endocrinol. 2011 Dec;27 Suppl 1:(pp 1114-9). doi: 10.3109/09513590.2012.637341.
https://pubmed.ncbi.nlm.nih.gov/22182054

Wolfe, HL., (1998). Managing Menopause Naturally with Chinese Medicine. Blue Poppy Press. Inc. Boulder, Colorado. USA.

Maciocia, G. (1989). The Foundations of Chinese Medicine. First edition. Churchill Livingston Elsevier, London, UK.

Nicole, W., (2014). A Question for Women's Health: Chemicals in Feminine Hygiene Products and Personal Lubricants, PMC US National Library of Medicine, National Institutes of Health. Ehp Environmental Health Perspectives: Environ Health Perspect. 2014 Mar; 122(3): A70–A75. Published online 2014 Mar 1. doi: 10.1289/ehp.122-A70
https://www.ncbi.nlm.nih.gov/pmc/articles/PMC3948026

Van Eijk, AM., Zulaika, G., Lenchner, M., et al, (2019). Menstrual cup use, leakage, acceptability, safety, and availability: a systematic review and meta-analysis, PMC US National Library of Medicine, National Institutes of Health, The Lancet. Public Health: Lancet Public Health. 2019 Aug; 4(8): e376–e393. Published online 2019 Jul 16.
doi: 10.1016/S2468-2667(19)30111-2
https://www.ncbi.nlm.nih.gov/pmc/articles/PMC6669309

Kaur, R., Kaur, K., Kaur, R., (2018). Menstrual Hygiene, Management, and Waste Disposal: Practices and Challenges Faced by Girls/Women of Developing Countries, PMC US National Library of Medicine, National Institutes of Health, Journal of Environmental and Public Health: J Environ Public Health. 2018; 2018: 1730964. Published online 2018 Feb 20. doi: 10.1155/2018/1730964
https://www.ncbi.nlm.nih.gov/pmc/articles/PMC5838436/

FDA, US Food & Drug Administration. (1995). CPG Sec. 345.300 Menstrual Sponges, FDA: Docket Number: FDA-2020-D-0957 Issued by: Center for Devices and Radiological Health Office of Regulatory Affairs.
https://www.fda.gov/regulatory-information/search-fda-guidance-documents/cpg-sec-345300-menstrual-sponges

4.6 Low Libido and Sexual Dysfunction

The term 'libido' or 'sex drive' describes a person's overall desire for sexual activity. It is intricately linked with physical and mental arousal, sexual pleasure, and orgasm.

The physiological mechanisms underlying libido are complex and not yet fully understood. However, it is apparent that a combination of neurological, endocrine, and genetic factors are involved. Societal and cultural beliefs, attitude, personal experience and sexual history, partner availability, self-confidence, and mood play a critical role.

From a neurological point of view, numerous brain structures are thought to be responsible for libido and arousal, including the brainstem, thalamus, hypothalamus, amygdala, septal region, prefrontal cortex, cingulate cortex, and insula. The reward system also plays an integral role, primarily through activity in the dopaminergic system. Meanwhile, the spinal cord and peripheral nerves bridge the gap between physical and mental stimulation.

In addition to dopamine, several other neurochemicals are involved in libido and sexual function, including serotonin, noradrenaline, acetylcholine, histamine, and endogenous opioids. Androgen and estrogen levels also have a significant impact.

Many peri and postmenopausal women report decreased sexual desire and reduced frequency of orgasm. For some, this does not cause any distress and may even be welcome in some cases. However, for many, low libido and sexual dysfunction are problematic. They can contribute to mood disorders and relationship issues, as well as decreasing one's overall quality of life and self-confidence.

Sexual Dysfunction

Sexual dysfunction can be subclassified as follows. However, it is essential to note that a reduction in or lack of sexual activity does not necessarily constitute a disorder.

Hypoactive Sexual Desire Disorder

Persistent deficiency or absence of sexual thoughts, fantasies, desire, or receptivity to sexual activity, which causes personal distress.

Sexual Aversion Disorder

Persistent aversion to and avoidance of sexual activity with a partner, which causes personal distress.

Sexual Arousal Disorder

Persistent lack of sufficient sexual arousal. It may manifest as a lack of subjective excitement or physiological responses (lubrication/swelling), which causes personal distress.

Orgasmic Disorder

Persistent difficulty or delay in reaching, or absence of, orgasm, which causes personal distress.

Sexual Pain Disorders

Including dyspareunia (painful intercourse), vaginismus (involuntary spasm of the vagina, interfering with penetration), and non-coital pain disorders (conditions that interfere with penetration), which cause personal distress.

Pathophysiology

Female sexual function is highly complex and relies on a combination of hormonal, physical, and psychological factors. It is also affected by some medications, including those commonly taken throughout the menopausal period.

Hormonal

Reduced estrogen levels result in urogenital dysfunction, including loss of pelvic muscle tone, thinning and atrophy of the vaginal tissue, reduced circulation, and reduced lubrication. All of these factors can lead to sexual pain and avoidance of intercourse. However, there is evidence that remaining sexually active can ameliorate some of these effects. (See Chapter 5.4 Sexual Activity).

Testosterone levels also decrease following menopause, leading to reductions in desire. This decline is exacerbated by some forms of oral hormonal contraception and MHT, which increase SHBG levels, thus reducing free testosterone.

There is also evidence of a link between increased age and decreased clitoral cavernosal erectile tissue, which may contribute to age-related sexual dysfunction in women.

Physical

In addition to the above, several physical factors can reduce desire and sexual satisfaction for menopausal women. They include:

- Other menopause symptoms (hot flashes etc.)
- Lack of sleep and tiredness
- A decline in general physical health
- Prolapse
- Osteoarthritis
- Diabetes
- Neurological conditions

Psychological

Sexual function and mental health are closely interrelated. On one hand, sexual dysfunction can lead to depression and anxiety. On the other hand, it can also be a symptom of these mood disorders.

The same goes for relationships. Sexual dysfunction can strain a relationship, especially if one partner desires sexual activity more frequently than the other. Equally, being in an unhappy relationship is likely to decrease one's desire considerably.

Furthermore, people are often faced with numerous stressors as they transition through the menopausal period. They include aging parents, children growing up and leaving home, career and employment changes, and more. All of these factors can reduce their ability to relax and enjoy sexual activity.

Cultural values, religious beliefs, body image, and sexual history also play a role in one's confidence and desire for sex.

Medical

Some medications commonly taken by menopausal women can lower libido, including:

- Selective serotonin reuptake inhibitors (SSRIs)
- Cardiovascular medications
- Neuroleptics

Risk Factors

Surgical Menopause

Women who undergo surgical menopause are more likely to experience sexual dysfunction as a result of the sudden interruption to hormone production.

Menopause Symptoms

Women with more severe menopause symptoms are more likely to experience sexual dysfunction.

Mood Disorders

Depression is a significant cause of low libido. It may perpetuate a vicious cycle of low self-worth, relationship issues, and sexual dysfunction.

Relationship Discord

Women who are in unsatisfactory relationships are more likely to experience sexual dissatisfaction and dysfunction. Problems such as poor communication and long-standing resentment may all play a role, especially for those who have been in the same relationship for many years.

Availability of a Sexual Partner

Changes in sexual partner status also influence sexual function. Initiating relations with a new partner may have a positive effect, while the loss of a former partner is more likely to have a negative impact.

History of Sexual Abuse

Women with a history of sexual abuse are more likely to experience sexual dysfunction at all stages of life, including during the menopausal transition. As one of the key Gates of Life, menopause is an opportunity for women to heal past traumas with the support of a compassionate therapist.

TCEAM Viewpoint

As well as being a manifestation of underlying deficiencies, these particular symptoms can also give rise to further imbalances. This may be the case if a woman has sexual desire but feels unable to act on it, for example, due to a fear of pain during intercourse.

The reason for this is that sexual desire is a product of Kidney yang and ministerial fire. It generates an accumulation of yang qi, which is released upon orgasm, promoting the free flow of qi.

If this release is obstructed, the ministerial fire becomes disturbed. It also affects the Heart and Pericardium due to their association with the uterus (which contracts during orgasm) via the *baomai*. The result is qi stagnation or Blood heat.

However, if a woman lacks sexual desire, then abstinence from sex should not cause a significant problem because there is no imbalance between desire and action.

Pattern Differentiation

1. Kidney yang deficiency
2. Liver qi stagnation
3. Blood heat

1. Kidney Yang Deficiency			
Kidney yang plays a crucial role in sexual desire and a deficiency can significantly reduce libido. It often occurs in conjunction with Kidney yin deficiency, increasing the chance of severe menopausal symptoms, which further interfere with sexual activity.			
Clinical Manifestations			
Hot flashes, hot sensation in the face, night sweats, lower backache, feeling cold, cold knees, back and feet, weak legs, bright white complexion, low libido, tiredness, lassitude, clear urination, nocturia, apathy, odema in the legs, loose stools, depression.			
Tongue	**Pulse**	**Treatment Principle**	**Points***
Pale	Deep-weak	Tonify Kidney yang	Mingmen DU-4 Shenshu BL-23 Guanyuan REN-4 Taixi KID-3 Zusanli ST-36 Baihui DU-20 Sishencong EX-HN 1 Shenmen HT-7 Hegu LI-4 Sanyinjiao SP-6 Shuidao ST-28 Qixue KID-13
Prescription			
Jin Gui Shen Qi Wan For Kidney yang deficiency with decline of fire in the *mingmen*: You Gui Wan			

* In addition, cupping over the navel or moxa on salt at Shenque REN-8 can help extract cold and warm yang in the lower *jiao*. Moxibustion on the sacrum is also effective.

Table 4.6a: Kidney yang deficiency.

2. Liver Qi Stagnation			
Sexual desire that is suppressed can cause Liver qi stagnation due to accumulated yang qi not being released via orgasm. The pattern may be exacerbated by emotional problems, including frustration, resentment, and repressed anger, which further impede the flow of qi.			
Clinical Manifestations			
Hypochondriac pain and distension, sighing, hiccups, nausea, vomiting, epigastric pain or pulsation, poor appetite, acid reflux, belching, difficulty swallowing, churning sensation in the stomach, abdominal distension, borborygmi, diarrhea, depression, mood swings, irritability, irregular or painful periods, premenstrual breast distension, premenstrual syndrome.			
Tongue	**Pulse**	**Treatment Principle**	**Points**
Normal body color, possibly with red tip or sides	Wiry, especially on the left side	Disperse the Liver and regulate qi	Neiguan P-6 Taichong LIV-3 Sanyinjiao SP-6 Zhangmen LIV-13 Zusanli ST-36 Xingjian LIV-2 Zhigou SJ-6 Yanglingquan GB-34 Baihui DU-20 Sishencong EX-HN 1 Shenmen HT-7 Hegu LI-4 Diji SP-8 Shuidao ST-28 Qixue KID-13
Prescription			
For stagnation without heat: Xiao Yao San For stagnation with heat: Dan Zhi Xiao Yao San, Yue Ju Wan For stronger Liver qi stagnation: Chai Hu Shu Gan San			

Table 4.6b: Liver qi stagnation.

3. Blood Heat			
When sexual desire is suppressed or does not have an appropriate outlet, the ministerial fire can become pathological. This generates depressed fire, which enters the Blood leading to Blood heat. This pattern can also occur with a diet that is rich in spicy foods, contracting heat from the external environment, or yin deficiency generating internal heat. Heat agitates the Blood and causes it to escape the vessels, causing symptoms such as bleeding and skin eruptions. In this pattern, yin is insufficient to contain the flaring fire.			
Clinical Manifestations			
I. General: Feeling of heat, skin disease with red eruptions, dry mouth, bleeding. **II.** Heart Blood heat: Anxiety, mood disorders, mouth ulcers. **III.** Liver Blood heat: Skin diseases with itching, heat, and redness. **IV.** Blood heat in uterus and *chongmai*: Heavy menstrual or vaginal bleeding with fresh red or dark blood.			
Tongue	**Pulse**	**Treatment Principle**	**Points***
Red with a dry body and sparse, dry, yellow coating or no coating if yin is damaged	Rapid, forceful	Direct yin fire downwards and tonify yin	Rangu KID-2 Xingjian LIV-2 Sanyinjiao SP-6 Xuehai SP-10 Daling P-7 Shenmen HT-7 Quze P-3 Quchi LI-11 Geshu UB-17 Baihui DU-20 Zhongji REN-3 Qichong ST-30 Dahe KID-12 Neiting ST-44
Prescription			
Huang Lian Jie Du Tang			

* Moxa is contraindicated.

Table 4.6c: Blood heat.

Patient Advice

> Manage stress and anxiety as much as possible.
> Seek sexual or psychotherapy where appropriate.
> Use a gentle, water-based lubricant to reduce discomfort during intercourse.
> Experiment with different positions to find one that is comfortable for both partners.
> Get tested for underlying conditions that may affect sexual function, such as heart disease, diabetes, thyroid disorders, or cancer.
> Discuss with a doctor whether sexual dysfunction could be a medication side effect.
> Reduce usage of alcohol and other recreational drugs.

References

Calabrò, RS., Cacciola, A., Bruschetta, D., et al. (2019). Neuroanatomy and function of human sexual behavior: A neglected or unknown issue? PMC US National Library of Medicine, National Institutes of Health, Brain and Behaviour: Brain Behav. 2019 Dec; 9(12): e01389. Published online 2019 Sep 30. doi: 10.1002/brb3.1389 https://www.ncbi.nlm.nih.gov/pmc/articles/PMC6908863

Boston University School of Medicine, Sexual Medicine, (sourced January 2021). Female Genital Anatomy, https://www.bumc.bu.edu/sexualmedicine/physicianinformation/female-genital-anatomy

Maciocia, G. (sourced January 2021). Sexual Life in Chinese Medicine, https://giovanni-maciocia.com/sexual-life-in-chinese-medicine

Wolfe, HL., (1998). Managing Menopause Naturally with Chinese Medicine. Blue Poppy Press. Inc. Boulder, Colorado. USA.

Maciocia, G. (1989). The Foundations of Chinese Medicine. First edition. Churchill Livingston Elsevier, London, UK.

4.7 Musculoskeletal Pain

Musculoskeletal pain is a common problem among women and its incidence tends to increase during and after menopause. There are many different types of musculoskeletal pain, and it may originate in a variety of structures, including:

- Muscle
- Bone
- The bursa (the fluid sac which provides cushioning for joints)
- The enthesis (the attachment point of ligaments or tendons)
- Joints

Generally speaking, musculoskeletal pain can be classified as either:

- Myalgia (muscle pain)
- Arthralgia (joint pain without inflammation)
- Arthritis (joint pain with inflammation)

These problems can stem from numerous underlying causes, including:

- Osteoarthritis
- Inflammatory arthritis (e.g. rheumatoid arthritis, psoriatic arthritis, systemic lupus erythematosus)
- Fibromyalgia
- Endocrine disorders (e.g. hypothyroidism, hyperparathyroidism)
- Nutritional deficiencies (e.g. vitamin D deficiency, anemia)
- Liver or kidney disease
- Infections
- Malignancy
- Medication (e.g. aromatase inhibitors, statins, bisphosphonates, diuretics)

The most commonly affected areas are the spine, knees, hips, hands, and shoulders. Frozen shoulder is an especially widespread issue. Musculoskeletal pain often occurs in combination with other menopausal symptoms, especially fatigue, mood disorders, and sleep problems.

Pathophysiology

The precise pathophysiology of musculoskeletal pain in menopause depends on the underlying cause and a detailed discussion of each condition is beyond the scope of this publication. However, reductions in estrogen levels may be a contributing factor in many cases.

Estrogen is synthesized in the connective tissues by the enzyme aromatase. These tissues also contain estrogen receptors. Estrogen appears to have several functions in the musculoskeletal system. They include promoting cartilage growth and protection, as well as anti-inflammatory and immunosuppressive properties.

Estrogen may also play a role in the perception of pain, as receptors are present in neurons, as well as the hypothalamus, limbic system, and dorsal root ganglion regions of the brain. Together with testosterone, the hormone appears to have an inhibitory action on pain pathways. It may also contribute to the activation of the endogenous opioid system.

Risk Factors

Genetics

Genetic factors may play a role in the development of certain painful conditions, especially those of an autoimmune nature.

Body Mass Index

Having a high body mass index is associated with greater strain on the weight-bearing joints, such as the knees and hips. Therefore, overweight and obese individuals are at increased risk of developing degenerative joint diseases like osteoarthritis. There is also a strong correlation between obesity and chronic inflammation.

Exercise

Lack of physical activity is associated with increased body mass index and reduced joint mobility and muscle strength.

Mood Disorders

There appears to be some correlation between musculoskeletal pain and mood disorders, such as stress and anxiety. Depending on the underlying condition, this could be due to a combination of factors, including neurotransmitter imbalances or chronic inflammation.

Smoking

Smoking is a pro-inflammatory activity and, therefore, increases the risk of painful, inflammatory conditions.

TCEAM Viewpoint

There are so many potential causes of musculoskeletal pain that it is beyond the scope of this book to discuss each one in detail. These are the patterns most often associated with pain during the menopausal period.

Pattern Differentiation

1. Kidney yin deficiency
2. Kidney yang deficiency with exterior syndromes
3. Liver Blood deficiency

1. Kidney Yin Deficiency			
The yin fluids produced by the Kidney are responsible for nourishing the joints and muscles. When they become deficient, there will be stiffness and pain.			
Clinical Manifestations			
Night sweats, sensations of heat, dry mouth and throat at night, hot flashes, cold feet, frequent-pale urination, dizziness, vertigo, tinnitus, poor memory, hearing problems, lower backache, aching bones, tiredness, lassitude, depression, and slight anxiety.			
Tongue	**Pulse**	**Treatment Principle**	**Points***
Normal color without coating, or rootless coating (red in severe cases)	Rapid and thin	Nourish Kidney yin, invigorate water, enrich yin	Shenshu BL-23 Guanyuan REN-4 Taixi KID-3 Zhaohai KID-6 Sanyinjiao SP-6 **Additional points:** Baihui DU-20 Shenting DU-24 Shenmen HT-7 Hegu LI-4 Taichong LIV-3 Yanglingquan GB-34 Qihai REN-6 Zusanli ST-36
Prescription			
Zhi Bai Di Huang Wan Zuo Gui Wan			

* Plus local points as required.

Table 4.7a: Kidney yin deficiency.

Attention: Chronic painful obstruction can lead to deficiency of the Liver and Kidney.

Clinical tip from Brian Grosam: Du Huo Ji Sheng Tang is for musculoskeletal pain due to Kidney and Liver deficiency. It is the most important formula to treat arthralgia, especially in chronic situations.

Actions: Disperse wind-dampness to stop arthralgia, benefit the Liver and Kidney, and tonify qi and Blood.

Indications: Arthralgia with deficiency of Liver and Kidney and deficiency of qi and Blood.

Root Pattern Formulas:

1. Kidney and Liver Essence Deficiency: Liu Wei Di Huang Wan
2. Kidney and Liver Yang Deficiency: Jin Gui Shen Qi Wan
3. Liver Yang Rising Patterns: Tian Ma Gou Teng Yin
4. Qi and Blood Deficiency: Ba Zhen Tang
5. Damp Heat Accumulation: Long Dan Xie Gan Tang
6. Damp Phlegm Accumulation: Er Chen Tang

2. Kidney Yang Deficiency with Exterior Syndromes			
Kidney yang has an association with *wei* qi, and when it becomes deficient, the body's defences are weakened. Therefore, there is greater potential for exterior syndromes to take hold and cause *bi* syndrome (see below), including: **I.** Dampness **II.** Wind **III.** Cold **IV.** Heat **V.** Blood stasis			
Clinical Manifestations			
Hot flashes, hot sensation in face, night sweats, lower backache, feeling cold, cold knees, back, and feet, weak legs, bright white complexion, low libido, tiredness, lassitude, clear urination, nocturia, apathy, odema in legs, loose stools, depression.			
Tongue	**Pulse**	**Treatment Principle**	**Points***
Pale	Deep-weak	Tonify Kidney yang, clear exterior pathogenic factors	Mingmen DU-4 Shenshu BL-23 Guanyuan REN-4 Taixi KID-3 Zusanli ST-36 **Additional points:** Baihui DU-20 Shenting DU-24 Shenmen HT-7 Hegu LI-4 Taichong LIV-3 Yanglingquan GB-34 Qihai REN-6
Prescription			
Gui Zhi Tang Du Huo Ji Sheng Tang			

* Plus local points as required.

Table 4.7b: Kidney yang deficiency with exterior syndromes.

2.1. Bi Syndrome

Bi syndrome is one of the most common causes of musculoskeletal pain. It occurs as a result of a pathogenic factor obstructing the free flow of qi and blood in the channels, leading to pain or numbness.

The word *bi* (痹) can be translated as impediment, although the term is most often translated as 'obstruction syndrome' or 'painful obstruction syndrome.'

"Bu tong ze tong, tong ze bu tong"
"Pain results without movement, with movement there is no pain"

The Tissues in TCEAM

Sinews (Tendons, Ligaments, and Cartilage) = Liver	Connect muscle to bone Connect bone to bone The Liver maintains smooth and unimpeded articulation Liver Blood nourishes the tendons Affected by emotions
Muscles = Spleen	The Spleen and Stomach break down food and drink which nourishes the muscles The Spleen and Stomach generate fuel (qi) Affected by diet
Bones = Kidney	Kidney *jing* fills the bones with marrow Affected by work and rest
Qi = Lung	The Lung generates qi Affected by exercise
Blood = Heart	The Heart generates Blood Affected by all other aspects of pathology and five *zang* interaction

Table 4.7c: The tissues in TCEAM.

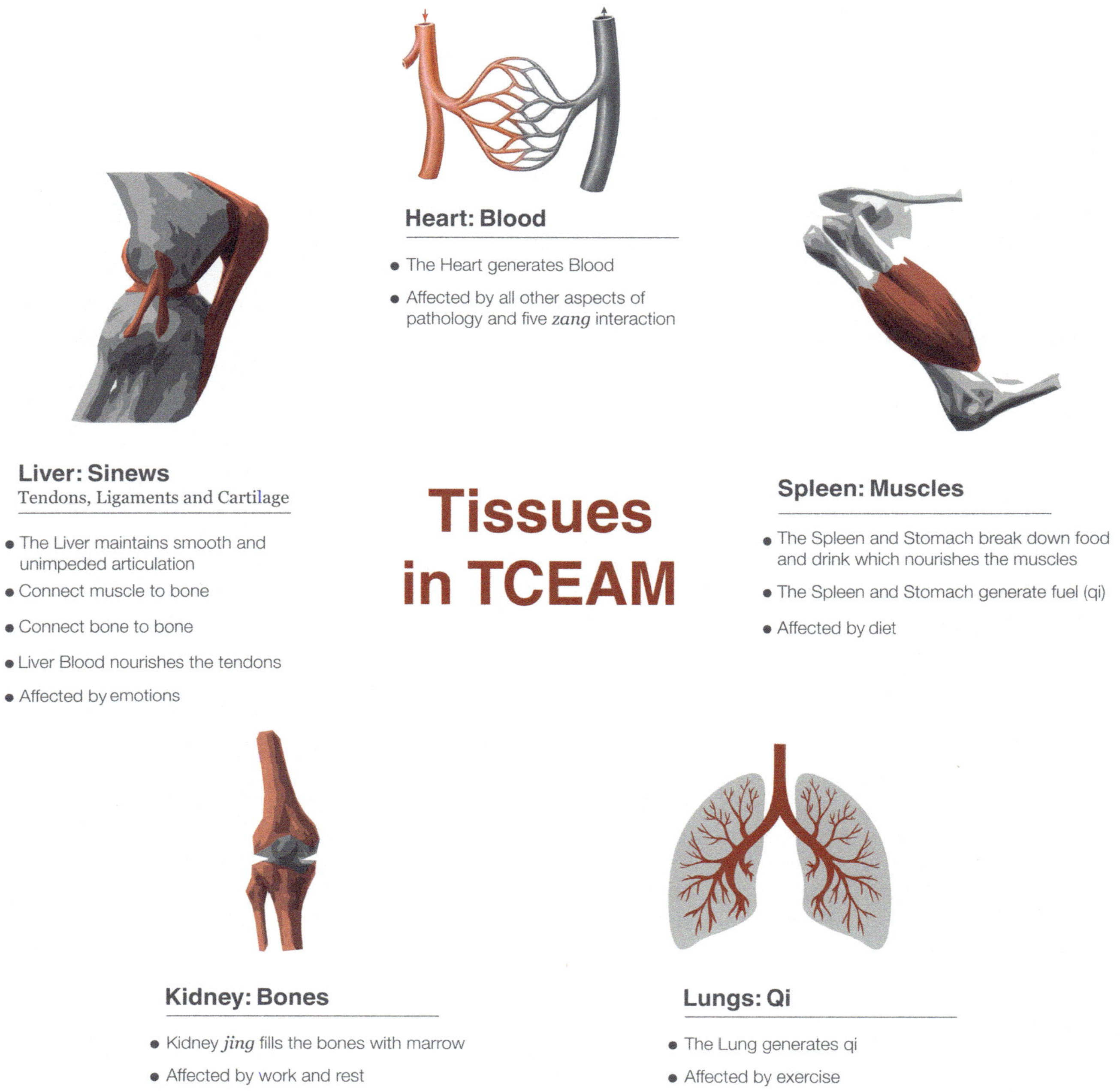

Figure 4.7: Tissues in TCEAM.

Healing Rates:

- **Muscles:** Heal fast (filled and rich with blood vessels)
- **Bones:** Heal fast (large blood supply)
- **Tendons and ligaments:** Heal slower (no direct blood supply)
- **Cartilage:** Heal Slowest (no direct blood supply)

The main treatment principle is to remove the obstruction and restore the circulation of qi and Blood in the affected area. Therefore, *bi* syndrome is frequently treated with local points, with those listed below being considered particularly appropriate. These local points can be paired with points that function to expel the specific pathogenic factor that is causing the obstruction.

Local points

Neck	Lower back
Yuzhen BL-9 Tianzhu BL-10 Dazhu BL-11 Fengmen BL-12 Fufen BL-41 Gaohuang BL-43 Tianrong SI-17 Tianchuang SI-16 Jianzhongshu SI-15 Jianwaishu SI-14 Guyuan SI-13 Bingfeng SI-12 Tianzong SI-11 Fengchi GB-20 Jianjing GB-21 Jianyu LI-15 Tutu LI-18 Fengfu DU-16 Dazhui DU-14	Shenshu BL-23 Qihaishu BL-24 Dachangshu BL-25 Guanyuansh BL-26 Xiaochangshu BL-27 Shangliao BL-31 Ciliao BL-32
Extra Points	
Jingbailao EX-HN 15 Cervical *jiaji* paravertebral points (lateral to the spinous processes of the vertebrae) *Ashi* points: tender areas lateral to C6-C7	Lumbar *jiaji* paravertebral points (M-BW-35): L2-S1 / adjacent to painful areas

Table 4.7d: Local points, neck, lower back, and extra points.

Upper Limb

Shoulder	Elbow	Wrist
Jianyu LI-15 Jianliao SJ-14 Jianzhen SI-9 Naoshu SI-10 Jianqian (M-UE-48) Taijian (below the acromion and lateral to the coracoid process)	Shousanli LI-10 Shouwuli LI-13 Shaohai HT-3 Chize LU-5 Tianjing SJ-10	Yangchi SJ-4 Waiguan SJ-5 Yangxi LI-5 Wangu SI-4 Hegu LI-4

Table 4.7e: Local points for upper limb.

Lower Limb

Hip	Knee	Ankle
Zhibian BL-54 Huantiao GB-30 Waiqiu GB-36 Juliao GB-29 Jingkua (midway between the greater trochanter and the crest of the ilium)	Ququan LIV-8 Xiyan (M-LE-16) Dubi St-35 Liangqiu ST-34 Yanglingquan GB-34 Xuehai SP-10 Yinlingquan SP-9 Zusanli ST-36	Kunlun BL-60 Shenmai BL-62 Qiuxu GB-40 Shangqiu SP-5 Jiexi ST-41 Taixi KID-3 Zhaohai KID-6

Table 4.7f: Local points for lower limb.

2.1.i. Damp *Bi*

Dampness is a yin pathogenic factor and is detrimental to yang. It is heavy and sticky, tending to accumulate in the joints and cause swelling and aching pain. The pain tends to be worse on cloudy or rainy days.

Clinical Manifestations

Sensations of heaviness, fixed pain in joints, local swelling, numbness, fatigue, loss of appetite, discomfort in chest/epigastrium, sticky taste, urinary difficulty, cloudy urine, white-sticky vaginal discharge.

Tongue	Pulse	Treatment Principle	Points*
White, greasy or sticky coating	Slippery-full, slow	Dispel dampness, dissipate wind, expel cold, supplement the Spleen, move qi	Fengchi ST-40 Yinlingquan SP-9 Zusanli ST-36 Shangqiu SP-5

Prescription

Juan Bi Tang
For extensive dampness add Yi Yi Ren (Semen Cocois) 30g, Cang Zhu (Rhizoma Atractylodis) 12g

* Plus local points as required. Moxa recommended.

Table 4.7g: Damp *bi*.

2.1.ii. Wind *Bi*			
Wind is a yang pathogenic factor and damages Blood and yin. It is fast-moving and travels around the body causing wandering pain that may be intermittent in nature. It may also combine with dampness to cause body aches with stiff or swollen joints.			
Clinical Manifestations			
Wandering pain with no fixed location, aversion to wind.			
Tongue	**Pulse**	**Treatment Principle**	**Points***
White or greasy coating	Floating	Dispel wind, dispel cold, disinhibit dampness, tonify qi and Blood	Baihui DU-20 Zhongting REN-16 Geshu UB-17 Xuehai SP-10 Sanyinjiao SP-6
Prescription			
Du Huo Ji Sheng Tang Gui Zhi Tang			

* Plus local points as required.

Table 4.7h: Wind *bi*.

2.1.iii. Cold *Bi*			
Cold is a yin pathogenic factor. It slows the circulation, contracts the muscles, and causes pain which is aggravated by cold conditions and relieved by warmth.			
Clinical Manifestations			
Severe, stabbing pain with a fixed location, pale and watery discharges.			
Tongue	**Pulse**	**Treatment Principle**	**Points***
White coating	Tight	Warm the channels, dissipate cold, course wind, dispel dampness	Shenshu BL-23 Mingmen DU-4 Guanyuan REN-4 Shenque REN-8 (moxa)
Prescription			
Xiao Huo Luo Dan Wu Ji San			

* Plus local points as required. Moxa recommended.

Table 4.7i: Cold *bi*.

2.1.iv. Heat *Bi*			
Heat is a yang pathogenic factor. It rises in the body, causing sensations of heat with thirst and mental restlessness. It can easily combine with either dampness or wind to cause inflammation, swelling, and pain.			
Clinical Manifestations			
Pain with local redness, swelling, or burning sensations, fever, sweating, thirst.			
Tongue	**Pulse**	**Treatment Principle**	**Points***
Red with yellow and greasy fur	Rapid	Clear heat, dispel dampness, diffuse impediment, relieve pain	Dazhui DU-14 Hegu LI-4 Quchi LI-11
Prescription			
Xuan Bi Tang Gui Zhi Shao Yao Zhi Mu Tang			

* Plus local points as required.

Table 4.7j: Heat *bi*.

2.1.v. Blood Stasis *Bi*			
Over time, pathogenic factors can transform into Blood stasis *bi*. Therefore, this type of *bi* syndrome is most often observed in patients with chronic pain.			
Clinical Manifestations			
Pain is chronic but may be intermittent, swelling, joint stiffness and deformity, numb limbs.			
Tongue	**Pulse**	**Treatment Principle**	**Points***
Dull purple with ecchymosis, white or greasy coating	Thready and unsmooth, or wiry	Remove stasis and restore the free flow of qi and Blood	Xuehai SP-10 Geshu BL-17 Taichong LIV-3
Prescription			
Shen Tong Zhu Yu Tang Huo Luo Xiao Ling Dan (strong formula)			

* Plus local points as required.

Table 4.7k: Blood stasis *bi*.

3. Liver Blood Deficiency			
Liver Blood is responsible for nourishing and moistening the sinews. It has a close relationship with Liver yin and Kidney yin. Therefore, this substance can easily become deficient during the menopausal period, leading to muscle weakness, stiffness, and pain. The condition is aggravated by poor diet or Spleen deficiency as these factors will further impair the formation of Blood.			
Clinical Manifestations			
Dizziness, numb limbs, insomnia, blurred vision, floaters, scant menstruation/ amenorrhea, dull-pale complexion and lips, muscle weakness, spasm, cramps, dry nails, hair, and skin.			
Tongue	**Pulse**	**Treatment Principle**	**Points***
Dry and pale, especially at the sides	Choppy or fine	Tonify the Liver, Kidneys, and Spleen, nourish Blood	Ganshu BL-18 Pishu BL-20 Geshu BL-17 Qimen LIV-14 Taichong LIV-3 Sanyinjiao SP-6 Zusanli ST-36 Guanyuan REN-4 Qihai REN-6
Prescription			
Tao Hong Si Wu Tang			

* Plus local points as required.

Table 4.7l: Liver blood deficiency.

Patient Advice

> > Remain as physically active as possible and maintain a healthy body weight, but avoid overexertion and muscle strain (see Chapter 5.1, Metabolism, Weight Management, and Exercise).
> > Ensure that workspaces are set up in a comfortable and ergonomic fashion.
> > Check that no everyday activities, such as carrying heavy bags, are causing misalignment of the body.
> > Eat an anti-inflammatory diet (see Chapter 6.3, Diet, Lifestyle, and Disease Prevention).
> > Use heat or cold packs as appropriate to relieve localized pain.
> > Apply topical pain-relief products to affected areas.
> > Schedule regular massages or learn self-massage techniques.
> > Consider pain-focused mindfulness and meditation practices.
> > If taking non-steroidal anti-inflammatory drugs, avoid doing so on an empty stomach.

References

Wolfe, HL., (1998). Managing Menopause Naturally with Chinese Medicine. Blue Poppy Press. Inc. Boulder, Colorado. USA.

Maciocia, G., (1989). The Foundations of Chinese Medicine. First edition. Churchill Livingston Elsevier, London, UK.

Zhang, E-Q., (2010). Bi Syndrome (Arthralgia Syndrome), Research Gate : June 2010 Journal of Traditional Chinese Medicine 30(2): (pp 145-52). DOI:10.1016/S0254-6272(10)60032-5 Source PubMed https://www.researchgate.net/publication/45284133_Bi_Syndrome_Arthralgia_Syndrome

Berry, K., (2019). Cupping and Adjunct Therapies for Menopause. Treating Women Academy, Healthy Hormones Naturally: Online Menopause Masterclass. https://www.treatingwomen.com/store/5tpUJ3Fk

4.8 Osteopenia, Osteoporosis, and Hyperkyphosis

Bones consist of rigid tissue that provides structure and mobility to the musculoskeletal system. With a complex internal and external structure, they are lightweight, yet strong and hard. Bones protect the internal organs and serve multiple other functions, including the production of red and white blood cells and storing minerals.

Bone mineral density (BMD) is the measurement of calcium and phosphorus contained in a certain volume of bone. Maintaining bone health is an important part of the aging process.

Osteopenia and Osteoporosis

Menopause increases the risk of osteopenia and osteoporosis. Both conditions describe reduced BMD, with osteoporosis being the more severe of the two.

Both conditions can increase the risk of fractures, especially of the wrist, hip, and vertebrae. Hip fractures are especially problematic as they are associated with a high mortality rate within the first year following the fracture.

Pathophysiology

Estrogen plays a crucial role in bone remodeling. This is the process by which old bone is continually being replaced by new. It relies on two different types of cells; osteoclasts and osteoblasts.

- **Osteoclasts** are responsible for creating an acidic environment on the surface of bones and dissolving their mineral content, a process known as resorption, resulting in a transfer of calcium from bone tissue into the blood.
- **Osteoblasts** are responsible for depositing collagen, which becomes mineralized to form new bone, a process known as formation.

Resorption increases in the presence of several different cytokines, and these cytokines are downregulated by estrogen. Therefore, as estrogen levels decrease, resorption activity overtakes formation, causing a net loss of bone.

Furthermore, age alters the body's ability to absorb calcium. For example, the intestines become increasingly resistant to circulating 1,25-dihydroxyvitamin D (calcitriol), which is necessary for calcium absorption. Meanwhile, the kidneys reduce their production of calcitriol, leading to further reductions in calcium. These changes may also contribute to hyperparathyroidism.

Risk Factors

Age of Menopause

Menopause before the age of 45 increases the risk of osteopenia and osteoporosis. The same is true for individuals who undergo medically-induced menopause.

Interestingly, decreases in calcium levels are far more dramatic during the first stages of menopause. They eventually taper off to a far steadier rate of loss 5–10 years post-menopause.

Ethnicity and Genetics

Ethnicity and genetics both play a role, with Caucasians being at the highest risk.

Reproductive Status

Nulliparous women appear to have a higher risk of hip and spine, but not wrist, fractures. This is despite there being no apparent difference in BMD between parous and nulliparous women.

Medical Conditions

Several different medical conditions are associated with an increased risk of osteopenia and osteoporosis, including:

- Rheumatoid arthritis
- Hyperthyroidism
- Hyperparathyroidism
- Type 1 diabetes
- Celiac disease and other malabsorption disorders
- Liver disease
- Chronic obstructive pulmonary disease (COPD)
- Organ transplant

Medication

Certain medications can increase the risk of osteopenia and osteoporosis. For example, long-term glucocorticoid use inhibits bone formation by directly and indirectly reducing the activity of osteoblasts.

Lifestyle Factors

Numerous lifestyle factors can also increase the rate of bone loss, including:

- Insufficient intake of vitamin D, vitamin K, calcium, magnesium, silicon, or boron
- Poor nutrition/excessive dieting or eating disorders such as anorexia nervosa
- Low body mass index
- Smoking
- Alcohol use
- Sedentary lifestyle
- Lack of weight-bearing exercise
- Lack of sunlight
- Vitamin D deficiency

Hyperkyphosis (Dowager's Hump)

The term 'hyperkyphosis' describes an exaggerated curvature of the thoracic spine. Some degree of curvature, or kyphosis, is normal in the thoracic spine. It is generally assessed by a measure known as the Cobb angle.

In young adults, a Cobb angle of up to around 40 degrees can be considered normal. Anything above this is classified as hyperkyphosis. It is a common issue among older people, especially women. For example, the average Cobb angle for women in their late 50s is approximately 43 degrees. The figure rises to 52 degrees in women in their late 70s.

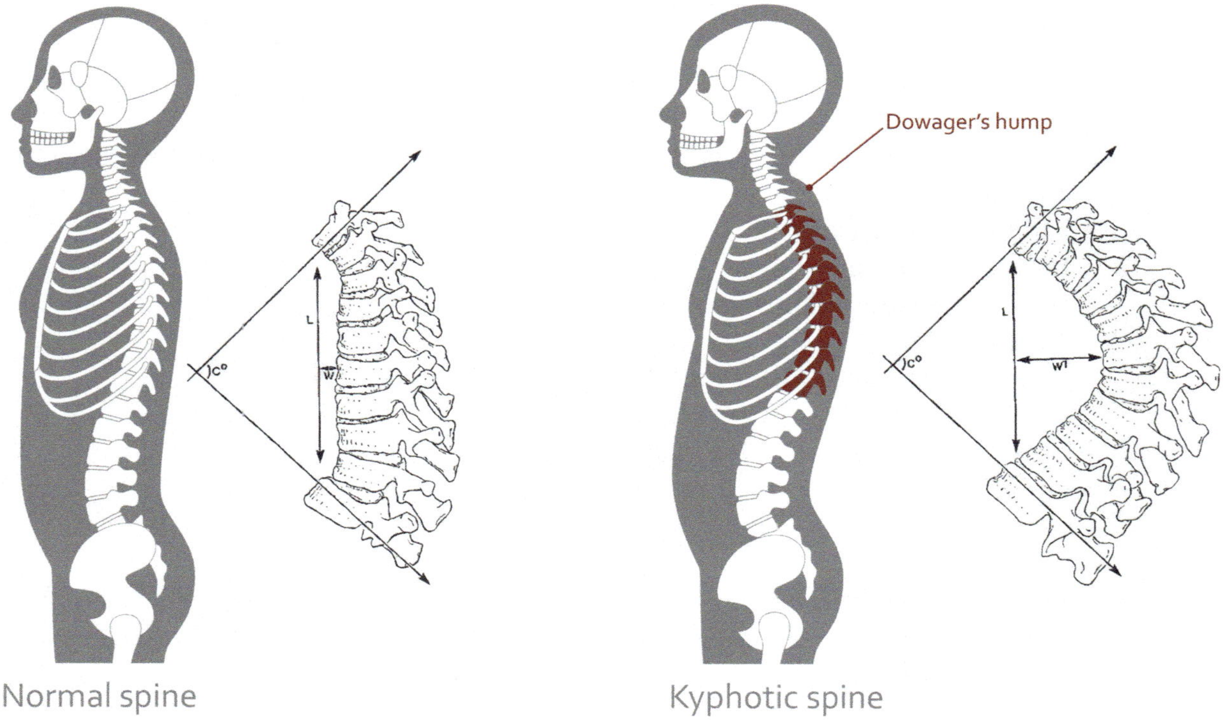

Figure 4.8: Hyperkyphosis (Dowager's Hump).

There are several serious problems associated with hyperkyphosis. Apart from esthetic concerns, it can negatively impact mobility, balance, gait, and overall quality of life. It increases the risk of falls and fractures and is also associated with decreased lung capacity and pulmonary death.

Pathophysiology

There is a clear relationship between decreased bone mineral density, vertebral fractures, and hyperkyphosis. Firstly, vertebral fractures increase the curvature of the spine leading to hyperkyphosis. Secondly, hyperkyphosis increases the risk of falls and fractures, thus worsening the original problem.

Several other conditions also play a role. They include degenerative disc disease and muscle weakness. Another factor is that as people age, there is a natural decrease in vision and vestibular function. This makes it more difficult to perceive a correct vertical posture, leading to a stooped head position. This forward head posture (FHP) is made worse by driving a car, working on computers, and reading mobile phones and other devices.

Risk Factors

Bone Mineral Density

Women with low BMD, osteopenia, or osteoporosis are more likely to experience vertebral fractures, leading to hyperkyphosis.

Degenerative Disc Disease

There is a significant correlation between degenerative disc disease and hyperkyphosis, with decreases in disc height leading to increased kyphosis.

Muscle Weakness

There is a relationship between the strength of the spinal extensor muscles and the degree of kyphosis experienced by postmenopausal women. There is also an association with shortened pectoral and hip flexor muscles, although it is unclear whether this is a cause or an effect of the condition.

TCEAM Viewpoint

These conditions are all related to softening of the bones, which occurs as a result of declining Kidney *jing*.

Pattern Differentiation

1. Kidney *jing* deficiency

1. Kidney *Jing* Deficiency

The Kidney, specifically Kidney *jing*, is responsible for filling the marrow and strengthening the bones and teeth. While *jing* is primarily a yin substance, it also has a yang aspect. This means that *jing* deficiency can occur alongside Kidney yin or yang predominant patterns.

Furthermore, there is often stagnation of qi and Blood and wind-dampness in the joints, which, if not cleared, prevent the bones from regenerating. Therefore, it may be necessary to simultaneously tonify and move qi and Blood.

Clinical Manifestations

Soft and weak bones, weak aching knees and legs, sore lower back, loose teeth, memory loss, graying or falling hair, sexual dysfunction, persistent and debilitating tiredness, exhaustion and weakness of mind and body, depression, dull eyes, flat affect. May have night sweats.

Tongue	Pulse	Treatment Principle	Points*
Pale, swollen	Deep, thready, weak	Supplement the Liver, Spleen, and Kidneys, Nourish yin, yang, and *jing*	Taixi KID-3 Zhaohai KID-6 Guanyuan REN-4 Shenshu BL-23 Mingmen DU-4 Xuanzhong GB-39 Baihui DU-20 Dazhui DU-14 Xinshu BL-15 Dashu BL-11 Zusanli ST-36 Sanyinjiao SP-6

Prescription

Gui Lu Er Xian Jiao
For predominant Kidney yang deficiency: Jin Gui Shen Qi Wan
Du Huo Ji Sheng Tang + Shu Jing Huo Xue Tang

* A meta-analysis of studies using Chinese herbs for osteoporosis found that, in postmenopausal women, Chinese herbal medicine produced an insignificantly higher increase in bone mineral density (BMD) than the Western drug regimes taken by the control groups. Whether the trial duration was under or over six months, BMDs were comparable between the two therapies. Given the incidence of side effects from the pharmaceutical medications for osteoporosis, Chinese herbal medicine may be worth using postmenopausally. Whichever treatments are used need to be long-term as cessation of treatment results in a deterioration of BMD.

Table 4.8a: Kidney *jing* deficiency.

Local points for the neck:
Fengfu DU-16
Tianzhu BL-10
Dazhu BL-11

Local points for the spine:
Huatuo *jiaji* paravertebral points
Lingtai DU-10
Geshu UB-17

Local points for the lower back:
Mingmen DU-4
Shenshu BL-23 to Dachangshu BL-25
Shangliao BL-31

Local points for the hips:
Zhibian BL-54
Huantiao GB-30

Moxa or warm acupuncture is applicable except in cases of yin deficiency with empty heat.

Care should be taken when needling very depleted people not to retain needles for a long time and not to use too many needles.

Patient Advice

> Maintain good posture during exercise.
> Strengthen the core stabilizer muscles but avoid crunches, curl-ups, or traditional sit-ups (flexed position).
> Keep the spine in neutral when lifting objects by bending the hips and knees (hip hinging), pulling in the abdominal muscles, and keeping objects close to the body.
> Stabilize the trunk when coughing or sneezing by hugging a pillow or placing the hands on the knees while hip hinging.
> Roll onto one side before sitting up when getting out of bed.
> Imagine lengthening through the crown of the head while sitting and standing.
> Adjust the height of walking sticks or frames to avoid reaching forward or pushing.
> Consider treatment with physiotherapy, manual or mobilization therapy, taping, MHT, or antiresorptive medication.
> *Jing* depletion is difficult to reverse, so much careful long-term treatment is necessary. Encourage a Kidney nourishing diet and limit exhausting work and exercise.

Key Nutrients for Bone Health

There is some evidence that the consumption of calcium supplements post-menopause can injure heart function and precipitate heart disease. Therefore, increasing one's dietary intake of calcium may be more appropriate. For example, dairy products (for those who can tolerate them), calcium-set tofu, fish with edible bones, bone soups, almonds, tahini, chia seeds, dark leafy greens.

Nutrient	Recommended Dietary Allowance	Median Intake	Authors' Prefered Supplementation
Vitamin D	600-800 IU	150-300 IU	400-1000 IU
Calcium	1000-1200 mg	735 mg	500 mg
Magnesium	320-420 mg	243 mg	250-350 mg
Silicon	40 mg for bone health	21 mg	20-40 mg
Vitamin K	90-120 mcg	70-80 mcg	50-150 mcg
Boron	3 mg for bone health	1 mg	1-3 mg
Vitamin C	75-90 mg	103 mg	50-100 mg
Copper	0.9 mg	1.1 mg	None
Zinc	8-11 mg	9.6 mg	None unless vegetarian or elderly
Manganese	1.8-2.3 mg	2.8 mg	None

Table 4.8b: Key nutrients for bone health.

References

Katzman, WB., Wanek, L., Shepherd, JA., et al. (2010). Age-Related Hyperkyphosis: Its Causes, Consequences, and Management, PMC US National Library of Medicine, National Institutes of Health, HHS Public Access, Author Manuscript: J Orthop Sports Phys Ther. 2010 Jun; 40(6): (pp 352–360).doi: 10.2519/jospt.2010.3099
https://www.ncbi.nlm.nih.gov/pmc/articles/PMC2907357

Price, CT., Langford, JR., Liporace, FA., (2012). Essential Nutrients for Bone Health and a Review of their Availability in the Average North American Diet, PMC US National Library of Medicine, National Institutes of Health, Bentham open, The Open Orthopaedics Journal: Open Orthop J. 2012; 6: (pp 143–149). Published online 2012 Apr 5. doi: 10.2174/1874325001206010143.
https://www.ncbi.nlm.nih.gov/pmc/articles/PMC3330619

Maciocia, G., (1989). The Foundations of Chinese Medicine. First edition. Churchill Livingston Elsevier, London, UK.

Jin, Y.X., Wu P., Mao, Y.F., Wang, B., Zhang, J.F., Chen, W.L., Liu, Z., Shi, X.L. (2017) Chinese Herbal Medicine for Osteoporosis: A Meta-analysis of Randomized Controlled Trials, Journal of Clinical Densitometry, Volume 20, Issue 4, Pages 516-525, ISSN1094-6950,
https://doi.org/10.1016/j.jocd.2017.07.003

Reid, IR., Birstow, SM., Bolland, MJ., (2017). Calcium and Cardiovascular Disease, NIH, National Library of Medicine, National Center for Biotechnology Information: EnM Endocrinology and Metabolism: Endocrinol Metab (Seoul). 2017 Sep; 32(3): 339–349.Published online 2017 Sep 18. doi: 10.3803/EnM.2017.32.3.339.
https://www.ncbi.nlm.nih.gov/pmc/articles/PMC5620030

Cormick, G., Belizán, M., (2019). Calcium Intake and Health, NIH, National Library of Medicine, National Center for Biotechnology Information, Nutrients: Nutrients. 2019 Jul; 11(7): 1606. Published online 2019 Jul 15. doi: 10.3390/nu11071606.
https://www.ncbi.nlm.nih.gov/pmc/articles/PMC6683260

Office of the Surgeon General (US). Rockville (MD), (2004). Bone Health and Osteoporosis: A Report of the Surgeon General. Table 7-2 Selected Food Sources of Calcium, NIH, National Library of Medicine, National Center for Biotechnology Information
https://www.ncbi.nlm.nih.gov/books/NBK45523/table/ch7.t2

4.9 Metabolic Syndrome, Diabetes, and Cardiovascular Disease

The term 'metabolism' describes the chemical reactions that occur within the body to convert food and drink into energy. This includes the breakdown of carbohydrates into glucose and its transportation into cells for conversion to adenosine triphosphate (ATP). This process relies heavily upon the hormone insulin, which is secreted by beta cells in the pancreas.

Metabolic syndrome is the blanket term used to describe a group of disorders involving obesity, insulin resistance, dyslipidemia, and hypertension. Its incidence in women increases significantly in the years following menopause, raising the risk of cardiovascular disease, type 2 diabetes, and stroke.

The key features of metabolic syndrome include:

- Central obesity, defined as a waist-hip ratio of >0.85
- High fasting blood glucose (> 100mg/dL)
- High serum triglycerides (> 150mg/dL)
- High low-density lipoprotein (LDL) cholesterol (> 130mg/dL)
- Low high-density lipoprotein (HDL) cholesterol (< 50 mg/dL for women is considered low)
- Hypertension (blood pressure > 130/80 mmHg)
- Microalbuminuria

Metabolic syndrome has a complex interrelationship with oxidative stress, chronic inflammation, and associated disorders. It may also play a role in the development of non-alcoholic fatty liver disease and obstructive sleep apnea.

Pathophysiology

Throughout the reproductive years, estrogen exerts a protective influence over the cardiovascular system. Reduced levels of this hormone mean that postmenopausal women are at increased risk of cardiovascular diseases, including hypertension and atherosclerosis.

Furthermore, female body fat distribution changes after menopause, with a greater tendency towards abdominal obesity. This increases the risk of dyslipidemia and insulin resistance, which in turn contributes to sodium and water retention, further increasing blood pressure.

Risk Factors

Age of Menarche

Women who experience menarche before the age of 10 or after the age of 16 are more likely to have irregular menstrual cycles. In later life, this is associated with a higher risk of obesity and high triglyceride levels.

Age of Menopause

Women who undergo early or medically induced menopause are at increased risk of developing diabetes and metabolic syndrome.

Family History

A genetic component is involved in developing metabolic syndrome, diabetes, and cardiovascular disease.

Body Weight and Fat Distribution

Women with a body mass index over 30 are more prone to metabolic syndrome and have a higher risk of developing cardiovascular disease and diabetes. The highest risk is in women with central obesity, defined as a waist-hip ratio of >0.85.

Physical Activity

There is a strong relationship between sedentary lifestyles, obesity, insulin resistance, and metabolic syndrome.

Diet

High-fat, high-calorie, high-sugar, and high-salt diets are all associated with an increased risk of metabolic syndrome, hypertension, and cardiovascular disease. Vitamin D deficiency also plays a role.

Postmenopausal women should increase their intake of fresh fruit and vegetables, whole grains, oily fish, and other healthy fats. Diets such as the DASH diet and Mediterranean diet are ideal.

See Section 6. Diet and Nutrition for more information.

TCEAM Viewpoint

Metabolic syndrome is a highly complex disorder; its underlying patterns can vary greatly depending on its predominant symptoms. Although the underlying pattern may involve qi or yang deficiency, diabetes, in particular, is considered a form of yin deficiency, which can result in empty heat. This can make diagnosis challenging, as the symptoms (heat, yin deficiency) may appear at odds with the root cause (qi or yang deficiency).

It is beyond the scope of this chapter to discuss all of the patterns associated with metabolic syndrome in detail, and further information on their diagnosis and treatment can be found elsewhere in the text or in various other sources (see References page 196). However, we have provided a brief overview.

Diabetes

In Chinese, diabetes is known as *xiaoke*, or dispersion thirst. It is a pathological condition that involves an increased intake of fluids (polydipsia), increased intake of food (polyphagia), increased urination (polyuria), and weight loss.

Pattern Differentiation

The early development of diabetes could present as the following patterns:

1. Qi stagnation due to Liver depression
2. Liver and Stomach heat stagnation
3. Phlegm and heat stasis
4. Excess heat in the Stomach and intestines
5. Intestinal damp and heat syndromes

These differing patterns lead to dryness in the lower *jiao* affecting the Kidney and heat attacking the three *jiao*, injuring the Lung, Spleen, and Kidney, and causing further deficiency.

There are five distinct stages in its development:

I. Yin deficiency (with or without hyperactive Liver yang or Liver fire)
II. Heat transmission (symptoms include aversion to heat, lassitude, polydipsia, polyphagia, polyuria, increased blood and urine sugars)
III. Dryness impairing yin
IV. Yin, yang, and qi deficiency and obstruction of the channels
V. Severe stage

This pathology is aggravated by poor diet and improper eating habits, combined with a lack of exercise.

Pattern Differentiation

There are seven classical patterns associated with diabetes:

1. Yin deficiency
2. Hyperactive fire due to yin deficiency
3. Qi and yin deficiency
4. Qi and yin deficiency with hyperactive fire
5. Yin and yang deficiency
6. Yin and yang deficiency with hyperactive fire
7. Blood stasis

> Suzanne Cochrane clinical commentary: "Most of these conditions begin as excess patterns and only after prolonged neglect become deficiencies. Qi stagnation and Stomach heat are especially common in the onset of diabetes and evident in metabolic syndrome".

Hypertension

Hypertension is another key feature of metabolic syndrome. There are several possible underlying patterns that can lead to unhealthy increases in blood pressure, including:

1. Hyperactive Liver yang ascending due to Kidney/Liver yin deficiency
2. Yin deficiency
3. Liver fire
4. Damp-phlegm accumulation (due to qi deficiency)

Cardiovascular Disease

Cardiovascular disease is often associated with what TCEAM practitioners refer to as 'chest impediment.' It occurs as a result of phlegm stagnation and Blood stasis congealing in the chest to prevent the diffusion of yang.

Pattern Differentiation

Some of the most common associated patterns are:

1. Damp-phlegm stagnation and/or
2. Blood stasis
3. Qi deficiency (yang qi deficiency)

Patient Advice

Although genetics play a role in the development of metabolic syndrome, diabetes, and cardiovascular disease, they are also frequently considered 'lifestyle diseases'. Therefore, they can be prevented or controlled to a certain extent by making behavioral modifications, including:

> Maintaining a healthy body weight.
> Eating a nutritious, low-glycemic index, anti-inflammatory diet.
> Reducing fat, sugar, and salt intake.
> Reducing alcohol intake.
> Not smoking.
> Exercising regularly.
> Taking medication on time and attending all medical appointments.
> Having blood glucose, blood pressure, and cholesterol levels checked regularly.
> Patients with diabetes and prediabetes should eat regularly and monitor blood glucose levels throughout the day.
> Patients with diabetes should have regular eye and foot check-ups to reduce the risk of complications.

References

Lee, T-C., Lo, L-C., Wu, F-C., (2016). Traditional Chinese Medicine for Metabolic Syndrome via TCM Pattern Differentiation: Tongue Diagnosis for Predictor. Hindawi: Evidence-Based Complementary and Alternative Medicine: Volume 2016 Article ID 1971295 https://doi.org/10.1155/2016/1971295
https://www.hindawi.com/journals/ecam/2016/1971295

Guo, J., Chen, H., Song, J., Wang, J., Zhao, L., & Tong, X. (2014). Syndrome Differentiation of Diabetes by the Traditional Chinese Medicine according to Evidence-Based Medicine and Expert Consensus Opinion. Evidence-Based Complementary and Alternative Medicine, 2014, 492193. doi:10.1155/2014/492193
https://www.ncbi.nlm.nih.gov/pmc/articles/PMC4123514/

Yin, J., Zhang, H., Ye, J., (2008). Traditional Chinese Medicine in Treatment of Metabolic Syndrome, PMC US National Library of Medicine, National Institutes of Health, HHS Public Access, Author Manuscript: Endocr Metab Immune Disord Drug Targets. Author manuscript; available in PMC 2009
https://www.ncbi.nlm.nih.gov/pmc/articles/PMC2467395

Huang, L-W., Chen, I-J., Hsu, C-H., (2016). Influence of traditional Chinese medicine syndrome groups on quality of life in women with metabolic syndrome, Journal of Traditional and Complementary Medicine, Volume 6, (Issue 4, October 2016), (pp 404-408).
https://www.sciencedirect.com/science/article/pii/S222541101500111X

Xia, S., Cai, J., Chen, J., et al. (2020). Factor and Cluster Analysis for TCM Syndromes of Real-World Metabolic Syndrome at Different Age Stage, Hindawi: Evidence-Based Complementary and Alternative Medicine: Volume 2020 Article ID 7854325 https://doi.org/10.1155/2020/7854325.
https://www.hindawi.com/journals/ecam/2020/7854325

Dharmananda, S., (2003). Treatment of Diabetes with Chinese Herbs and Acupuncture, Internet Journal of The Institute for Traditional Medicine and Preventive Health Care.
http://www.itmonline.org/journal/arts/diabetes.htm

HealthCMi: Healthcare Medicine Institute, (2014). Laser Acupuncture Metabolic Weight Loss Study.
https://www.healthcmi.com/Acupuncture-Continuing-Education-News/1359-laser-acupuncture-metabolic-weight-loss-new-study

Yu, A., Adelson, D., Mills, D., (2018). Chinese Herbal Medicine Versus Other Interventions in the Treatment of Type 2 Diabetes. A Systematic Review of Randomized Controlled Trials, Journal of Evidence-Based Integrative Medicine: J Evid Based Integr Med. 2018; 23: 2515690X18781519. Published online 2018 Jul 19. doi: 10.1177/2515690X18781519
https://www.ncbi.nlm.nih.gov/pmc/articles/PMC6053856

Covington, MB., (2001). Traditional Chinese Medicine in the Treatment of Diabetes. American Diabetes Association. Diabetes Spectrum: Diabetes Spectr 2001;14(3): (pp 154–159). https://doi.org/10.2337/diaspect.14.3.154.
https://spectrum.diabetesjournals.org/content/14/3/154

Wang, J., Xiong, X., (2012). Control Strategy on Hypertension in Chinese Medicine: Hindawi Evidence-Based Complementary and Alternative Medicine, Volume 2012, Article ID 284847. https://doi.org/10.1155/2012/284847.
https://www.hindawi.com/journals/ecam/2012/284847

Wang, J., Xiong, X., (2013). Evidence-Based Chinese Medicine for Hypertension, NIH National Library of Medicine, National Center for Biotechnology Information, Hindawi, Evid Based Complement Alternat Med. 2013; 2013: 978398. Published online 2013 Jun 3. doi: 10.1155/2013/978398.
https://www.ncbi.nlm.nih.gov/pmc/articles/PMC3686073

Yang, M., Lao, L., (2019). Emerging Applications of Metabolomics in Traditional Chinese Medicine Treating Hypertension: Biomarkers, Pathways and More, Frontiers in Pharmacology Ethnopharmacology: Front. Pharmacol., 08 March 2019. https://doi.org/10.3389/fphar.2019.00158.
https://www.frontiersin.org/articles/10.3389/fphar.2019.00158/full

Wiseman, N., Feng, Y. (2014). A Practical Dictionary of Chinese Medicine. Third edition. Paradigm Publications, Taos, New Mexico, USA.

Hao, P., Jiang, F., Cheng, J., et al. (2017). Traditional Chinese Medicine for Cardiovascular Disease: Evidence and Potential Mechanisms, Science Direct, Elsevier, Journal of the American College of Cardiology, Volume 69 (issue 24) 20 June 2017, (pp 2952-2066).
https://www.sciencedirect.com/science/article/pii/S0735109717371711

Chen, R., Xiao, Y., Chen, Minghao., et al. (2018). A traditional Chinese medicine therapy for coronary heart disease after percutaneous coronary intervention: a meta-analysis of randomized, double-blind, placebo-controlled trials, Portland Press: Biosci Rep (2018) 38 (5): BSR20180973.
https://doi.org/10.1042/BSR20180973. https://portlandpress.com/bioscirep/article/38/5/BSR20180973/87521

4.10 Cognitive Decline

The term cognition can be defined as a group of mental processes, including thinking, learning, memory, awareness, and judgement. It has been described by some as "the ultimate function of the brain."

Numerous neural networks and neurochemicals are involved in the process of cognition. The dopaminergic, serotonergic, cholinergic, and glutaminergic systems are all thought to play a fundamental role. However, scientists still do not fully understand the complex interactions between these systems and how dysfunctions in them can lead to cognitive decline.

From early perimenopause onward, many women experience a gradual but progressive state of cognitive decline. It may begin as temporary episodes of forgetfulness, such as an inability to recall specific words or misplacing objects. In some cases, this may progress to failure to remember appointments or events, and eventually dementia.

Dementia can be defined as significant cognitive decline that impairs one's ability to function in daily life. It includes conditions such as Alzheimer's disease and vascular dementia.

Pathophysiology

Estrogen has both direct and indirect effects on neuronal function. High concentrations of estrogen receptors exist in the hippocampus and prefrontal cortex, regions of the brain associated with episodic and working memory.

It appears that the hormone influences the activity of neurotransmitters, including serotonin and acetylcholine. Deficits in acetylcholine, especially, play a role in the development of dementia. Meanwhile, serotonin helps mood regulation, which can be adversely affected by cognitive decline.

Estrogen also promotes neuronal growth and the formation of new synapses, displays antioxidant activity, and regulates calcium homeostasis, a mechanism that is implicated in the development of Alzheimer's disease. The hormone also protects the small blood vessels of the brain to prevent vascular dementia.

Alzheimer's disease is the most common cause of dementia. Three of the most significant risk factors are advanced age, apolipoprotein-E (APOE)-4 genotype, and female sex.

As women transition through menopause, they undergo a series of neuroendocrine changes. One of these is the uncoupling of estrogen from the brain's bioenergetic system, leading to a hypometabolic state.

Sometimes described as a "brain bioenergetic crisis," this state promotes the aggregation of harmful amyloid-beta and tau proteins, causing amyloid plaques and neurofibrillary tangles, the hallmark characteristics of Alzheimer's disease. Although the precise role of these structures in the disease's pathology is unclear, they are thought to interfere with nervous transmission within the brain.

Another link between memory and menopause relates to vasomotor symptoms. Hot flashes can cause a temporary spike in cortisol levels, which can reversibly impair verbal memory. These symptoms may be more pronounced in women suffering from stress, anxiety, or depression.

Risk Factors

Body Mass Index

Women between the ages of 40 and 50 years with a high body mass index may be at increased risk of developing dementia. Conversely, those with increased body mass index later in life (over 65 years) appear to have a lower risk.

Metabolic Syndrome

Women with cardiovascular disease, type 2 diabetes, high cholesterol, and high blood pressure are at increased risk of developing dementia.

Physical Activity

Low levels of physical activity are associated with an increased risk of cognitive decline during and following menopause.

Diet

A diet rich in omega-3 fatty acids (especially DHA) and antioxidants (e.g. vitamin E) may offer some protection against cognitive decline.

Smoking

Women who smoke are at increased risk of developing dementia later in life.

TCEAM Viewpoint

Cognitive decline, including mild cognitive impairment, memory loss, and Alzheimer's disease are the result of Kidney, Heart, and Spleen deficiency. Cognitive decline becomes most evident in withdrawal into somnolence, an inability to stay alert during the day, and/or forgetfulness which may or may not be accompanied by agitation.

The Kidney is the sea of marrow and provides the substance of the brain, while the Heart regulates its activity. The Spleen's involvement stems from its function of transforming fluids. When the Spleen becomes deficient, the result is dampness and phlegm. These substances accumulate in the channels, making the sea of marrow turbid and obstructing the orifices that connect the Heart and brain.

Somnolence

Generally, this condition results from clear yang not reaching the head or insufficient yang. The following patterns may be involved:

Pattern Differentiation

1. Dampness encumbering the Spleen
2. Phlegm obstruction
3. Blood stasis
4. Spleen qi (and Blood) deficiency
5. Spleen and Kidney yang deficiency

1. Dampness Encumbering the Spleen			
Dampness interferes with the normal circulation of yang qi, especially to the head where it fails to invigorate the brain and brighten the eyes, resulting in mental dullness, difficulty thinking, and difficulty keeping the eyes open.			
Clinical Manifestations			
Sleepiness, particularly after eating, variable fatigue which is better for movement and exercise, heavy sensations, poor appetite with loss of taste, loose stools.			
Tongue	**Pulse**	**Treatment Principle**	**Points**
Swollen with thick, white greasy coat	Soft and soggy or slippery	Dry dampness, strengthen the Spleen	Fenglong ST-40 Taibai SP-3 Baihui DU-20 Shenmai BL-62 Zhaohai KID-6 Yinlingquan SP-9 Sanyinjiao SP-6 Zhongwan REN-12 Zusanli ST-36 Fengchi GB-20
Prescription			
Ping Wei San			

Table 4.10a: Dampness encumbering the Spleen.

2. Phlegm Obstruction			
Similar to dampness encumbering the Spleen, phlegm obstructs the rise of yang through the same pathological mechanism but can become a more chronic and stubborn condition.			
Clinical Manifestations			
Chronic and continuous somnolence, heavy sleep, difficult to rouse, tendency to obesity, glossy or greasy skin, sensations of heaviness.			
Tongue	**Pulse**	**Treatment Principle**	**Points**
Flabby with a thick greasy coat	Slippery	Transform phlegm, open the channels to the head	Fenglong ST-40 Taibai SP-3 Baihui DU-20 Yinlingquan SP-9 Sanyinjiao SP-6 Tianshu ST-25 Zhongwan REN-12 Pishu BL-20 Zusanli ST-36 Taichong LIV-3 Fengchi GB-20 Zhaohai KID-6 Shenmai BL-62
Prescription			
Di Tan Tang Er Chen Wan			

Table 4.10b: Phlegm obstruction.

3. Blood Stasis			
Blood stasis could arise from head injury or from other chronic conditions such as prolonged qi stagnation failing to move the Blood.			
Clinical Manifestations			
Persistent daytime drowsiness, recurrent fixed headache, other signs of Blood stasis such as broken blood vessels, darkish complexion, purplish lips and nail beds, perhaps mood swings and hair loss.			
Tongue	**Pulse**	**Treatment Principle**	**Points**
In chronic cases, dark or purplish body with brown or purple spots In acute cases tongue may be unremarkable	Choppy or wiry and thready	Invigorate Blood circulation, open channels and collaterals	Local points on head + Xinshu BL-15 Hegu LI-4 Geshu BL-17 Sanyinjiao SP-6 Xuehai SP-10 Fengchi GB-20 Shenmai BL-62 Houxi SI-3 Zhaohai KID-6 Taichong LIV-3 Sishencong M-HN-1
Prescription			
Tong Qiao Huo Xue Tang Xue Fu Zhu Yu Tang			

Table 4.10c: Blood stasis.

4. Spleen Qi (and Blood) Deficiency			
Qi deficiency prevents the brain and senses from receiving sufficient qi.			
Clinical Manifestations			
Daytime drowsiness and desire to sleep (worse for exertion or eating), perhaps Blood deficient insomnia at night, mental and physical fatigue, weakness and tiredness in limbs, loose stools, pale and sallow complexion.			
Tongue	**Pulse**	**Treatment Principle**	**Points**
Pale and swollen with tooth marks and thin white coat	Deficient and weak	Strengthen the Spleen and tonify qi	Baihui DU-20 Sanyinjiao SP-6 Zhongwan REN-12 Shenmai BL-62 Zhaohai KID-6 Fenglong ST-40 Taibai SP-3 Zusanli ST-36 Pishu BL-20 Sishencong M-HN-1
Prescription			
Xiang Sha Liu Jun Zi Tang			

Table 4.10d: Spleen qi (and Blood) deficiency.

5. Spleen and Kidney Yang Deficiency			
Yang being the dynamic force of all physiology, its lack will show as an excess of yin with dulled senses and drowsiness. Yang deficiency is more pronounced in the daytime.			
Clinical Manifestations			
Constant drowsiness and desire to sleep, physical and mental exhaustion, apathy and depression, forgetfulness, reluctance to speak, digestive weakness, low libido, cold intolerance with cold extremities.			
Tongue	**Pulse**	**Treatment Principle**	**Points***
Pale or bluish and swollen with a thin moist coat	Deep, thready and weak	Benefit qi, warm yang, strengthen the Spleen and Kidney	Shenshu BL-23^ Pishu BL-20^ Mingmen DU-4^ Taixi KID-3 Zhishi BL-52 Qihai REN-6^ Baihui DU-20 Shenmai BL-62 Zhaohai KID-6 Zusanli ST-36^
Prescription			
Fu Zi Li Zhong Wan Jin Gui Shen Qi Wan			

* Consider adding moxa on some of the points marked with ^

Table 4.10e: Spleen and Kidney yang deficiency.

Forgetfulness

A functioning memory relies upon the balanced interaction of aspects of the Heart, Spleen, and Kidney function. Disordered memory or memory loss could result from Heart Blood and Spleen qi deficiency, the Heart and Kidney not communicating fully, the decline of *jing*, or Blood stasis and phlegm stagnation.

Pattern Differentiation

1. Heart Blood and Spleen qi deficiency
2. Heart and Kidney yin deficiency
3. Kidney *jing* deficiency
4. Blood stasis and phlegm stagnation

1. Heart Blood and Spleen Qi Deficiency			
When Heart Blood is weak, the *shen* becomes unanchored and unstable. With Spleen qi deficiency the *yi* will be weak. The symptoms displayed depend on whichever pattern dominates - Heart Blood weakness results in more forgetfulness, Spleen qi deficiency in an inability to concentrate or pay attention.			
Clinical Manifestations			
Forgetfulness, poor memory, absentmindedness, inability to concentrate, insomnia with difficulty falling to sleep, dream disturbed sleep, palpitations with or without anxiety, anxiety, postural dizziness, blurred vision, fatigue and tiredness, poor appetite, pale complexion, easy bruising.			
Tongue	**Pulse**	**Treatment Principle**	**Points**
Pale with thin white coat	Thready and weak	Strengthen and nourish the Heart and the Spleen, tonify qi and Blood, calm the *shen*	Baihui DU-20 Zhishi BL-52 Shaohai HT-3 Shenmen HT-7 Xinshu BL-15 Geshu BL-17 Pishu BL-20 Yintang M-HN-3 Sanyinjiao SP-6 Zusanli ST-36 Guanyuan REN-4
Prescription			
Gui Pi Tang			

Table 4.10f: Heart Blood and Spleen qi deficiency.

2. Heart and Kidney Yin Deficiency			
Heart and Kidney yin deficiency type forgetfulness develops when the mind loses stability as the Kidney yin fails to nourish the Heart yin and balance Heart fire which blazes out of control. As well as being acquired slowly over time it also can be a result of trauma or shock.			
Clinical Manifestations			
Forgetfulness, insomnia with frequent waking or feeling hot and sweaty, restlessness, palpitations, anxiety, sensation of heat in palms and soles, night sweats, dry mouth and throat, low backache, dizziness and tinnitus.			
Tongue	**Pulse**	**Treatment Principle**	**Points**
Red with scant coating	Thready and rapid	Nourish Heart and Kidney yin, clear heat, calm the *shen*	Neiguan P-6 Daling P-7 Taixi KID-3 Shenmen HT-7 Shaofu HT-8 Zhishi BL-52 Baihui DU-20 Xinshu BL-15 Shenshu BL-23 Jueyinshu BL-14 Taichong LIV-3 Yintang M-HN-3
Prescription			
Tian Wang Bu Xin Dan			

Table 4.10g: Heart and Kidney yin deficiency.

3. Kidney *Jing* Deficiency			
Most common in the elderly as the *jing* declines with aging or in those with a history of multiple pregnancies, chronic illness, drug use, and other factors that deplete *jing*.			
Clinical Manifestations			
Poor memory which may lead to loss of recognition of those who are familiar and short-term memory loss, dulled senses, generalized weakness perhaps with emaciation, graying, falling lifeless hair or balding, weak lower back and lower limbs, poor libido, nocturia and frequent urination, loss of hearing, decreased eyesight.			
Tongue	**Pulse**	**Treatment Principle**	**Points***
Pale with thin white coat	Thready and weak	Nourish and tonify the Kidney, qi and Blood, consolidate *jing*	Taixi KID-3^ Shenshu BL-23^ Baihui DU-20 Zhishi BL-52 Guanyuan REN-4^ Mingmen DU-4^ Shenmen HT-7 Xinshu BL-15^ Zhaohai KID-6 Shenmai BL-62 Yongquan KID-1
Prescription			
Ren Shen Yang Rong Tang			

* Consider adding moxa on some of the points marked with ^

Table 4.10h: Kidney *jing* deficiency.

4. Blood Stasis and Phlegm Stagnation			
Blood stasis and phlegm stagnation are a complication of chronic disease common in the elderly. Traumatic head injury can also cause a progression to this pattern. Clear yang is impeded in its circulation hence poor mental functioning.			
Clinical Manifestations			
Forgetfulness, poor memory, absentmindedness, short attention span, inability to concentrate, slow speech, dulled senses, blank expression.			
Tongue	**Pulse**	**Treatment Principle**	**Points**
Dark or pale purple with brown or purple stasis spots and greasy white coat; sublingual veins distended and dark	Generally slippery or thready and choppy	Transform phlegm, invigorate Blood and eliminate stagnant Blood	Xinshu BL-15 Shenshu BL-23 Zhishi BL-52 Geshu BL-17 Jianshi P-4 Sanyinjiao SP-6 Hegu LI-4 Baihui DU-20 Sishencong M-HN-1 Fenglong ST-40 Taibai SP-3
Prescription			
Shou Xing Wan			

Table 4.10i: Blood stasis and phlegm stagnation.

Patient Advice

The major modifiable risk factors for cognitive decline and Alzheimer's disease are primarily related to either cardiovascular risk factors (diabetes, hypertension, and obesity) or lifestyle habits (e.g. smoking, physical inactivity, poor diet, and a lack of mental and social stimulation). Therefore advice to patients is to improve modifiable lifestyle factors:

- Preventing the onset of diabetes mellitus.
- Not smoking.
- Managing mood and treating depression.
- Maintaining mental activity.
    - Mind strengthening exercises: puzzles, crosswords, etc.
    - Promoting neural plasticity: learning an instrument or new language.
- Engaging in regular physical activity.
- Consuming a balanced, antioxidant-rich diet and nutritional supplements.

References

Scheyer, O., Rahman, A., Hristov, H., et al. (2018). Female Sex and Alzheimer's Risk: The Menopause Connection, SpringerLink: The Journal of Prevention of Alzheimer's Disease volume 5, (pp 225–230). https://link.springer.com/article/10.14283/jpad.2018.34

Robbins, TW., (2011) Cognition: The Ultimate Brain Function, PMC US National Library of Medicine, National Institutes of Health, Neuropsychopharmacology: Neuropsychopharmacology. 2011 Jan; 36(1): 1–2. Published online 2010 Nov 30. doi: 10.1038/npp.2010.171. https://www.ncbi.nlm.nih.gov/pmc/articles/PMC3055511

Kametani, F., Hasegawa, M., (2018). Reconsideration of Amyloid Hypothesis and Tau Hypothesis in Alzheimer's Disease, PMC US National Library of Medicine, National Institutes of Health. Frontiers in Neuroscience: Front Neurosci. 2018; (pp 12: 25). Published online 2018 Jan 30. doi: 10.3389/fnins.2018.00025. https://www.ncbi.nlm.nih.gov/pmc/articles/PMC5797629

Kong, M., Yuan, S., Liu, J., et al. (2014). History and Experience: A Survey of Traditional Chinese Medicine Treatment for Alzheimer's Disease: Hindawi: Evidence-Based Complementary and Alternative Medicine: Volume 2014, Article ID 642128 https://doi.org/10.1155/2014/642128. https://www.hindawi.com/journals/ecam/2014/642128

Yan, H., Li, L., Tang, XC., (2007). Treating senile dementia with traditional Chinese medicine, PMC US National Library of Medicine, National Institutes of Health. Dovepress, Clinical Interventions in Aging: Clin Interv Aging. 2007 Jun; 2(2): (pp 201–208). Published online 2007 Jun. PMC2684515. https://www.ncbi.nlm.nih.gov/pmc/articles/PMC2684515

Dharmananda. S., (1996). Alzheimer's Disease: Treatment with Chinese Herbs, ITM Online.. http://www.itmonline.org/arts/alzheimers.htm

Crous-Bou, M., Minguillón, C., Gramunt, N., et al. (2017). Alzheimer's disease prevention: from risk factors to early intervention, Springer Link: Alzheimer's Research & Therapy volume 9, Article number: 71 (2017). https://link.springer.com/article/10.1186/s13195-017-0297-z

Clavey, S., (2020). Fluid Physiology and Pathology in Traditional Chinese Medicine. Third Edition, Eastland Press Inc. Seattle, Washington, USA.

Maclean, W. & Lyttleton, J. (1998) Clinical Handbook of Internal Medicine Vol.1. University of Western Sydney, Macarthur, Australia.

Maclean, W., Lyttleton, J., Bayley, M. & Taylor, K. (2019) Clinical Handbook of Internal Medicine. Redwing Book Co. 2nd edition.

SECTION 5 - Lifestyle

5.1 Metabolism, Weight Management, and Exercise

"Exercise is a journey, not a destination. It must be continued for the rest of your life. We do not stop exercising because we grow old - we grow old because we stop exercising". [15]

Metabolism

Metabolism is the process by which the body converts everything a person eats and drinks into energy. During this series of complex biochemical reactions, calories from food and beverages are combined with oxygen to release the energy the body needs to function in the form of adenosine triphosphate (ATP).

Even at rest, the body requires energy for all its autonomic functions, such as breathing, circulating blood, adjusting hormone levels, and cell growth and repair. The number of calories the body uses to carry out these basic functions is known as the basal metabolic rate (BMR), or what some people might refer to as 'metabolism.'

Energy requirements for an individual's basic functions stay fairly consistent and are not easily altered. Several factors determine BMR, including:

Body Mass and Composition

People who are larger burn more calories, even at rest. Furthermore, muscle burns more calories than adipose tissue, meaning that those with increased muscle mass have a higher BMR than those with a high percentage of body fat.

Gender

Men usually have less body fat and more muscle mass than women of the same age and weight, meaning men generally burn more calories.

Age

Muscle mass tends to decrease with age (sarcopenia) and fat accounts for more of our overall weight, thus slowing down calorie burning.

Other factors

In addition to BMR, two other factors determine how many calories the body burns each day:

Food Processing (Thermogenesis)

The digestion, absorption, transportation, and storage of nutrients from food also require energy. Approximately 10% of the calories from the carbohydrates and protein a person consumes are used during these complex processes.

[15] This quote is widely attributed to Dr. Kenneth H Cooper who pioneered the benefits of aerobic exercise in the US in the 1970s.

Physical Activity

Physical activity and exercise are by far the most variable of the factors that determine how many calories an individual burns each day. Most experts recommend that adults engage in 150 minutes of moderate or 75 minutes of vigorous exercise each week. They also advocate performing strengthening exercises for each of the major muscle groups twice weekly.

Although this is solid advice, it offers a somewhat simplistic view. There are five types of exercise and each has unique effects. Therefore, to truly reap the benefits, it is critical to take part in a variety of different activities on a regular basis.

Types of Exercise

The five types of exercise are as follows:

1. Aerobic (cardio)

Aerobic exercise, also known as cardio training, utilizes oxygen as an energy source. The term 'aerobic' refers to how the body uses oxygen to meet its energy demands during exercise.

The key features of aerobic exercise are that it uses the large muscle groups, is rhythmic in nature, and can be maintained continuously for at least 10 minutes. It strengthens the heart and lungs and benefits the entire cardiovascular system to deliver oxygen more efficiently throughout the body.

The benefits of aerobic exercise include:

- Improving circulation and helping the body utilize oxygen more efficiently
- Increasing energy
- Increasing endurance, making it possible to work out for longer
- Reducing the risk of cardiovascular disease
- Reducing the risk of type 2 diabetes
- Helping to reduce body fat
- Helping individuals reach and maintain a healthy weight
- Assisting in the reduction of stress, tension, anxiety, and depression
- Improving sleep

This form of exercise includes any physical activity that induces sweating, stimulates deeper breathing, and increases heart rate. Examples of aerobic exercise include:

- Brisk walking
- Jogging
- Racket sports
- Dancing
- Cycling or using an exercise bike
- Swimming
- Manual labor (digging, raking, gardening, etc.)
- Climbing stairs

TCEAM Viewpoint
Aerobic exercise engages both the respiratory and cardiovascular systems. Therefore, from a TCEAM perspective, the benefits of aerobic exercise include:
- Benefiting the Heart and Lung systems
- Tonifying qi and yang
- Improving qi and Blood circulation

However, excessive aerobic exercise is not recommended. Sweating means the loss of yin and body fluids, which is something that our menopausal patients will want to avoid. Furthermore, putting too much strain on the joints and tendons can divert Blood away from the Liver causing deficiency in the long run. Therefore, regular, moderate exercise is preferable to high-intensity cardio workouts.

2. Endurance Training

Like aerobic exercise, endurance training involves repeated movements of the large muscle groups. However, it is performed at an intensity below maximum capacity in order to progressively increase the anaerobic threshold, at which cells begin producing energy independent of oxygen. While anaerobic exercise does have some advantages, it leads to the buildup of lactic acid and muscle fatigue. Therefore, it is only possible to perform it for short durations.

By increasing the anaerobic threshold, individuals are able to exercise for longer periods, thus maximising the benefits of their chosen activity. Furthermore, endurance training induces positive changes in muscle tissue, including alterations in fiber type, increased density of capillaries, mitochondria, and the oxidative enzymes that produce ATP.

The benefits of endurance training include:
- Reducing body mass index and body fat percentage
- Lowering resting heart rate
- Improving oxygen uptake
- Reducing triglycerides and LDL cholesterol
- Increasing HDL cholesterol

Examples of endurance training include:
- Long-distance running, swimming, or cycling
- Cross-country skiing

High-intensity endurance training may result in inflammation of the airways and should be avoided.

TCEAM Viewpoint
Endurance training has somewhat similar benefits to aerobic exercise from a TCEAM perspective. However, since it is performed at a lower intensity, it is less likely to injure yin and body fluids.

3. Strength Building

Sarcopenia is the involuntary loss of muscle mass that occurs with age. Muscle mass decreases in both men and women by approximately 3–8% every decade after the age of 30 and the rate of decline is even higher after the age of 60. This increases the rate of falls and fractures and is a major contributor to disability among the elderly.

Muscle loss is also associated with increases in body fat and the risk of insulin resistance, diabetes, and metabolic disorder. For women, there is also a critical relationship between skeletal muscle and the changes in bone mechanosensitivity that occur with estrogen loss during menopause.

There are three types of muscle: cardiac, smooth, and skeletal. Skeletal muscle is the most abundant tissue in the human body and is composed of different types of fibers which vary in terms of their form, biochemical composition, and function.

Interestingly, there are key differences in the way that these fibers are expressed in males and females. Muscle function is closely linked to a protein called myosin, which is influenced by hormones, including thyroid hormone (triiodothyronine-T3), estrogen, and testosterone. This explains, in part, how estrogen affects the cardiovascular and musculoskeletal systems both pre and post-menopause.

Furthermore, progesterone and testosterone appear to have the effect of stimulating the growth of skeletal muscle. Therefore, reduced levels of these hormones potentially contribute to post-menopausal muscle loss. However, the exact role of these hormones in the process of sarcopenia is still unclear.

What we do know is that strength training is the best exercise for preventing sarcopenia and reducing the rate at which muscle mass deteriorates. These exercises promote muscle strength and increase bone density, thus reducing the risk of osteoporosis.

The benefits of strength training include:
- Increasing muscle mass
- Strengthening the bones
- Improving joint flexibility
- Improving balance and stability
- Helping individuals maintain a healthy weight

Examples of strength training:
- Lifting free weights
- Using resistance machines at the gym
- Using resistance bands to build strength by leveraging body weight
- Bodyweight exercises such as push-ups, crunches, lunges, and squats

TCEAM Viewpoint

The muscles have a close, two-way relationship with the Spleen. One of the Spleen's primary functions is controlling the muscles and the four limbs. Good Spleen function is essential in order to extract *gu* qi from food and build strong, healthy muscles.

Equally, since muscles burn more calories than adipose tissue, they play a critical role in metabolism and maintaining optimal Spleen function. The role of exercise in reducing worry and preoccupation will relieve the Spleen qi of the depleting influence of excess rumination and anxiety, hence reducing the impact on the muscles.

4. Flexibility and Stretching

The entire body is united by a web of connective tissue known as the fascia. It is a soft, collagen-containing substance that forms either loose or dense fibrous tissue depending upon its location. The fascia covers every structure in the body, not only wrapping, supporting, and separating them, but also creating continuity throughout the organism. The fascia also facilitates movement by reducing friction and allowing muscles, nerves, and blood and lymph vessels to slide over one another freely.

Some experts believe the fascia also plays a role in emotional function. This tissue contains a wide and diverse network of nerve cells, including those that control proprioception (awareness of physical position and movement), nociception (detection of potentially harmful stimuli), and interoception (awareness of internal signals, such as hunger or thirst). Afferent pathways of interoceptive nerves, in particular, may influence emotionality via their connection with the autonomic and medullary centers, as well as the brainstem. Therefore, it has been suggested that dysfunction in the fascial system could alter a person's emotional state.

Finally, one of the most critical functions of the fascia is its role in muscle building. It adapts to short and long-term mechanical stress by stimulating fibroblasts (collagen-producing cells). For this reason, stretching the fascia is one of the best ways to improve muscle flexibility and function and increase the range of motion of individual joints.

The benefits of stretching include:
- Improving range of motion
- Improving posture
- Reducing pain

There are three different types of stretching: static, dynamic, and pre-contraction stretching. The most common form of pre-contraction stretching is proprioceptive neuromuscular facilitation (PNF). Stretching also includes practices such as yoga, which has the additional benefits of improving respiratory and cardiovascular function, improving sleep, and enhancing mood.

Static Stretching
Static stretching can be performed alone or with a partner. It involves moving a muscle or joint into a lengthened (stretched) position and holding for an extended period of 15–30 seconds. The stretch can be repeated 2–4 times for optimal results. In the past, static stretching was recommended as a warm-up before exercise. However, the current evidence suggests that it reduces muscle power immediately after being performed. Therefore, it is more appropriate for post-exercise recovery or rest days, unless specifically recommended for rehabilitation by a healthcare professional.

Dynamic Stretching
Dynamic stretching involves moving muscles and joints through their full range of motion and repeating several times. This type of stretching is useful as a pre-exercise warm-up and may increase power for activities such as running and jumping. It is essential to perform these stretches carefully to avoid injury or muscle soreness, and to avoid 'bouncing' the muscle at the end-range of motion.

Proprioceptive Neuromuscular Facilitation (PNF) Stretching
This type of stretching involves contracting a muscle or its antagonist while stretching. There are three different types of PNF: Contract relax (CR), hold relax (HR), and contract-relax antagonist contract (CRAC). For optimal effects, the muscle should be contracted at 75–100% of its maximum and held for 6 seconds before relaxing. PNF can be performed with a partner or using a band or strap for resistance. It effectively improves range of motion but should not be performed prior to high-intensity activities. Furthermore, PNF should not be carried out more than twice per week due to the risk of muscle damage.

TCEAM Viewpoint
The sinews, including the tendons, are controlled by the Liver and stiff, inflexible joints can point to Liver Blood deficiency. However, the relationship between the Liver and the sinews is not one-way. Just as a healthy Liver ensures that the sinews remain flexible, regular stretching assists the Liver in its function of circulating qi and Blood.

5. Balance Training

Good balance control is fundamental to a person's ability to move and live independently. It relies upon several different factors, including gait stability, postural awareness and response, and sensory orientation (visual, vestibular, and whole-body sensation).

Unfortunately, balance control reduces with age, potentially leading to falls, fractures, and disability. Furthermore, the fear of falls can cause individuals to become less physically active, thus speeding their rate of physical decline and increasing their risk of chronic disease. Therefore, balance training is essential for older adults, especially those over the age of 65.

The benefits of balance training include:

- Improving muscle strength, especially the core muscles
- Reducing the risk of falls and fractures
- Maintaining activity levels and independence
- Increasing walking speed

Examples of balance training include:

- Heel-to-toe walking
- Standing on one foot
- Sitting on an exercise ball
- Yoga
- Tai chi
- Qi gong

Since many falls happen when a person's attention is divided, it may be useful to perform motor and cognitive tasks during balance training. For example, throwing and catching or kicking a ball, or reading silently or aloud while seated on an exercise ball.

TCEAM Viewpoint

From a TCEAM perspective, qi gong and tai chi, specifically, are associated with both physical and emotional balance. By incorporating slow, deliberate movements with deep breathing, they aim to still the mind and aid the cultivation of qi. Although they are not traditionally viewed in the same sense, other forms of balance training could be seen as having similar effects. They forge a connection between body and mind, helping to improve focus and maintain mobility and independence.

Exercise Considerations for Menopausal Women

The ideal exercise regime for menopausal and postmenopausal women will comprise a combination of aerobic, strength, flexibility, and balance exercises. The primary objectives are to maintain fitness, increase muscle mass, and increase bone mass and strength.

The most effective regime should include resistance/weight training three days per week, performed on alternate days, and focusing on rotating muscle groups. This should preferably be done under the supervision of a professional trainer to avoid injury.

Some especially beneficial exercises are those which strengthen the hips and spine, the areas most prone to osteoporotic fractures. They include:

- Wall or Smith machine[16] squats (with barbell)
- Lat pulldowns (with barbell)
- Leg press

[16] Named after Rudy Smith, a gym owner who invented the Smith Machine with a fixed rail for squatting: movement up and down in a vertical line.

- One arm military press
- Seated row
- Back extensions

The remaining days should include some moderate exercise, to a total of 150 minutes per week. People who have not exercised in some time should start slowly and gradually build up to this target.

The type of exercise is less important than finding an activity that is enjoyable and sustainable in the long-term. Brisk walking, using a treadmill, cycling, dancing, and gardening are all acceptable examples.

The 'talk test' can be used to gauge whether the level of exercise is appropriate. During moderate exercise, participants should be able to talk but not sing, and should not be out of breath. During more intense exercise, they should be able to say a few words but not hold a conversation.

Stretching and flexibility exercises should be performed daily. It is also critical to warm up and cool down sufficiently pre and post-exercise as flexibility reduces with age.

Cautions and Contraindications

Osteoporosis
Women with osteoporosis should avoid high-impact exercises and activities that increase the risk of falls. They should also avoid repeated trunk flexions (such as sit-ups or toe-touches) as these increase pressure on the spine.

Cardiovascular disorders
Women with the following cardiovascular disorders should seek medical advice before starting a new exercise regime:

- Hypertension
- Cardiomyopathy
- Valvular heart disease
- Complex ventricular ectopy
- Uncontrolled metabolic disorder

Furthermore, exercise may be contraindicated in the following circumstances:

- Recent ECG or heart attack
- Uncontrolled arrhythmia
- Unstable angina
- Third-degree heart block
- Acute progressive heart failure

Summary

Physical activity is one of the most crucial components of a healthy lifestyle and becomes especially important with advanced age. It not only helps to maintain optimal body weight and reduce the risk of chronic disease but also counters the muscle loss that occurs naturally with age and improves cardiovascular, respiratory, and bone health.

There are several safety considerations to keep in mind when recommending an exercise regime to older patients. In fact, it is preferable that they consult with a personal trainer who can work with them to develop a program that is safe and suited to their individual needs.

That said, encouraging patients to become more active is one of the most effective ways to support your treatments and improve their general wellbeing.

References

NCBI, (2004). Bone Health and Osteoporosis: A Report of the Surgeon General. 7. Lifestyle Approaches to Promote Bone Health, Office of the Surgeon General (US). Rockville (MD): Office of the Surgeon General (US). https://www.ncbi.nlm.nih.gov/books/NBK45523

Conti, FF., de Oliveira Brito, J., Bernardes, N., et al. (2015). Positive effect of combined exercise training in a model of metabolic syndrome and menopause: autonomic, inflammatory, and oxidative stress evaluations, American Journal of Physiology-Regulatory, Integrative and Comparative Physiology, Vol. 309, (No. 12). 15 Dec 2015 https://doi.org/10.1152/ajpregu.00076.2015. (https://journals.physiology.org/doi/full/10.1152/ajpregu.00076.2015)

Morici, G., Gruttad'Auria, CI., Baiamonte, P., et al. (2016). Endurance training: is it bad for you? PMC US National Library of Medicine, National Institutes of Health, Breathe, Practice-Focused Education for Respiratory Professionals: Breathe (Sheff). 2016 Jun; 12(2): (pp 140–147). doi: 10.1183/20734735.007016/. https://www.ncbi.nlm.nih.gov/pmc/articles/PMC4933620

Patel, H., Alkhawam, H., Madanieh, R., et al. (2017). Aerobic vs anaerobic exercise training effects on the cardiovascular system, PMC US National Library of Medicine, National Institutes of Health, WJC: World Journal of Cardiology: World J Cardiol. 2017 Feb 26; 9(2): (pp 134–138). Published online 2017 Feb 26. doi: 10.4330/wjc.v9.i2.134. https://www.ncbi.nlm.nih.gov/pmc/articles/PMC5329739

Baker, JS., McCormick, MC , Robergs, RA., (2010). Interaction among Skeletal Muscle Metabolic Energy Systems during Intense Exercise, PMC US National Library of Medicine, National Institutes of Health, Journal of Nutrition and Metabolism: J Nutr Metab. 2010; 2010: 905612. Published online 2010 Dec 6. doi: 10.1155/2010/905612 https://www.ncbi.nlm.nih.gov/pmc/articles/PMC3005844

Bordoni, B., Mahabadi, N., Varacallo. M., (2021). Anatomy, Fascia, NCBI, StatPearls [Internet] Treasure Island (FL): StatPearls Publishing; 2021 Jan- . https://www.ncbi.nlm.nih.gov/books/NBK493232

Gatt, A., Agarwal, S., Zito, PM., (2021). Anatomy, Fascia Layers, NCBI, StatPearls [Internet]. Treasure Island (FL): StatPearls Publishing; 2021 Jan-. https://www.ncbi.nlm.nih.gov/books/NBK526038

Page, P., (2012). Current Concepts in Muscle Stretching for Exercise and Rehabilitation, PMC US National Library of Medicine, National Institutes of Health, IJSPT, International Journal of Sports Physical Therapy: Int J Sports Phys Ther. 2012 Feb; 7(1): (pp 109–119). PMID: 22319684.
https://www.ncbi.nlm.nih.gov/pmc/articles/PMC3273886

Hindle, KB., Whitcomb, TJ., Briggs, WO., et al. (2012). Proprioceptive Neuromuscular Facilitation (PNF): Its Mechanisms and Effects on Range of Motion and Muscular Function, PMC US National Library of Medicine, National Institutes of Health, Sciendo, Journal of Human Kinetics: J Hum Kinet. 2012 Mar; 31: (pp 105–113). Published online 2012 Apr 3. doi: 10.2478/v10078-012-0011-y.
https://www.ncbi.nlm.nih.gov/pmc/articles/PMC3588663

Kim, DJ., Cho, ML., Park, YH., et al. (2015). Effect of an exercise program for posture correction on musculoskeletal pain, PMC US National Library of Medicine, National Institutes of Health, Journal of Physical Therapy Science: J Phys Ther Sci. 2015 Jun; 27(6): (pp 1791–1794). Published online 2015 Jun 30. doi: 10.1589/jpts.27.1791.
https://www.ncbi.nlm.nih.gov/pmc/articles/PMC4499985

Woodyard, C., (2011). Exploring the therapeutic effects of yoga and its ability to increase quality of life, PMC US National Library of Medicine, National Institutes of Health, IJoY, International Journal of Yoga: Int J Yoga. 2011 Jul-Dec; 4(2): (pp 49–54). doi: 10.4103/0973-6131.85485.
https://www.ncbi.nlm.nih.gov/pmc/articles/PMC3193654

Haizlip, KM., Harrison, BC., Leinwand, LA., (2015). Sex-Based Differences in Skeletal Muscle Kinetics and Fiber-Type Composition, PMC US National Library of Medicine, National Institutes of Health, American Physiological Society, Physiology: Physiology (Bethesda). 2015 Jan; 30(1): (pp 30–39). doi: 10.1152/physiol.00024.2014.
https://www.ncbi.nlm.nih.gov/pmc/articles/PMC4285578

Volpi, E., Nazemi, R., Fujita, S., (2004). Muscle tissue changes with aging, PMC US National Library of Medicine, National Institutes of Health, HHS Public Access Author Manuscript: Curr Opin Clin Nutr Metab Care. Author manuscript; available in PMC 2010 Jan 12. Published in final edited form as: Curr Opin Clin Nutr Metab Care. 2004 Jul; 7(4): (pp 405–410). https://www.ncbi.nlm.nih.gov/pmc/articles/PMC2804956

Smith, GI., Yoshino, J., Reeds, DN., et al. (2014). Testosterone and Progesterone, But Not Estradiol, Stimulate Muscle Protein Synthesis in Postmenopausal Women, JCEM, The Journal of Clinical Endocrinology & Metabolism: The Journal of Clinical Endocrinology & Metabolism, Volume 99, Issue 1, 1 January 2014, (pp 256–265),
https://doi.org/10.1210/jc.2013-2835. https://academic.oup.com/jcem/article/99/1/256/2836325

The American Cancer Society, (2019). 5 Benefits of Strength Training.
https://www.cancer.org/latest-news/five-benefits-of-strength-training.html

Halvarsson, A., Dohrn, I-M., Ståhle, A., (2015). Taking balance training for older adults one step further: the rationale for and a description of a proven balance training programme, PMC US National Library of Medicine, National Institutes of Health, Sage Clinical Rehabilitation: Clin Rehabil. 2015 May; 29(5): (pp 417–425). doi: 10.1177/0269215514546770.
https://www.ncbi.nlm.nih.gov/pmc/articles/PMC4419050

Jahnke, R., Larkey, L., Rogers, C., et al. (2011). A Comprehensive Review of Health Benefits of Qigong and Tai Chi, PMC US National Library of Medicine, National Institutes of Health, HHS Public Access Author Manuscript: Am J Health Promot. Author manuscript; available in PMC 2011 Jul 1. Published in final edited form as: Am J Health Promot. 2010 JUL-AUG; 24(6): e1–e25. doi: 10.4278/ajhp.081013-LIT-248.
https://www.ncbi.nlm.nih.gov/pmc/articles/PMC3085832/

Nalini Mishra, N., Mishra, VN., Devanshi. (2011). Exercise beyond menopause: Dos and Don'ts. PMC US National Library of Medicine, National Institutes of Health, Journal of Mid-Life Health, Indian Menopause Society,: J Midlife Health. 2011 Jul-Dec; 2(2): (pp 51–56). doi: 10.4103/0976-7800.92524.
https://www.ncbi.nlm.nih.gov/pmc/articles/PMC3296386/

5.2 Stress, Trauma, and Stress Resistance

Stress is a natural and healthy response to a potentially threatening situation. However, when it becomes chronic, it can have a severe negative impact on a person's health.

The primary stress hormone is cortisol, which is secreted by the adrenal glands along with adrenaline. Its functions include increasing glucose in the bloodstream, providing a quick burst of energy that could be lifesaving in a fight or flight situation. It also curbs nonessential functions in the immune, digestive, and reproductive systems. While these actions are beneficial in acute, genuinely dangerous circumstances, they are highly damaging in the long-term.

The Impact of Chronic Stress on Health and Hormones

Increased cortisol levels are associated with HPA activation[16], decreased insulin secretion and sensitivity, and obesity. Furthermore, stress is a major contributing factor to chronic inflammation and its associated diseases, including diabetes, cardiovascular disease, Alzheimer's disease, and some cancers. Therefore, reducing stress and learning how to cope with it are among the most essential things we can do to protect our health. In many instances, we can educate our patients to do the same.

It is especially important to support adrenal health as these glands are the primary site of hormone synthesis following menopause. Potential issues include stress causing the hormonal precursor pregnenolone to convert directly into cortisol rather than intermediary progesterone. Furthermore, trauma has been known to trigger early menopause in some individuals.

Factors associated with psychological symptoms during menopause are listed in Table 5.2 page 226.

[16] The hypothalamic-pituitary-adrenal axis, or HPA axis, describes the interaction between the hypothalamus, pituitary gland and the adrenal glands in response to stress. The HPA axis mediates the sympathetic nervous system and the secretion of adrenaline and noradrenaline, which are responsible for the rapid physiological responses like increased heart rate and perspiration.

Stressor	Description
Children	Dealing with teenagers or young adults at home Loss of identity with changing roles when children leave home: 'empty nest syndrome' Educational, financial, or marital difficulties of young adult offspring Grief about end of fertile years
Partner	Loss of a partner through death, separation, or divorce Caring for a partner who is unwell / dependent Lack of intimacy and sexlessness in long-term relationship Adjusting to dating or sexual intimacy with a new partner
Parents	Caring for aging parents and their possible dependency Bereavement and death of parent(s)
Social	Lack of social support Death or illness of a friend or sibling Coming to terms with aging in a culture that values youth and fertility Loss of confidence Adverse response to alcohol and other drugs which may have previously been used as 'social lubricants' to reduce inhibition
Employment	Financial stress Increased responsibilities and workload due to increased seniority The threat of redundancy or being side-lined in the workplace Lack of confidence seeking promotions or new employment opportunities
Ill health	Vasomotor instability leading to sleep problems and fatigue Changes in mood, cognition, memory, and confidence
Self-Image	Negative attitudes toward menopause and aging Feeling less desirable or attractive due to physical changes Uncertainty regarding identity and role in society

Table 5.2: Factors associated with psychological symptoms during menopause.

Trauma and Menopause

Domestic Abuse, Intimate Partner Violence (IPV) and Sexual Assault

An estimated 25% of women experience emotional or physical intimate partner violence (IPV), or sexual assault during their lifetime. These women may be more likely to develop severe menopausal symptoms. For example, IPV has been linked with clinically significant sleep disorders, night sweats, and painful intercourse. Meanwhile, sexual assault is associated with vaginal symptoms, including dryness, irritation, and painful intercourse. It is essential for clinicians to recognize the impact of these factors when caring for their menopausal patients.

Childhood Abuse or Neglect

Childhood maltreatment, including neglect, emotional, physical, and sexual abuse, is associated with adverse health outcomes later in life. Mental health disorders, cardiovascular disease, and metabolic syndrome are just a few examples. Childhood abuse and neglect are also associated with an increased incidence of vasomotor symptoms, especially during sleep.

Post Traumatic Stress Disorder (PTSD)

An estimated 1 in 10 women develop PTSD as a result of the above or other traumatic experiences. PTSD has been linked with clinically significant sleep disorders, vasomotor symptoms, and vaginal symptoms.

PTSD is notoriously challenging to treat. However, according to the Gates of Life theory discussed in Chapter 3.3, menopause presents an opportunity to heal past traumas and take on a new lease of life. In this case, a combination of acupuncture and intensive psychotherapy may be the most effective course of action.

Divorce

A significant proportion of marriages end in divorce. This presents a variety of unique stressors that can have a detrimental effect on the mental health of both partners and any children they may have. This stress may greatly exacerbate the challenges of menopause when it occurs concurrently. Some of the many difficulties that can arise as a result of divorce include:

- Co-parenting during conflict and worrying about its impact on children
- Financial insecurity plus the high cost of an acrimonious divorce
- Dealing with lawyers and the legal system, often for the first time
- Moving out of the family home
- Friends taking sides
- Using social media for revenge
- Loneliness when the children are with the other parent

Poverty

In general, women earn significantly less than men, accrue smaller pension funds, and have less capital. The Whitehall II[17] study was a longitudinal study that followed male and female civil servants aged 35-55 for over 15 years. It showed that women were more likely to be employed in lower-grade positions than men (clerical and support staff rather than executives) and that this directly correlated with decreased physical functioning.

A higher proportion of women are also unemployed (often invisibly so, if they have a partner who is working) and are often less able to achieve fair financial settlements from divorce and separation. This can lead to insecure housing and even homelessness, major stressors that can contribute to decreased psychological and physical wellbeing.

Reducing Stress and Increasing Resilience

Relaxation

One of the best ways to combat the negative effects of stress is by minimizing external stressors. This could include creating planners to aid in time management, prioritizing tasks and delegating if possible, and sometimes, simply saying "no."

However, this is not always as easy as it sounds. Therefore, it is beneficial to build relaxing activities into one's routine in order to increase resilience. It is especially important to relax before meals as the parasympathetic nervous system is responsible for the body's 'rest and digest' function. Therefore, eating in a calm and relaxed state is critical for digestive health and optimal nutrient absorption.

Some helpful practices include meditation, mindfulness, breathing exercises, yoga, qi gong, tai chi, exercise, walking, acupuncture, and massage. In cases of chronic stress, behavioral therapies, such as cognitive behavioral therapy (CBT), may be beneficial.

Meditation, Mindfulness, and Breathing

The terms meditation and mindfulness are often used interchangeably, although there are subtle differences in their meanings.

Meditation describes a formal practice aimed at enhancing one's connection to their deep, inner-self, which is separate from the mind, intellect, and ego. It can encompass a broad range of different techniques, including contemplation, concentration, guided meditations, the use of sound, mantras, breathing awareness, and more.

---

[17] Marmot, M., Brunner, E., (2005). Cohort Profile: The Whitehall II study, International Journal of Epidemiology, International Journal of Epidemiology, Volume 34, (Issue 2), (pp 251–256), https://doi.org/10.1093/ije/dyh372. https://academic.oup.com/ije/article/34/2/251/746997

Meanwhile, mindfulness is a practice that aims to increase one's awareness of the present moment. While meditation is one key way of doing this, it is also possible to perform everyday activities mindfully (i.e. with awareness). For example, paying attention to the sensation of warm water on the hands and the smell of soap can transform a task as mundane as washing the dishes into a moment of mindfulness.

What both of these practices have in common is that they place great emphasis on the breath. The breath can be used as an anchor during meditation practices, helping to focus one's attention on sensations in the body rather than distracting thoughts. Deep, diaphragmatic breathing may be especially useful as it reduces respiratory frequency and activates the parasympathetic nervous system.

The many benefits of meditation, mindfulness, and breathing practices include:

- Reduced stress, anxiety, depression, and PTSD
- Reduced physical and psychological pain
- Improved memory and attention
- Reduced blood pressure and heart rate
- Reduced cortisol levels

Consistent practice can help an individual to react more calmly to external influences, thus increasing their stress resistance. Regular meditation may also help to counteract age-related reductions in neuron-rich gray matter in the brain.

For a simple breathing exercise by Peter Deadman, see Chapter 7.1, Yang Sheng (page 323).

Yoga, Tai Chi, and Qi Gong

Yoga, tai chi (*taiji*), and qi gong aim to promote self-healing by uniting the body, mind, and breath. Many people consider them to be forms of moving meditation, and they share many characteristics with the practice.

Yoga was developed in India approximately 3000 years ago as a way to reduce or alleviate structural, physiological, spiritual, and emotional pain. Although many people associate yoga with performing specific stretches and poses, there are many different forms. Some have a more physical focus, such as ashtanga or hatha yoga. Others are more mental or meditative, such as yoga nidra.

Tai chi and qi gong both developed in China, with qi gong being the more ancient of the two. Although the two practices have shared roots and many other similarities, there are some fundamental differences too. Tai chi tends to involve long, choreographed sequences of movements, whereas qi gong tends to be simpler, more repetitive, and easier to learn. Like yoga, there are numerous forms of tai chi and qi gong that have developed over the years, although all have similar features.

Generally speaking, the benefits of these mind-body practices include:
- Improved cardiovascular and respiratory function
- Reduced blood pressure and heart rate
- Improved physical function (balance, flexibility, strength)
- Increased bone mineral density, reduced risk of fractures
- Reduced stress, anxiety, and depression
- Improved quality of life and self-efficacy

Exercise and Movement

The physical benefits of exercise are numerous and are discussed in detail in Chapter 5.1. However, exercise has many psychological benefits too.

It can help to relieve stress by regulating HPA axis activity, influencing the serotonergic system, and releasing endogenous opioids, such as beta-endorphin. It can also provide a welcome distraction from everyday worries and negative thoughts. Even gentle activities such as walking can be beneficial. Walking has the additional advantage of taking individuals outdoors and into nature, and can also be seen as a social activity when done with friends or as part of a walking group.

Unfortunately, some people tend to become less physically active during stressful periods, creating a vicious cycle of low mood and inactivity. Therefore, it may be necessary to remind patients of the benefits of exercise and encourage them to find an activity that they will continue to enjoy even when motivation is reduced.

Acupuncture, Massage, and Other Therapies

Booking a treatment with a therapist is a significant act of self-care on both a physical and mental level. Simply taking time out from one's normal routine can help to reduce stress levels. However, massage and acupuncture also have specific physiological effects that can help to reduce stress, anxiety, and depressive symptoms.

The benefits of massage include:
- Reduced cortisol levels
- Reduced diastolic blood pressure and heart rate

The benefits of acupuncture include:
- Regulating sympathetic and parasympathetic nervous system activity
- Reducing corticosterone levels (this hormone is measured in some animal studies and is similar to cortisol in humans)
- Regulating neurotransmitter levels, including serotonin, noradrenaline, dopamine, gamma-aminobutyric acid (GABA), neuropeptide Y, adrenocorticotropic hormone (ACTH)
- Increasing serotonin receptor expression in several brain regions
- Promoting endogenous opioid release
- Reducing inflammation

Nutrition

Deficiencies in certain nutrients, including magnesium, zinc, and vitamin C may have a significant impact on stress levels (see Chapter 6.2, Vitamins, Minerals, and Micronutrients). Furthermore, some nutritional supplements may provide benefits.

Adaptogens

Adaptogens are herbs that are said to support adrenal function and enhance resilience against stress and fatigue. The key features of adaptogens are having non-specific effects and regulating homeostasis without harming the normal physiological functions of the body. They act upon the neuroendocrine-immune system and HPA axis, exhibiting neuroprotective, anti-fatigue, antidepressant, anxiolytic, nootropic, and CNS stimulating activity.

Many different herbs are classified as adaptogens, including several common Chinese herbal medicines like Ren Shen (*Panax ginseng*), Xi Yang Shen (*Panax quinquefolius*), and Wu Wei Zi (*Schisandra chinensis*). Other herbs that are commonly considered adaptogens include ashwagandha (*Withania somnifera*), eleuthero or Siberian ginseng (*Eleutherococcus senticosus*), and Hong Jing Tian or rhodiola (*Rhodiola rosea*). However, since the precise definition of the term 'adaptogen' is open to interpretation, many other herbs are listed as such in various sources.

Due to the fact that some adaptogens nourish the adrenals while others stimulate them, they should only be used under the supervision of a qualified professional.

Summary

Stress and trauma can have an overall adverse effect on health and wellbeing as well as impacting menopausal symptoms. Therefore, it is highly beneficial to find ways to manage stress levels and clear trauma, although there is no one-size-fits-all approach for doing so.

Acupuncture can play a significant role in moving beyond past traumas by utilizing menopause as a Gate of Life and catalyst for positive change. However, it may be necessary to employ multiple approaches depending on the complexity, severity, and duration of the individual's symptoms.

References

Gibson, CJ., Huang, AJ., McCaw, B., et al. (2019). Associations of Intimate Partner Violence, Sexual Assault, and Posttraumatic Stress Disorder With Menopause Symptoms Among Midlife and Older Women, JAMA Network, JAMA Internal Medicine: JAMA Intern Med. 2019;179(1):(pp 80-87). doi:10.1001/jamainternmed.2018.5233. https://jamanetwork.com/journals/jamainternalmedicine/article-abstract/2715160

Carson, MY., Thurston, RC., (2020). Childhood abuse and vasomotor symptoms among midlife women, PMC US National Library of Medicine, National Institutes of Health, HHS Public Access, Author Manuscript: Menopause. Author manuscript; available in PMC 2020 Oct 1. Published in final edited form as: Menopause. 2019 Oct; 26(10): (pp 1093–1099). doi: 10.1097/GME.0000000000001366. https://www.ncbi.nlm.nih.gov/pmc/articles/PMC6768766

Midei, AJ., Matthews, KA., Chang, Y-F., et al. (2013). Childhood physical abuse is associated with incident metabolic syndrome in mid-life women, APA PsycNet, American Psychological Association: Health Psychology, 32(2), (pp 121–127). https://doi.org/10.1037/a0027891.
https://psycnet.apa.org/record/2012-17656-001

Thurston, RC., Bromberger, J., Chang, Y., et al. (2008). Childhood abuse or neglect is associated with increased vasomotor symptom reporting among midlife women, Menopause, The Journal of the North American Menopause Society: Menopause: January 2008 - Volume 15 (Issue 1), (pp 16-22). doi: 10.1097/gme.0b013e31805fea75
https://journals.lww.com/menopausejournal/Abstract/2008/15010/Childhood_abuse_or_neglect_is_associated_with.7.aspx

Marmot, M., Brunner, E., (2005). Cohort Profile: The Whitehall II study, International Journal of Epidemiology, International Journal of Epidemiology, Volume 34, (Issue 2), (pp 251–256), https://doi.org/10.1093/ije/dyh372.
https://academic.oup.com/ije/article/34/2/251/746997

Sharma, H., (2015). Meditation: Process and effects, PMC US National Library of Medicine, National Institutes of Health, AYU, An International Quarterly Journal of Research in Ayurveda: Ayu. 2015 Jul-Sep; 36(3): (pp 233–237). doi: 10.4103/0974-8520.182756.
https://www.ncbi.nlm.nih.gov/pmc/articles/PMC4895748

Ma, X., Yue, Z-Q., Gong, ZQ., et al. (2017). The Effect of Diaphragmatic Breathing on Attention, Negative Affect and Stress in Healthy Adults, PMC US National Library of Medicine, National Institutes of Health, Frontiers in Psychology: Front Psychol. 2017; 8: 874. Published online 2017 Jun 6. doi: 10.3389/fpsyg.2017.00874.
https://www.ncbi.nlm.nih.gov/pmc/articles/PMC5455070

Woodyard, C., (2011). Exploring the therapeutic effects of yoga and its ability to increase quality of life, PMC US National Library of Medicine, National Institutes of Health, AYU, An International Quarterly Journal of Research in Ayurveda: Ayu: Int J Yoga. 2011 Jul-Dec; 4(2): (pp 49–54). doi: 10.4103/0973-6131.85485.
https://www.ncbi.nlm.nih.gov/pmc/articles/PMC3193654

Jahnke, R., Larkey, L., Rogers, C., et al. (2011). A Comprehensive Review of Health Benefits of Qigong and Tai Chi, PMC US National Library of Medicine, National Institutes of Health, HHS Public Access, Author Manuscript: Am J Health Promot. Author manuscript; available in PMC 2011 Jul 1. Published in final edited form as: Am J Health Promot. 2010 Jul-Aug; 24(6): e1–e25. doi: 10.4278/ajhp.081013-LIT-248.
https://www.ncbi.nlm.nih.gov/pmc/articles/PMC3085832

Lu, Y-H., Rosner, B., Chang, G., et al. (2016). Twelve-Minute Daily Yoga Regimen Reverses Osteoporotic Bone Loss, PMC US National Library of Medicine, National Institutes of Health, Lippincott Williams & Wilkins, Open Access, Topics in Geriatric Rehabilitation: Top Geriatr Rehabil. 2016 Apr; 32(2): (pp 81–87). Published online 2015 Nov 5. doi: 10.1097/TGR.0000000000000085.
https://www.ncbi.nlm.nih.gov/pmc/articles/PMC4851231

Anderson, E., Shivakumar, G., (2013). Effects of Exercise and Physical Activity on Anxiety, PMC US National Library of Medicine, National Institutes of Health, Frontiers in Psychiatry: Front Psychiatry. 2013; 4: 27. Published online 2013 Apr 23. doi: 10.3389/fpsyt.2013.00027.
https://www.ncbi.nlm.nih.gov/pmc/articles/PMC3632802

Stults-Kolehmainen, MA., Sinha, R., (2014). The Effects of Stress on Physical Activity and Exercise, PMC US National Library of Medicine, National Institutes of Health, HHS Public Access, Author Manuscript: Sports Med. Author manuscript; available in PMC 2015 Jan 1. Published in final edited form as: Sports Med. 2014 Jan; 44(1): (pp 81–121). doi: 10.1007/s40279-013-0090-5. https://www.ncbi.nlm.nih.gov/pmc/articles/PMC3894304

Hanson, S., Jones, A., (2015). Is there evidence that walking groups have health benefits? A systematic review and meta-analysis, PMC US National Library of Medicine, National Institutes of Health, Open Access from BMJ, British Journal of Sports Medicine: Br J Sports Med. 2015 Jun; 49(11): (pp 710–715). Published online 2015 Jan 19. doi: 10.1136/bjsports-2014-094157.
https://www.ncbi.nlm.nih.gov/pmc/articles/PMC4453623

Moraska, A., Pollini, RA., Boulanger K., et al. (2010). Physiclogical Adjustments to Stress Measures Following Massage Therapy: A Review of the Literature, PMC US National Library of Medicine, National Institutes of Health, Hindawi: Evid Based Complement Alternat Med. 2010 Dec; 7(4):(pp 409–418). Published online 2008 May 7. doi: 10.1093/ecam/nen029.
https://www.ncbi.nlm.nih.gov/pmc/articles/PMC2892349

Wild, B., Brenner, J., Joos, S., et al (2020). Acupuncture in persons with an increased stress level—Results from a randomized-controlled pilot trial, PMC US National Library of Medicine, National Institutes of Health, PLoS One: PLoS One. 2020; 15(7): e0236004. Published online 2020 Jul 23. doi: 10.1371/journal.pone.0236004.
https://www.ncbi.nlm.nih.gov/pmc/articles/PMC7377446

Lee, M-J., Ryu, J-S, Won, S-K., et al. (2019). Effects of Acupuncture on Chronic Stress-Induced Depression-Like Behavior and Its Central Neural Mechanism, PMC US National Library of Medicine, National Institutes of Health, Frontiers in Psychology: Front Psychol. 2019; 10: 1353. Published online 2019 Jul 5. doi: 10.3389/fpsyg.2019.01353.
https://www.ncbi.nlm.nih.gov/pmc/articles/PMC6625224

Cuciureanu, MD., Vink, R., (2011). Magnesium and Stress, NCBI, Magnesium in the Central Nervous System [Internet]. Adelaide (AU): University of Adelaide Press;
https://www.ncbi.nlm.nih.gov/books/NBK507250

Wang, J., Um, P., Dickerman, BA., et al (2018). Zinc, Magnesium, Selenium and Depression: A Review of the Evidence, Potential Mechanisms and Implications, PMC US National Library of Medicine, National Institutes of Health, MDPI, Nutrients: Nutrients. 2018 May; 10(5): 584. Published online 2018 May 9. doi: 10.3390/nu10050584.
https://www.ncbi.nlm.nih.gov/pmc/articles/PMC5986464

Padayatty, SJ., Doppman, JL., Chang, R., et al. (2007). Human adrenal glands secrete vitamin C in response to adrenocorticotrophic hormone, The American Journal of Clinical Nutrition, Volume 86,(Issue 1), July 2007, (pp 145–149), https://doi.org/10.1093/ajcn/86.1.145
https://academic.oup.com/ajcn/article/86/1/145/4754397

de Oliveira, IJL., de Souza, VV., Motta, V., et al, (2015). Effects of Oral Vitamin C Supplementation on Anxiety in Students: A Double-Blind, Randomized, Placebo-Controlled Trial, NIH, National Library of Medicine, National Center for Biotechnology Information, Pak J Biol Sci. 2015 Jan;18(1):11-8. doi: 10.3923/pjbs.2015.11.18.
https://pubmed.ncbi.nlm.nih.gov/26353411

Panossian, A., Wikman, G., (2010). Effects of Adaptogens on the Central Nervous System and the Molecular Mechanisms Associated with Their Stress—Protective Activity, MDPI, Pharmaceuticals (Basel). 2010 Jan; 3(1): (pp. 188–224). Published online 2010 Jan 19. doi: 10.3390/ph3010188.
https://www.ncbi.nlm.nih.gov/pmc/articles/PMC3991026

Liao, L-Y., He, Y-F., Li, L., et al, (2018). A preliminary review of studies on adaptogens: comparison of their bioactivity in TCM with that of ginseng-like herbs used worldwide, PMC US National Library of Medicine, National Institutes of Health, BMC Chinese Medicine: Chin Med. 2018; 13: 57. Published online 2018 Nov 16. doi: 10.1186/s13020-018-0214-9.
https://www.ncbi.nlm.nih.gov/pmc/articles/PMC6240259

5.3 Sleep, Energy, and Fatigue

Sleep is an extraordinary in-built recovery and repair system that many people take for granted, until it is disrupted. Adults are advised to sleep 7-9 hours per night.

There are four stages in a sleep cycle, with two sub-categories: rapid eye movement (REM) and non-REM sleep. Typically a person will go through four to five sleep cycles over an 8 hour period. Each cycle takes 70-120 minutes.

Sleep Cycles

Non-REM Activity

The first three stages of the sleep cycle are non-REM activity, these are:
Stage N1 (transition to sleep): A brief period of time during which an individual dozes off to sleep.
Stage N2 (settling in to sleep): The brain waves slow and become synchronized.
Stage N3 (deep or 'delta slow wave' sleep): Characterized by high-amplitude, low-frequency waves with 'spindles.' These bursts of high-frequency activity are linked to cognitive function and memory. This is considered the most important phase. It is when the body regenerates and repairs its tissues, builds muscle and bone, and strengthens the immune system. Older people tend to spend less time in the N3 sleep phase and more time in N2.[18]

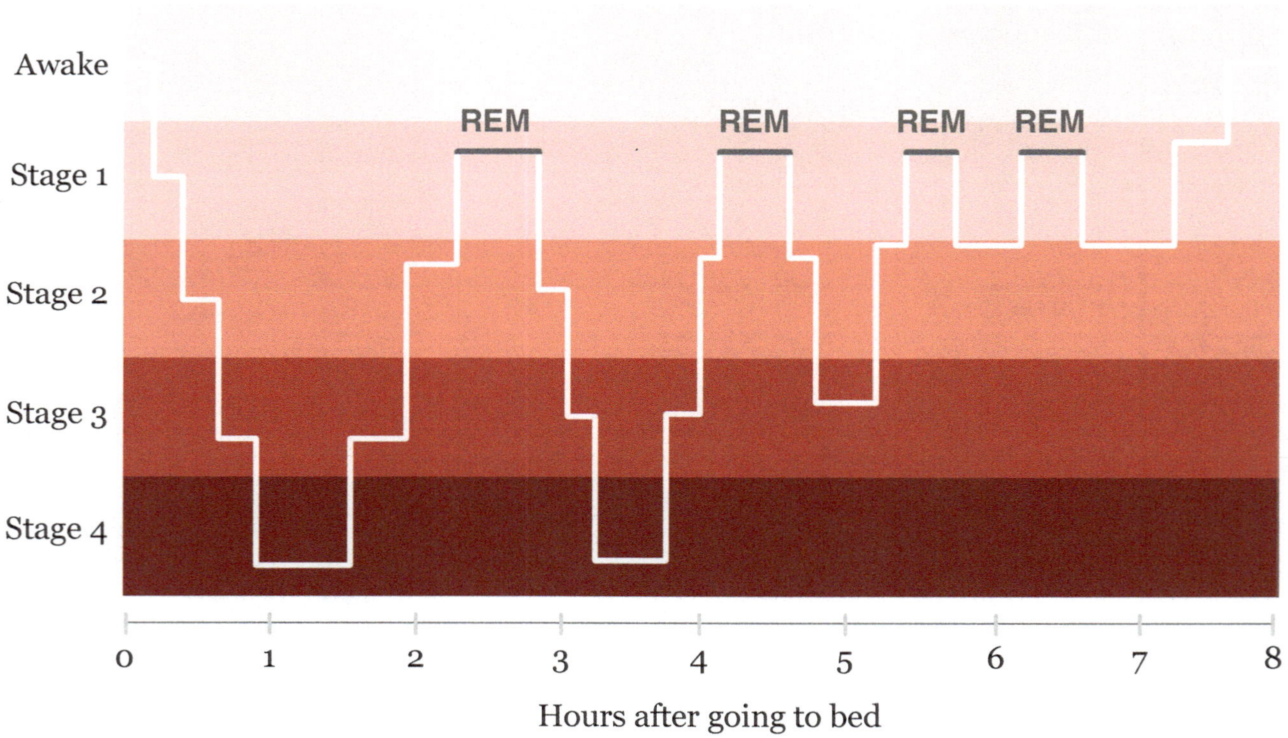

Figure 5.3a: A typical 8 hour sleep cycle.

[18] Note: It is easiest to be awoken during the first two stages.

REM Activity

Stage 4: Rapid Eye Movement (REM) 'Active sleep': Characterized by low-amplitude, high-frequency brain waves, alpha rhythm, and eye movements which sleep experts believe are related to dreaming.

The Anatomy of Sleep

Several brain structures are involved in sleep and their activity changes as we cycle through the different phases.

The Hypothalamus

Neurons within the hypothalamus play a crucial role in the sleep-wake cycle. One especially important structure is the suprachiasmatic nucleus (SCN). It contains cells that receive information about light exposure from the eyes and controls our behavioral rhythms. Some people with SCN damage experience disrupted circadian rhythms and sleep erratically throughout the day.

The Pineal Gland

The pineal gland receives messages from the SCN in response to changing light levels, triggering the release of melatonin (see below).

The Brain Stem

The brain stem and hypothalamus communicate with one another to control transitions between wakefulness and sleep. The process relies upon the inhibitory neurotransmitter gamma-aminobutyric acid (GABA), which reduces hypothalamus and brain stem activity. The brain stem also signals the muscles to relax during REM sleep, preventing us from acting out our dreams.

The Thalamus

The thalamus relays information between the sense organs and the cerebral cortex. It is inactive during most phases of sleep, but becomes active during REM sleep, creating the images we see in our dreams.

The Basal Forebrain

The basal forebrain releases adenosine (a by-product of cellular energy consumption), which supports the sleep drive. Caffeine interferes with this process by blocking adenosine receptors and promoting wakefulness.

The Midbrain

Parts of the midbrain act as an arousal system, playing a significant role in our sleep-wake cycles.

The Amygdala

The emotional center of the brain, the amygdala, becomes increasingly active during REM sleep.

Sleep and Hormones

Melatonin

Melatonin is the hormone responsible for feelings of sleepiness. It plays an essential role in our diurnal rhythms and is produced by the pineal gland in the brain in the evenings, as a response to dimming light. Therefore, one of the best ways to promote good sleep is to create an environment with low light levels by using lamps or a dimmer switch rather than bright ceiling lights.

The blue light given off by electronic screens, including laptops, tablets, and smartphones, also interferes with melatonin production. Therefore, the use of these devices should be limited in the hours leading up to bedtime.

Melatonin production can also be reduced by a phenomenon known as the tryptophan steal, or tryptophan kynurenine pathway (TKP). Tryptophan is an amino acid and acts as a precursor to both melatonin and serotonin. However, when it is metabolized via the TKP it reduces the body's levels of these compounds.

Furthermore, tryptophan metabolism via the TKP generates inflammation and is associated with depression, neurodegenerative diseases, and tumorigenesis. This pathway appears to be induced by stress and immune activation. It may also be influenced by diet, gut health, and exercise.

Another factor that can affect melatonin production is vitamin B3 status. Tryptophan is a precursor for this micronutrient as well as melatonin. Therefore, adequate dietary B3 is essential to prevent tryptophan from being diverted to synthesize it endogenously.

Cortisol

Cortisol is released by the adrenal glands and is responsible for promoting wakefulness. Its release should peak during the early morning, supporting our circadian rhythms and acting as the yang to melatonin's yin. If cortisol levels remain elevated throughout the day, it can interfere with sleep, as well as contributing to other health issues. For a full discussion on cortisol, see Chapter 5.2 Stress, Trauma, and Stress Resistance.

Ghrelin and Leptin

Ghrelin and leptin are two hormones that play a role in appetite regulation. Ghrelin is a stomach-derived hormone that promotes hunger. Meanwhile, leptin is produced by adipocytes and promotes satiety.

Short sleep durations are associated with increases in ghrelin and reductions in leptin production. Therefore, people who routinely do not get enough sleep may experience increased appetite and tend to have higher body mass indexes.

Women and Sleep

Women experience sleep differently from men, and respond differently to sleep disorders, deficiencies, and deprivation.

Hormonal changes throughout the menstrual cycle and during pregnancy and menopause can all have a significant impact, increasing the incidence of sleep disturbances and subsequently raising the risk of negative health outcomes.

In addition to poor sleep quality in general, fluctuations in female reproductive hormones can also contribute to obstructive sleep apnea, restless legs syndrome, and insomnia. It is essential to understand these challenges and manage them appropriately as they arise.

Menopausal women often suffer from poor sleep, whether due to vasomotor symptoms, anxiety, or other causes. Lack of sleep leads to a variety of issues, ranging from fatigue to reduced concentration and increased risk of accidents. It can also cause metabolic and hormonal dysregulation and contribute to the development of chronic disease.

It appears that falling levels of estrogen and progesterone, coupled with increases in FSH may all play a role, although the precise mechanisms are not fully understood.

Snoring and Obstructive Sleep Apnea

The incidence of snoring and obstructive sleep apnea (OSA) increases significantly following menopause, contributing to poor sleep quality, daytime drowsiness, and cognitive impairment.

It seems that the tendency to gain weight following menopause, combined with age-related changes to the pharyngeal muscles, is responsible for this phenomenon. The use of exercises specifically for the mouth and throat muscles, alongside appropriate weight management, may help. For ongoing OSA symptoms, sleeping with a continuous positive airway pressure (CPAP) machine may be necessary.

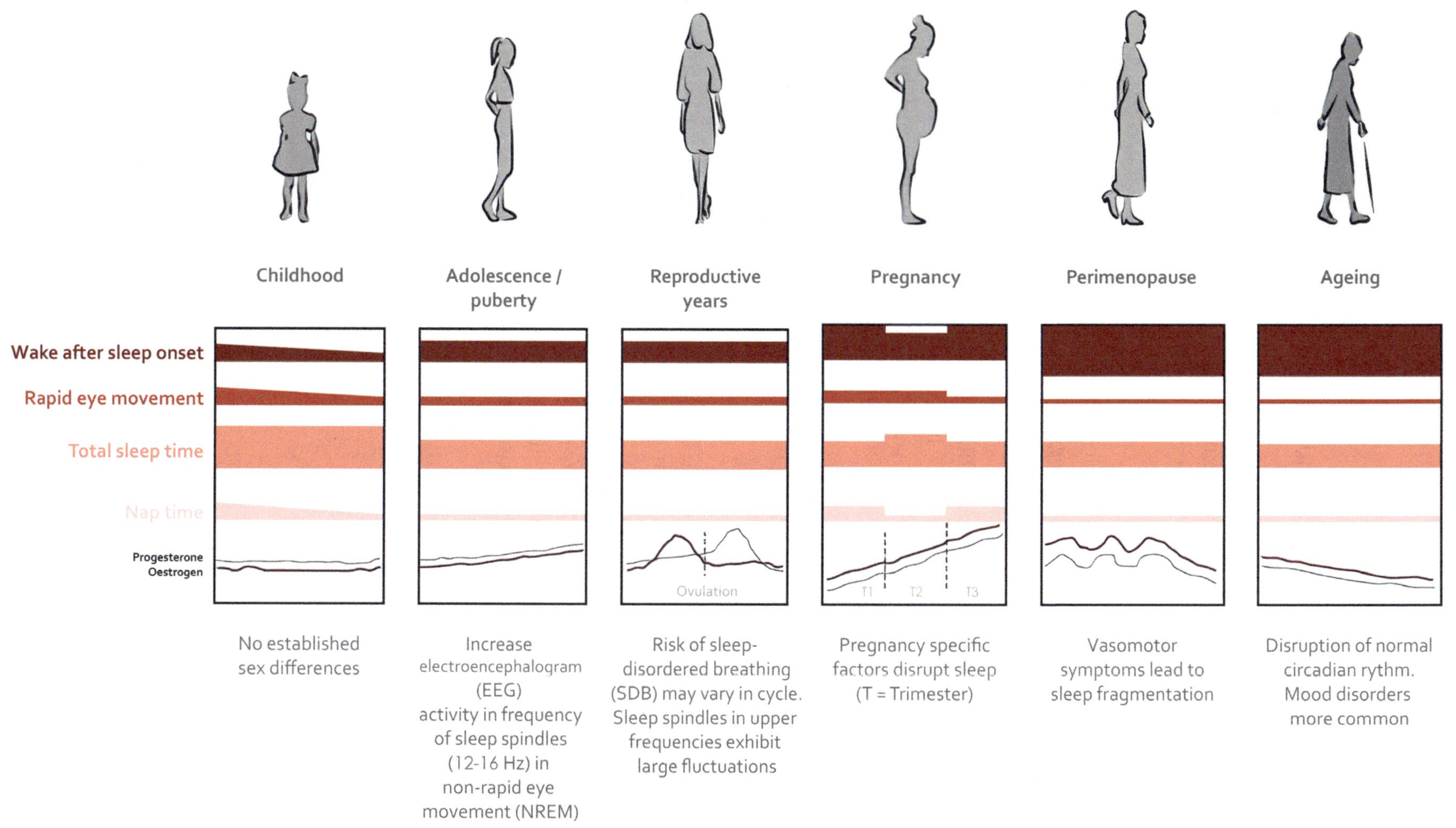

Figure 5.3b: Sleep in women across the lifespan.[19]

---

[19] Image Source Pengo, MF., Won, CH., Bourjeily, G., (2018). Sleep in Women Across the Lifespan, NIH, National Library of Medicine, National Center for Biotechnology Information: Chest: 2018 Jul;154(1): (pp. 196-206). doi: 10.1016/j.chest.2018.04.005. Epub 2018 Apr 19. https://pubmed.ncbi.nlm.nih.gov/29679598

Improving Sleep Quality

Sleep Hygiene

The basics of sleep hygiene include maintaining a regular bedtime and getting up at the same time each day. It is essential to stick to the same routine, even at weekends.

Bedrooms should be kept cool and comfortable, and reserved for sleep rather than other activities such as watching television or working. However, women who have difficulty relaxing may find reading in bed or listening to a guided meditation/audiobook helpful.

An electric fan, a comfortable mattress, cotton bedclothes, and blackout curtains are all worthwhile investments. Women who live in noisy areas may also benefit from purchasing a good pair of earplugs.

Avoid eating late at night and the consumption of stimulants.

Stimulants

Stimulants, including caffeine, sugar, and refined carbohydrates can all interfere with sleep and should be kept to a minimum or avoided completely, especially during the evening.

Alcohol

While some people may use alcohol as a relaxant to help initiate sleep, large quantities can lead to sleep disturbances, especially during the second half of the night.

Blood Sugar

Poorly regulated blood sugar can lead to nocturnal hypoglycemia, resulting in night sweats and poor sleep.

Improving Energy and Reducing Fatigue

Low energy levels and fatigue are often a direct result of poor sleep. However, there are many other potential causes, including chronic illness, poorly regulated blood sugar, circulatory disorders, mitochondrial dysfunction, or general lack of nutrition.

Regulating Blood Sugar

Glucose is the primary source of energy for our cells and they require a steady supply of it throughout the day. Eating high-sugar foods and simple carbohydrates causes blood sugar spikes, with a subsequent 'crash' and feelings of fatigue. This can lead to snacking, especially on high-calorie foods, and contribute to weight gain, further dysregulating insulin sensitivity and blood sugar control.

High-fiber, high-protein foods with a low glycemic index release their energy more steadily, providing longer-lasting satiety and preventing fatigue.

Circulation

Improving blood circulation will ensure that oxygen and nutrients are able to reach their target tissues and support effective energy production. Exercise, not smoking, and regulating blood sugar can all help to maintain a healthy circulatory system. Plant-based diets that are rich in antioxidants and low in saturated fats may also help to reduce blood viscosity and improve circulation.

Iron

Iron is a key component of hemoglobin, the protein responsible for binding oxygen to red blood cells. It also plays a role in DNA synthesis and energy production. Therefore, iron deficiency can result in fatigue as well as other symptoms of iron-deficiency anemia, including pale skin, palpitations, and shortness of breath.

Postmenopausal women often have higher iron levels than their premenopausal counterparts due to the cessation of menstruation. Therefore, it is important to establish the cause of iron deficiency in older women, whether it be due to blood loss, absorption issues, or parasites.

It has also been suggested that excess iron storage could cause health problems of its own, including an increased risk of cardiovascular disease, diabetes, neurodegenerative disorders, and cancer. Therefore, care should be taken with iron supplementation in postmenopausal women.

Mitochondrial Health

Mitochondria are the powerhouses of our cells and produce energy in the form of adenosine triphosphate (ATP). Some of the essential nutrients for mitochondrial health include vitamins B2, B3, B6, B7, B9, C, and K1, magnesium, and manganese.

Mitochondrial function also appears to be influenced by circadian rhythms. It appears that sleep deprivation may have a negative impact, although research in this area is in its infancy.

Hormesis

Hormesis describes a situation whereby minimal exposure to a stressor or toxin can prove beneficial to cells by priming them against larger amounts that would otherwise be harmful. Inducing hormesis may be beneficial to mitochondria and, therefore, energy production. Helpful practices include exercise, especially high-intensity interval training, fasting, saunas, cold showers, and cognitive stimulation.

Summary

Good quality sleep is essential for many reasons. However, menopausal patients can routinely find their sleep disturbed. They may also experience decreased energy levels and fatigue, either independently or as a direct result of poor sleep.

When treating patients living with sleep disorders or insomnia, there are several factors to consider. The most fundamental consideration is sleep hygiene, and discussing patients' bedtime routine can highlight any areas that may need improvement. If making adjustments here is insufficient, a deeper imbalance may be at play. Through effective questioning and good diagnostic skills, we can uncover clues that point us to the underlying cause and treat or refer as appropriate.

References

Schönauer, M., Pöhlchen, D., (2013). Sleep spindles, Current Biology Magazine: Current Biology 28, R1121–R1142, October 8, 2018 © 2018 Elsevier Ltd. R1129.
https://www.cell.com/current-biology/pdf/S0960-9822(18)30934-5.pdf

Pengo, MF., Won, CH., Bourjeily, G., (2018). Sleep in Women Across the Life Span, NIH, National Library of Medicine, National Center for Biotechnology Information: Chest: 2018 Jul;154(1): (pp. 196-206).
doi: 10.1016/j.chest.2018.04.005. Epub 2018 Apr 19.
https://pubmed.ncbi.nlm.nih.gov/29679598

Harvard Medical School. (2008). Natural Patterns of Sleep, A resource from the Division of Sleep Medicine at Harvard Medical School. Produced in partnership with WGBH Educational Foundation
http://healthysleep.med.harvard.edu/healthy/science/what/sleep-patterns-rem-nrem

Patel, AK., Reddy, V., Araujo, JF., (2021). Physiology, Sleep Stages, NCBI, StatPearls [Internet].: Treasure Island (FL): StatPearls Publishing; 2021 Jan
https://www.ncbi.nlm.nih.gov/books/NBK526132

NIH – National Institute of Neurological Disorders and Stroke, (2019). Brain Basics: Understanding Sleep. NIH Publication No. 17-3440c.
https://www.ninds.nih.gov/health-information/public-education/brain-basics/brain-basics-understanding-sleep

Taheri, S., Lin, L., Austin, D., et al. (2004). Short Sleep Duration Is Associated with Reduced Leptin, Elevated Ghrelin, and Increased Body Mass Index, PMC US National Library of Medicine, National Institutes of Health, PLOS Medicine, PLoS Med. 2004 Dec; 1(3): e62. Published online 2004 Dec 7. doi: 10.1371/journal.pmed.0010062
https://www.ncbi.nlm.nih.gov/pmc/articles/PMC535701

Jehan, S., Auguste, E., Zizi, F., et al, (2016). Obstructive Sleep Apnea: Women's Perspective, NIH, National Library of Medicine, National Center for Biotechnology Information: J Sleep Med Disord. Author manuscript; available in PMC 2017 Feb 23. Published in final edited form as: J Sleep Med Disord. 2016; 3(6): 1064. Published online 2016 Aug 25.
https://www.ncbi.nlm.nih.gov/pmc/articles/PMC5323064

Eikermann, M., Jordan, AS., Chamberlin, NL., et al, (2007). The Influence of Aging on Pharyngeal Collapsibility During Sleep, NIH, National Library of Medicine, National Center for Biotechnology Information: HHS Public Access, Chest. Author manuscript; available in PMC 2008 Apr 1.Published in final edited form as: Chest. 2007 Jun; 131(6): 1702–1709. Published online 2007 Apr 5. doi: 10.1378/chest.06-2653.
https://www.ncbi.nlm.nih.gov/pmc/articles/PMC2278166

Davis, I., Liu, A., (2015). What is the tryptophan kynurenine pathway and why is it important to neurotherapy? PMC US National Library of Medicine, National Institutes of Health, HHS Public Access, Author manuscript: Expert Rev Neurother. Author manuscript; available in PMC 2015 Oct 1. Published in final edited form as: Expert Rev Neurother. 2015 Jul; 15(7): (pp 719–721). Published online 2015 May 24. doi:10.1586/14737175.2015.1049999.
https://www.ncbi.nlm.nih.gov/pmc/articles/PMC4482796

Gostner, J.M., Geisler, S., Stonig, M., et al. (2020). Tryptophan Metabolism and Related Pathways in Psychoneuroimmunology: The Impact of Nutrition and Lifestyle, Neuropsychobiology: 2020;79: (pp 89–99).
https://doi.org/10.1159/000496293
https://www.karger.com/Article/Fulltext/496293

Fukuwatari, T., Shibata, K., (2013). Nutritional Aspect of Tryptophan Metabolism, PMC US National Library of Medicine, National Institutes of Health, International Journal of Tryptophan Research: Int J Tryptophan Res. 2013; 6(Suppl 1): 3–8. Published online 2013 Jul 21. doi: 10.4137/IJTR.S11588
https://www.ncbi.nlm.nih.gov/pmc/articles/PMC3729278

Stein, MD., Friedmann, PD., (2009) Disturbed Sleep and Its Relationship to Alcohol Use, PMC US National Library of Medicine, National Institutes of Health, HHS Public Access, Author manuscript: Subst Abus. Author manuscript; available in PMC 2009 Nov 10. Published in final edited form as: Subst Abus. 2005 Mar; 26(1): (pp 1–13).
https://www.ncbi.nlm.nih.gov/pmc/articles/PMC2775419

Naghedi-Baghdar, H., Nazari, S-M., Taghipour, A., et al, (2018). Effect of diet on blood viscosity in healthy humans: a systematic review, PMC US National Library of Medicine, National Institutes of Health, Electronic Physician, Excellence in Constructive Peer Review: Electron Physician. 2018 Mar; 10(3): (pp 6563–6570). Published online 2018 Mar 25. doi: 10.19082/6563.
https://www.ncbi.nlm.nih.gov/pmc/articles/PMC5942579

Jian, J., Pelle, E., Huang, X., (2009). Iron and Menopause: Does Increased Iron Affect the Health of Postmenopausal Women? PMC US National Library of Medicine, National Institutes of Health, Antioxidants & Redox Signaling: Antioxid Redox Signal. 2009 Dec; 11(12): (pp 2939–2943). doi: 10.1089/ars.2009.2576
https://www.ncbi.nlm.nih.gov/pmc/articles/PMC2821138

Rodrigues,NR., Macedo, GE., Martins, IK., et al. (2018). Short-term sleep deprivation with exposure to nocturnal light alters mitochondrial bioenergetics in Drosophila, NIH, National Library of Medicine, National Center for Biotechnology Information: Free Radic Biol Med. 2018 May 20;120: (pp 395-406). doi: 10.1016/j.freeradbiomed.2018.04.549. Epub 2018 Apr 12.
https://pubmed.ncbi.nlm.nih.gov/29655867

Schmitt, K., Grimm, A., Dallmann, R., et al. (2018). Circadian Control of DRP1 Activity Regulates Mitochondrial Dynamics and Bioenergetics, NIH, National Library of Medicine, National Center for Biotechnology Information: Cell Metab. 2018 Mar 6;27(3):657-666.e5. doi: 10.1016/j.cmet.2018.01.011. Epub 2018 Feb 22.
https://pubmed.ncbi.nlm.nih.gov/29478834

Mattson, MP., (2008). Hormesis Defined, PMC US National Library of Medicine, National Institutes of Health, HHS Public Access, Author manuscript: Ageing Res Rev. Author manuscript; available in PMC 2009 Jan 1. Published in final edited form as: Ageing Res Rev. 2008 Jan; 7(1): (pp 1–7). Published online 2007 Dec 5.
doi: 10.1016/j.arr.2007.08.007.
https://www.ncbi.nlm.nih.gov/pmc/articles/PMC2248601

Lee, Y-M., Lee, D-H., (2019). Mitochondrial Toxins and Healthy Lifestyle Meet at the Crossroad of Hormesis, PMC US National Library of Medicine, National Institutes of Health, Diabetes & Metabolism Journal: Diabetes Metab J. 2019 Oct; 43(5): (pp 568–577). Published online 2019 Oct 24. doi: 10.4093/dmj.2019.0143
https://www.ncbi.nlm.nih.gov/pmc/articles/PMC6834830

5.4 Sexual Activity and Sexual Function

Although menopause is often associated with reduced libido and sexual dysfunction, this is not always the case.

Approximately 52% of people aged 50-60, and 25% of over 60s still desire intercourse at least once a week. It appears that individuals who continue to work have increased desire, suggesting that remaining physically and mentally active plays a vital role.

Sexual Activity in Older Women: Benefits

There are several potential benefits to growing older when it comes to having a satisfactory sex life. For example, couples may have more privacy once their children have left home and a higher degree of intimacy having been together for many years. Likewise, singles may find dating and meeting potential new partners easier with increased confidence and a better sense of their relationship needs.

Moreover, there is evidence that remaining sexually active may help to mitigate some of the most common menopausal symptoms. Some experts have even suggested that married women experience menopause later than unmarried women. Although the evidence for this theory is somewhat inconclusive, there is some logic behind it. It is possible that remaining sexually active increases the body's investment of energy into ovulation and extends fecundity. Conversely, if there is no chance of conception, ovulation may cease so that more energy can be diverted into caring for one's existing offspring and grandchildren, a phenomenon known as the 'grandmother hypothesis.'

The Grandmother Hypothesis

Menopause is unique to just a handful of species; humans (*Homo sapiens*) and several aquatic mammals, including killer whales (*Orcinus orcas*), short-finned pilot whales (*Globicephala macrorhynchus*), beluga whales (*Delphinapterus leucas*), and narwhals (*Monodon monoceros*).

While these sea creatures may initially appear to have little in common with humans, they are social animals and tend to live in groups, known as pods. These pods can consist of several families which are, in many cases, matrilineally related.

Experts have suggested that menopause is an evolutionary phenomena that increases the chances of a mother passing on her genetics. It enables her to devote more energy to the family or pod's survival rather than continuing to reproduce.

Offspring born to older mothers have a lower survival rate than those born to younger individuals. Therefore, shutting off reproduction at middle age and assisting in the care of grandchildren preserves genetic lineage more efficiently than competing with younger descendants who are also reproducing.

This is known as the grandmother hypothesis of menopause. However, it is currently just that, a hypothesis. Although there is strong evidence to support it, some scientists argue that menopause is simply an evolutionary quirk that has persisted in our genes for no particular reason. However, if proven, the grandmother hypothesis would explain why humans and other species go through menopause, and why women's life spans can extend far beyond the reproductive years.

Sexual Activity in Older Women: Challenges

Older people may face challenges in maintaining regular and enjoyable intercourse. They may have to make adaptations to accommodate physical changes and other health-related issues.

Aside from the natural shortening and narrowing of the vagina that occurs throughout the menopausal transition, conditions such as arthritis, chronic pain, dementia, diabetes, and heart disease can all present difficulties. Depression, anxiety, and negative self-image due to one's changing body can also have an impact. However, many of these obstacles can be overcome by having open discussions with one's sexual partner, experimenting with different positions, and seeking appropriate medical treatment or psychological support where necessary.

Furthermore, the importance of good vaginal health cannot be overstated. Applying a specially formulated vaginal moisturizer every 2-3 days and using a lubricant during intercourse can help to combat issues such as vaginal dryness and discomfort.

Women with diabetes should take extra care to avoid *Candida albicans* infections (thrush) by keeping their blood glucose levels under control. Glucose control is also crucial for male partners with diabetes as uncontrolled diabetes is a frequent cause of erectile dysfunction. It is currently unclear whether diabetes affects female sexual function similarly, but it is possible that reduced blood flow to the sexual organs could impair sexual pleasure and orgasm.

Finally, older women may take longer to become sufficiently aroused to allow for comfortable penetration. Therefore, adequate foreplay can greatly enhance the sexual experience and increase the chances of achieving orgasm.

Silicon Versus Water-Based Lubricants

Lubricants are a useful adjunct to a healthy sex life. They decrease friction and make sex more pleasurable and enjoyable. Silicone lubricants are less likely to dry up than water-based lubricants (or saliva) and therefore should be encouraged as the prefered choice for women experiencing vaginal dryness.

Contraception and Menopause

Although female fertility declines from the mid-30s, it is still possible to conceive right up until menopause (i.e. 12 months after the last menstrual period). It is essential that perimenopausal women understand the risks associated with having unprotected intercourse, especially since late pregnancy is associated with several risks to both the mother and baby.

For example, the incidence of chromosomal abnormalities, miscarriage, pregnancy complications, and maternal morbidity increase significantly for women over 40.

Finding an appropriate method of contraception can be complex and women should carefully discuss all available options with a doctor or family planning nurse. No method is contraindicated on the basis of age alone, but it is necessary to consider various age-related comorbidities.

It is also important to note that condoms are the only method of contraception that provides protection against sexually transmitted infections. This remains relevant for post-menopausal women even once the risk of unplanned pregnancies has passed.

Female Anatomy and Sexual Pleasure

Female sexual physiology is a very new area of conventional medicine having first been described in Dickinson's textbook in 1949 and subsequently by Masters and Johnson in 1966[20] Therefore, there is still a lack of understanding surrounding the subject.

Many people consider vaginal and clitoral orgasm to be distinct, but this is incorrect from a physiological viewpoint. The vagina itself has little sensitivity and there is no anatomical evidence for the existence of the so-called 'G-spot.'

Clitoral stimulation plays the most significant role in female orgasm. However, the clitoris is much larger than most people realize, with the majority of the organ being hidden beneath the vulva. Clitoral response and female orgasm do not appear to be directly affected by aging. For a full discussion on the anatomy of the sexual organs, see Chapter 2.1.

Penetration of the vagina, with a penis, finger(s), or sex toy along with gentle repetitive motion or 'massage' increases the blood supply to the vaginal walls which are made of mucosal tissue similar to those in the digestive tract, mouth, and nose. Vaginal elasticity comes from the deeper layers of smooth muscle tissue, elastic fibers, and collagen which provide structure and flexibility.

Maintaining sexual activity, including coitus and masturbation, maintains the functionality of the circulatory, nervous, and muscular systems of the genitals. The vaginal deposition of semen may also instigate improvements in mood and increase the frequency of ovulatory cycles due to the combination of prostaglandins and hormones that it contains.

Sexual activity can also contribute to one's overall wellbeing by temporarily increasing heart rate, blood pressure, respiration, and muscular activity. Some researchers have even proposed an inverse relationship between orgasm frequency and mortality.

---

[20] Puppo. V., (2009). Embryology and anatomy of the vulva: the female orgasm and women's sexual health, European Journal of Obstetrics & Gynecology and Reproductive Biology.
https://www.ejog.org/article/S0301-2115(10)00415-X/pdf

Masturbation

Often a taboo subject, female masturbation is gaining attention with the success of campaigns that promote self-pleasure, advances in sexual technology, and the burgeoning sex toy industry.

Although the stigma surrounding female masturbation has decreased in recent times, a proportion of women still report negative emotions when masturbating, including guilt, shame, and "feeling ridiculous." These feelings likely stem from the outdated and culturally-constructed belief that masturbation is sinful, immoral, and unhealthy.

Female masturbation, in particular, is a topic that is seldom discussed and is frequently omitted from medical texts and sex education curriculums. However, emerging research suggests that masturbation plays a vital role in the development of sexuality and has numerous benefits, including:

- Reclamation of personal pleasure
- Learning about one's individual sexual response and preferences
- Increased bodily awareness
- Increase in overall desire and sexual fantasies
- Greater ease of arousal and orgasm
- Increased self-esteem and self-confidence
- Increased independence and reduced reliance on a sexual partner

Aside from these social and personal gains, there are physiological benefits to consider, particularly for menopausal and post-menopausal women. Interestingly, women aged 47-56 report more positive and fewer negative feelings toward masturbation than those in other age groups, although the reason for this is unclear.

While there is currently little research exploring how masturbation influences women's experience of menopause, it is speculated that masturbating is beneficial because it increases blood flow to the genital area. This facilitates oxygenation of the surrounding tissues, thus assisting the maintenance of smooth muscle and countering atrophy.

It has been suggested that including vaginal penetration is more beneficial than clitoral stimulation only as it engages a broader range of structures. While clitoral stimulation transmits signals to the brain via the pudendal nerve, vaginal stimulation activates the pelvic, hypogastric, and possibly vagus nerves. Therefore, combining the two is likely to produce the greatest satisfaction and physiological benefit.

TCEAM Viewpoint

Much has been written in TCEAM texts regarding the perils of excessive sexual activity and its propensity to deplete *jing*. However, these warnings primarily apply to men since semen is seen as a form of *jing*, which is lost via ejaculation. For women, this loss of *jing* is more often associated with menstruation, pregnancy (especially multiple or late pregnancies), childbirth, and lactation.

In general, sexual intercourse is seen as a natural meeting of yin and yang and something to be embraced rather than avoided. Indeed, according to the classics of TCEAM, the suppression of sexual desire can lead to stagnation and disease, ultimately shortening one's life.

There are many ancient Chinese sex manuals, which suggest that sex should be an enjoyable and fulfilling experience. Many of these texts placed great emphasis on female pleasure, suggesting that it could stimulate qi and Blood, encouraging free flow. Some sources even suggest that women could use their partner's *jing* to nourish themselves and reverse the aging process!

Of course, having a healthy libido relies upon an abundance of Kidney yang and *jing* itself. Therefore, maintaining regular sexual activity has the potential to increase one's desire, while lack of sex may diminish it.

Sexual Tonics and Aphrodisiacs

Sexual tonics and aphrodisiacs are substances that are purported to increase desire and improve sexual function. The key difference is that sexual tonics are slower acting, whereas aphrodisiacs have a more rapid onset.

For women, the most effective aphrodisiacs are herbs that nourish yin and blood (see Chapter 4.6 Libido and Sexual Dysfunction for more detail). However, the existing literature has focused on aphrodisiacs for men and there is little evidence that any particular substance can enhance sexual function in women.

One possible exception is cannabis, which has been shown to increase sexual desire and orgasm satisfaction while reducing symptoms such as pain. Unfortunately, this information is of limited use to most women due to the plant's illegal status in the majority of places, although there is a growing trend toward legalization in several countries around the world.

References

U S. Department of Health and Human Services, NIH National Institute on Aging. (2017). Sexuality and Intimacy in Older Adults
https://www.nia.nih.gov/health/sexuality-and-intimacy-older-adults

Kalra, G., Subramanyam, A., Charles Pinto, C., (2011). Sexuality: Desire, activity and intimacy in the elderly, PMC US National Library of Medicine, National Institutes of Health, Indian Journal of Psychiatry: Indian J Psychiatry. 2011 Oct-Dec; 53(4): (pp 300–306). doi: 10.4103/0019-5545.91902.
https://www.ncbi.nlm.nih.gov/pmc/articles/PMC3267340/

Thornton, K., Chervenak, J., Neal-Perry, G., (2018). Menopause and Sexuality, PMC US National Library of Medicine, National Institutes of Health, HHS Public Access, Author manuscript: Endocrinol Metab Clin North Am. Author manuscript; available in PMC 2018 Jun 11. Published in final edited form as: Endocrinol Metab Clin North Am. 2015 Sep; 44(3): (pp 649–661). doi: 10.1016/j.ecl.2015.05.009.
https://www.ncbi.nlm.nih.gov/pmc/articles/PMC5994393/

Arnot, M., Mace, R., (2020). Sexual frequency is associated with age of natural menopause: results from the Study of Women's Health Across the Nation, The Royal Society Open Science:
https://doi.org/10.1098/rsos.191020. https://royalsocietypublishing.org/doi/10.1098/rsos.191020

Avis, NE., Brockwell, S., Randolph Jr. FJ., et al, (20010). Longitudinal Changes in Sexual Functioning as Women Transition Through Menopause: Results from the Study of Women's Health Across the Nation (SWAN), PMC US National Library of Medicine, National Institutes of Health, HHS Public Access, Author manuscript: Menopause. Author manuscript; available in PMC 2010 Jul 22. Published in final edited form as: Menopause. 2009 May–Jun; 16(3): (pp 442–452). doi: 10.1097/gme.0b013e3181948dd0.
https://www.ncbi.nlm.nih.gov/pmc/articles/PMC2908487/

Bakour, SH., Hatti, A., Susan Whalen, S., (2017). Contraceptive methods and issues around the menopause: an evidence update, TOG, The Obstetrician & Gynecologist: First published: 26 September 2017 https://doi.org/10.1111/tog.12416.
https://obgyn.onlinelibrary.wiley.com/doi/full/10.1111/tog.12416

Puppo, V., (2009). Embryology and anatomy of the vulva: the female orgasm and women's sexual health, European Journal of Obstetrics & Gynecology and Reproductive Biology.
https://www.ejog.org/article/S0301-2115(10)00415-X/pdf

Puppo, V., (2013). Anatomy and physiology of the clitoris, vestibular bulbs, and labia minora with a review of the female orgasm and the prevention of female sexual dysfunction, NIH, National Library of Medicine, National Center for Biotechnology Information: Clin Anat. 2013 Jan;26(1): (pp 134-52). doi: 10.1002/ca.22177. Epub 2012 Nov 21..
https://pubmed.ncbi.nlm.nih.gov/23169570/

Hoag, N., Keast, JR., O'Connell, HE., (2017). The «G-Spot» Is Not a Structure Evident on Macroscopic Anatomic Dissection of the Vaginal Wall, NIH, National Library of Medicine, National Center for Biotechnology Information: J Sex Med. 2017 Dec;14(12): (pp 1524-1532). doi: 10.1016/j.jsxm.2017.10.071.
https://pubmed.ncbi.nlm.nih.gov/29198508.

Leibel, I., (2021). Discourses of Female Masturbation in Human Sexuality Textbooks, MacEwan University, Department of Sociology: Vol. 6 No. 1 (2021):
https://journals.macewan.ca/studentresearch/article/view/2209

Levin, RJ., (2007). Sexual activity, health and well-being - The beneficial roles of coitus and masturbation, University of Sheffield, Department of Biomedical Science, Sexual and Relationship Therapy, Vol 22 (no. 1).
https://www.researchgate.net/publication/244887033_Sexual_activity_health_and_well-being_-_The_beneficial_roles_of_coitus_and_masturbation

Carvalheira, A., Leal, I., (2012). Masturbation Among Women: Associated Factors and Sexual Response in a Portuguese Community Sample, February 2012. Journal of Sex and Marital Therapy 39(4). DOI:10.1080/0092623X.2011.628440.
https://www.researchgate.net/publication/235668234_Masturbation_Among_Women_Associated_Factors_and_Sexual_Response_in_a_Portuguese_Community_Sample

Sokol, Al.., Shveiky, D., Clinical Anatomy of the Vulva, Vagina, Lower Pelvis, and Perineum, GLOWM, The Global Library of Women's Medicine's Welfare of Women Global Health Programme. Sokol, A, Shveiky, D, Glob. libr. women's med., (ISSN: 1756-2228) 2008; DOI 10.3843/GLOWM.10000
https://www.glowm.com/section-view/heading/clinical-anatomy-of-the-vulva-vagina-lower-pelvis-and-perineum/item/445#.Y0f11nZBzlV

Kaestle, C., Allen, K., (2011). The Role of Masturbation in Healthy Sexual Development: Perceptions of Young Adults. Springer Link, Archives of Sexual Behavior, 40(5), (pp 983–994).
https://doi.org/10.1007/s10508-010-9722-0.

Hogarth, H., Ingham, R., (2009). Masturbation among Young Women and Associations with Sexual Health: An Exploratory Study. Taylor Francis Online, The Journal of Sex Research, 46(6), (pp 558-567).
https://doi.org/10.1080/00224490902878993

Deadman, P., (2016). Live Well, Live Long: Teachings from the Chinese Nourishment of Life Tradition and Modern Research. The Journal of Chinese Medicine Ltd : Hove, England.

Kotta, S., Ansari, SH., Ali, J., (2013). Exploring scientifically proven herbal aphrodisiacs, PMC US National Library of Medicine, National Institutes of Health, Pharmacognosy Review: Pharmacogn Rev. 2013 Jan-Jun; 7(13): (pp 1–10). doi: 10.4103/0973-7847.112832.
https://www.ncbi.nlm.nih.gov/pmc/articles/PMC3731873/

Lynn, BK., López, JD., Miller, C., et al. (2019). The Relationship between Marijuana Use Prior to Sex and Sexual Function in Women, PMC US National Library of Medicine, National Institutes of Health, Sexual Medicine: Sex Med. 2019 Jun; 7(2): (pp 192–197). Published online 2019 Mar 2. doi: 10.1016/j.esxm.2019.01.003.
https://www.ncbi.nlm.nih.gov/pmc/articles/PMC6522945/

5.5 Alcohol, Tobacco and Other Drugs

Drugs (including alcohol and tobacco) are pharmacologically diverse. They have different psychotropic and physiological effects, likeability, abuse liability, and dependence potential. That is, they vary in the relative probability that they will become a social, psychological, or physical problem for an individual or for society.

Drugs alter perception, cognition, and mood by affecting chemical pathways in the brain. The interplay between menopause and drug and alcohol use is largely under studied. This chapter is a brief overview of some common drugs this population may use and considerations in your clinic.

Key Terms

Tolerance

Tolerance is a process of neuroadaptation whereby the body becomes accustomed to a substance over time, resulting in the need for increased doses in order to produce an identical effect. An escalation of dose, frequency, and change in route of administration (e.g. from smoking to injecting heroin) places someone at greater risk of developing dependence.

Withdrawal

Withdrawal is a physiological response that occurs in the absence of a substance, a decrease in dose, or reduced frequency of use. It is the body's homeostatic effort to remain balanced in the absence of a substance.

Withdrawal symptoms can vary significantly among individuals and depend greatly on the type of drug, quantity, duration of drug use, and route of administration. However, there are some commonalities, most notably depression, anxiety, sleep disorders, and intense cravings for the drug. Many people relapse and return to drug use because the withdrawal symptoms are unbearable.

Drug Dependence and Substance Use Disorders

Some drug users develop a physiological or psychological dependence on the substance that causes them to continue using it, despite the adverse impact it may be having on their lives. While some drugs are considered more likely to cause dependence than others, any misused substance has the potential to do so.

There are varying degrees of drug dependence, and the term 'substance use disorder' is now prefered as it reflects that fact that substance use can become problematic, even without complete physiological dependence.

According to the Diagnostic and Statistical Manual of Mental Disorders (DSM-5), the diagnostic criteria for substance use disorders include:

- Taking the substance in larger amounts over longer periods than intended
- A persistent desire or unsuccessful efforts to reduce or control use of the substance
- Spending a great deal of time engaged in activities required to obtain and use the substance, or recover from its effects
- Cravings or a strong desire to use the substance
- Failure to fulfil major obligations at work, school, or home due to continued substance use
- Reducing or giving up important social, occupational, or recreational activities due to use of the substance
- Recurrent use of the substance in physically hazardous situations
- Continuing use of the substance despite knowledge of persistent or recurrent physical or psychological problems caused or exacerbated by the substance
- Tolerance
- Withdrawal

Drug Classifications

1. **Central nervous system (CNS) stimulants**
2. **CNS depressants**
   - Opioid analgesics
3. **Psychedelics**
   - Cannabis
   - Hallucinogens
   - Dissociative Anesthetics

1. Central Nervous System (CNS) Stimulants

CNS stimulants work by releasing large amounts of dopamine into the neuroendocrine system. Examples include nicotine, caffeine, cocaine, amphetamines, and 3,4-methylenedioxymethamphetamine (MDMA), commonly known as ecstasy.

As an excitatory neurotransmitter, dopamine is similar to adrenaline and influences brain processes that control movement, emotional response, and the ability to experience pleasure and pain. Taking CNS stimulants results in euphoria, increased energy, and alertness, making them a popular choice for recreational drug users.

Nicotine in Tobacco (Cigarette Smoking)

Smoking and vaping are effective and rapid means of delivering a drug to the body. Drugs are introduced via the lungs and absorbed into the bloodstream within a few seconds of administration.

Smoking tobacco introduces over 4000 chemicals to the brain (250 are known to be harmful, including 43 known carcinogens) and the active ingredient is nicotine. The average cigarette contains about one gram of nicotine.

In recent years, vaping has been promoted as a safer alternative and many people use it as a means to reduce and cease tobacco smoking. However, the long-term health effects of vaping are still largely unknown and the thinning agents used in many products may cause issues of their own. It is likely that vaping is preferable to tobacco when used as a short-term solution to facilitate smoking cessation. However, individuals should make every effort to reduce their nicotine dosage and wean off vaping as early as possible.

Nicotine and Menopause

Smoking cigarettes activates nicotinic acetylcholine receptors and reduces circulating estrogen resulting in early onset of menopause. Furthermore, smoking nicotine reduces the effectiveness of MHT. Smoking cessation should be encouraged in menopausal patients with assistance from nicotine replacement therapies (NRT) when necessary.

Caffeine

Caffeine is the most widely used psychoactive substance and caffeine-containing beverages are consumed by almost every culture worldwide. Tea and coffee are the best known examples, but caffeine is also found in cocoa, chocolate, soft drinks, and energy drinks.

Caffeine and Menopause

Caffeine promotes awakeness and alertness by acting as a competitive antagonist at adenosine receptors in the CNS, thus increasing dopamine, noradrenaline, and glutamate release. High doses can cause side effects, including anxiety, agitation, restlessness, insomnia, gastrointestinal disturbances, tremors, and tachycardia. Therefore, it may exacerbate these symptoms in patients already experiencing them. There is also some inconclusive evidence that caffeine could contribute to hot flash severity.

That said, caffeine-containing beverages such as tea and coffee also contain antioxidant compounds, such as polyphenols. Furthermore, coffee beans contain lignans, which may have phytoestrogenic effects. Low doses of caffeine have been shown to improve cognitive performance and higher doses could aid functional performance during exercise. Caffeine may also provide some protection against neurodegenerative disorders, such as Alzheimer's disease.

Therefore, moderate caffeine consumption may be beneficial for some menopausal patients and should be considered on a case-by-case basis. Care should be taken with decaffeinated beverages as the solvents necessary for the process may have deleterious effects on one's health.

Cocaine

Cocaine is a CNS stimulant drug derived from the *Erythroxylon coca* plant and manufactured to form:

1. **Cocaine hydrochloride:** a white crystalline powder which is commonly consumed intranasally, although it may be taken orally or rectally.
2. **Crack:** rocks of 'free base' cocaine which is processed with ammonia or sodium bicarbonate and heated to produce a potent form of cocaine that can be smoked.

Cocaine binds to sites in areas of the brain that are rich in dopamine synapses resulting in a flood of dopamine in the neuroendocrine system. The consequence is an immediate and intense feeling of euphoria and pleasure. Additionally, cocaine increases dopamine levels by preventing its reuptake, leaving more dopamine in the synapses. With a half-life of 30 to 60 minutes, cocaine leaves a person craving more shortly afterwards, greatly increasing its abuse potential.

Cocaine and Menopause

Women are more susceptible to cocaine addiction compared with men. Studies of female rats implicate estradiol as a potential mechanism in developing an addicted phenotype.

A particularly under-studied area of human research is changes in women's response to cocaine use at menopause. However, there is some evidence that cocaine affects the production of reproductive hormones via the HPA axis and may alter hormone levels in women taking MHT.

Furthermore, medications typically used to treat acute myocardial infarction and heart arrhythmias such as beta blockers and anticoagulants may be fatal to a cocaine user. Cardiac medications work by lowering blood pressure. However, with cocaine induced vasoconstriction they have an inverse effect and increase blood pressure. A person with atherosclerotic (hardened) arteries is at greatest risk of cocaine related myocardial infarction.

Amphetamine Type Substances

Amphetamine type substances are CNS stimulants and increase the activity of the parts of the sympathetic nervous system which support 'fight and flight' adrenal responses. Amphetamines come in the form of tablets, capsules, powder, or a hard 'rock' substance. The tablet or capsule forms are usually swallowed but may be administered intranasally or crushed and injected. The powder or 'rock' is used intranasally, injected, and sometimes smoked.

Amphetamines have a rapid onset (within seconds) when smoked or injected, peaking after 30-60 minutes. The onset is slower with intranasal administration (3-10 minutes) or oral use (30-60 minutes). The effects of stimulants last from 2-24 hours depending on the dose, type, and route of administration. Methamphetamine is the most potent of the amphetamines and has the longest duration of action.

Amphetamines and Menopause

There is little research on how amphetamines affect menopausal women. However, as these substances stimulate not only the CNS but also the cardiovascular system, they could be dangerous in older populations. For example, side effects include increases in pulse rate, systolic blood pressure, and central pulse pressure (i.e. the carotid, femoral, and brachial pulses). Amphetamine use could also contribute to the development of atherosclerosis, hypertensive crises, cerebrovascular accidents, aneurysms, and tachyarrhythmias, including sudden cardiac death.

Some scientists have also speculated that long-term amphetamine use accelerates the overall aging process due to prolonged stress on the CNS and sympathetic overdrive.

2. CNS Depressants

By promoting the inhibitory physiological systems, CNS depressants lower the rate of arousal, with a reduction in motor and cognitive activity, and depression of cardiorespiratory centers. In short, they slow down activity in the CNS.

The brain contains over 10 billion neurons which control every bodily function. The transmission of electrical impulses or signals from one neuron to another depends on the action of certain chemicals known as neurotransmitters.

CNS depressants slow the system by affecting gamma-aminobutyric acid (GABA). GABA is the primary inhibitory neurotransmitter and an inability to produce it results in disorders such as anxiety, tension, insomnia, and epilepsy.

GABA works by decreasing brain activity. Although the different types of CNS depressants each have a unique mechanism of action, it is through their ability to increase GABA activity that they produce a relaxing effect.

Examples include alcohol and prescription medications commonly referred to as sedatives such as barbiturates and benzodiazepines; sleeping pills, anti-anxiety tranquillizers, and anticonvulsants.

Alcohol

Alcohol lowers the rate of arousal, with a reduction in motor and cognitive activity and depression of cardiorespiratory centers. Alcohol is often mistaken for a stimulant drug as a person may become talkative or more self-confident. However, these behaviors are the result of the suppression of the behavioral inhibitory centers in the cerebral cortex, the part of the brain responsible for consciousness and thought. Alcohol softens or depresses our normal social inhibitions. With continued use, shortly after the excitement phase, alcohol's dominant CNS depressant qualities become apparent, characterized by drowsiness, slurred speech, and loss of coordination and balance.

Long-Term Use

Long-term alcohol use causes numerous chronic health issues:

- Hypertension, stroke, liver and heart disease, and digestive issues
- Cancer, immunosuppression, and increased risk of other illnesses
- Mental and cognitive problems such as memory loss, dementia, depression, and anxiety

Absorption

Alcohol is absorbed directly into the bloodstream via the stomach (20%) and the small intestine (80%). The rate of alcohol absorption depends on:

- The concentration of alcohol in the drink: high concentration = fast absorption rate
- Whether the stomach is full or empty[21]; food slows down alcohol absorption
- The preparation (e.g. carbonation speeds up the absorption of alcohol)

---

[21] If a person has food in their stomach before drinking alcohol the absorption rate may be slowed. However, it does NOT prevent a person becoming intoxicated. Regardless of how much food is in the stomach before drinking, all of the alcohol consumed will reach the bloodstream eventually.

Excretion

- 91% of alcohol excretion takes place in the liver
- 6% in the lungs and skin (breath 3% & sweat 3%)
- 3% in the kidneys

As alcohol is metabolized by the liver at a fixed rate (one Standard Drink per hour), if a person drinks a lot of alcohol in one session (i.e. bingeing) then it is quite likely that alcohol will still be present in the bloodstream the following day. This may place someone at risk of associated harms such as traffic accidents (including as a pedestrian).

Alcohol and Menopause

Alcohol affects women differently to men. Women have lower levels of dehydrogenase enzymes, the enzymes that break down alcohol, and a higher water to body fat ratio. These factors increase women's vulnerability to the harmful effects of alcohol and the risk of alcohol-related diseases earlier in life compared to men. Age-related changes in body composition, stress, and depression may trigger the onset of heavy alcohol consumption or worsen established alcohol dependence in menopausal women.

Benzodiazepines

Benzodiazepines are CNS depressants prescribed by medical doctors for their sedative effects on sleep, muscle relaxation, restlessness, and anxiety, for example diazepam (Valium).

With a high risk of dependence, benzodiazepines are not ideal for chronic conditions. Tolerance develops quickly, resulting in a need for markedly increased amounts to achieve the desired effect. Benzodiazepine withdrawal can occur in people who have been taking therapeutic or higher doses on a regular basis for two or more weeks.

Benzodiazepines rarely cause fatal overdose when used in isolation. However, in combination with alcohol they are very dangerous, with a high risk of overdose. As an alternative to benzodiazepines, prolonged-release melatonin should be considered as a first-line treatment for insomnia given its good tolerability, safety, and efficacy in helping promote sleep, without harmful side effects.

Benzodiazepines and Menopause

Menopausal women often experience sleep disturbances including insomnia, night sweats, and mood changes, including anxiety. Therefore, benzodiazepine use may be especially prevalent within this population. However, there is little research on the subject of benzodiazepine use and menopause specifically. Patients should be made aware of the risks associated with long-term benzodiazepine use and encouraged to discuss alternatives with their prescribing doctor.

Opioid Analgesics

The term 'opioids' is a broad name given to a group of CNS depressants that bind to the body's opioid receptors, found principally in the CNS and the gastrointestinal tract. Opioids have strong analgesic and sedative effects. They may cause euphoria and disinhibition, and relieve discomfort from other drug withdrawal syndromes through effects on sleep, pain, muscle relaxation, restlessness, and anxiety.

Opioids tend to rapidly produce tolerance and have extremely unpleasant withdrawal symptoms. Therefore, short-term medical use can easily turn into misuse and dependence. This has led to significant issues in the past few decades due to the overprescribing of opioids for chronic pain conditions. The much publicized 'opioid epidemic' has led to many overdose deaths and can be considered one of the worst public health crises of the late 20th and early 21st centuries. The situation is steadily beginning to improve but the overprescribing of opioids remains an issue in many regions.

There are a number of broad classes:

1. **Natural opiates:** alkaloids contained in the resin of opium poppies (*Papaver somniferum*), e.g. morphine and codeine.
2. **Semi-synthetic opiates:** created from the natural opioids, e.g. oxycodone and heroin.
3. **Fully synthetic opioids:** e.g. pethidine and methadone.
4. **Endogenous opioid peptides:** produced naturally in the body, e.g. endorphins and enkephalins.

Opioids and Menopause

Women in midlife have shown the greatest increase in opioid use and overdose mortality of any demographic. Furthemore, women with menopausal symptoms are believed to have the highest odds of long-term use, long-term high doses, or long-term use alongside other prescription CNS depressants. This is thought to be a result of an altered pain experience coupled with comorbidities, making effective pain management challenging and increasing the incidence of polypharmacy.

Moreover, chronic pain may share some physiological mechanisms with symptoms such as hot flashes, mood, and sleep disorders, further exacerbating the issue. For example, estrogen has a regulatory effect on the endogenous opioid system and a low estrogen state is associated with increased vulnerability to pain.

Unfortunately, opioids have an adverse effect on the endocrine system, which could worsen menopausal symptoms. Long-term use appears to suppress hypothalamic gonadotropin releasing hormone (GnRH) secretion, leading to hypogonadism and a range of symptoms, including reduced libido, fatigue, depression, anxiety, reduced muscle mass and strength, and an increased risk of osteoporosis/fractures.

3. Psychedelics

Cannabis

The *Cannabis sativa* plant is the most widely used recreational drug in the world. The major biologically active chemical compound in cannabis is delta-9-tetrahydrocannabinol, commonly referred to as THC. THC is one of many chemicals known as cannabinoids. They share structural similarities with endogenously produced signaling chemicals (endocannabinoids), such as anandamide and 2-arachidonoyl (2-AG), and exert their effects by binding with cannabinoid receptors throughout the body.

In addition to THC, cannabis contains myriad other bioactive compounds, including secondary cannabinoids (CBD, CBG, CBC, THCV, etc.) and aromatic terpenes. The concentrations of these compounds vary significantly from plant to plant, meaning that different cultivars can produce a diverse range of effects.

Cannabis sits in two drug classes as it is a CNS depressant but may have hallucinogenic qualities in high doses. Cannabis varies in form and potency:

1. Marijuana: dried flowering heads (or 'buds') which contain a high concentration of THC, with relatively tiny amounts in the leaves and stems.
2. Hashish: hashish or cannabis resin is compressed THC made by separating resinous glands known as trichomes from the plant material to produce a powdery substance called kief. Kief may be consumed in its unprocessed state or pressed into solid blocks of hash.
3. Hash oil and concentrates: hash oil is a greasy viscous liquid extracted from cannabis plant material using a solvent. Hash oil is just one of many potent cannabis preparations known as concentrates. Other examples include a glass-like substance called shatter and the softer cannabis wax. Concentrates contain exceedingly high levels of THC, sometimes up to 90%.

Inhaled cannabis has a rate of onset of about 5-15 mins, peaking at 30-120 minutes, with a duration of 2-6 hours depending upon type, dose, and tolerance. When eaten or infused in a tea, the effects are delayed in onset, are prolonged, and tend to be more potent.

The effects of cannabis are unpredictable and vary from person to person. Factors influencing the effect of cannabis include:

Substance

- Amount, preparation, and potency (THC content: marijuana, hashish, hash oil)
- Route of administration (smoked in a joint or bong, oral as in a hash cookie)
- Whether the cannabis is taken with alcohol or other drugs

Set

- The person's weight and general health
- The person's mood, prior exposure, and previous experience
- Person's understanding of how the drug will affect them and their expectation or desired effects

Setting

- Whether the person is taking cannabis alone or with other people
- The location: at home or at a party, night club, or festival

Immediate Effects

Even a small dose of cannabis can produce the following immediate effects:

- Feelings of euphoria and wellbeing, relaxation
- Loss of inhibitions
- Tendency to giggle or laugh
- Loss of concentration
- Impaired balance and coordination
- Altered sense of time and space
- Heightened senses
- Increased appetite
- Conjunctival suffusion (red eyes)
- Nausea and/or vomiting
- Anxiety and paranoia

Longer Term Use

The following is a list of common findings from research regarding the long-term effects of cannabis use in frequent and heavy cannabis users:

- Increased risk of bronchitis, and respiratory disease (smoked cannabis)
- A change in motivation
- Decreased concentration, memory, and learning abilities
- Interference with libido and hormone production
- Psychological disturbances
- Heavy doses of cannabis can produce brief and sometimes severe psychotic behavior
- Cannabis dependence and withdrawal symptoms (anxiety, sleep disturbances, etc.)
- Sleep disorders

Cannabis is often mixed with tobacco, which contains the highly addictive nicotine. People trying to reduce their cannabis use or stop entirely may go through periods of withdrawal and not recognize this is in fact nicotine withdrawal, particularly in those that do not smoke tobacco.

Cannabis and Menopause

Once again, there is little evidence relating to cannabis and menopause, specifically. An increasing number of menopausal patients may self-medicate with cannabis to relieve symptoms such as chronic pain, sleep, and mood disorders. However, high doses and repeated use may exacerbate these symptoms in the long run. For example, while cannabis may aid relaxation in low doses, high doses can cause severe anxiety and paranoia. And while cannabis can reduce sleep latency and increase deep sleep, cessation of the drug causes rebound effects, such as insomnia and vivid dreams.

That said, there is a growing body of evidence that cannabis may be useful in the management of some chronic conditions and a trend for medical marijuana legalization around the world. Patients should be encouraged to use the minimum dosage required to manage their symptoms and choose administration methods other than smoking where possible.

Hallucinogens and Dissociative Anesthetics

The defining characteristic of psychedelic or hallucinogenic drugs is their ability to distort reality and markedly interfere with sensory and cognitive processing. Their effects vary considerably depending on the substance, set, and setting. However, generally speaking, they cause mood changes, including euphoria, spontaneous laughter or crying, an increased sense of connection with the self, other beings, or a higher power, anxiety, paranoia, and panic. They may also cause hallucinations, including altered perception of sounds and colors, or seeing, hearing, smelling, touching, and tasting things that may not exist.

There are several major classes of hallucinogens:

1. **Tryptamines:** also known as 'classic hallucinogens,' this drug class includes lysergic acid diethylamide (LSD), psilocybin or psilocin (the active components of 'magic mushrooms'), and N, N-dimethyltryptamine (DMT). Ayahuasca is a psychedelic drink made by combining the DMT-containing plant *Psychotria viridis* with *Banisteriopsis caapi vine*, which contains chemicals that inhibit DMT breakdown and prolong its effects. There are also numerous synthetic tryptamines which are sold as 'research chemicals' and fall under the category of 'new psychoactive substances' (NPS). They primarily exert their effects by binding with serotonin receptors in the brain.
2. **Phenethylamines:** this category includes mescaline (from the hallucinogenic peyote or San Pedro cacti), MDMA, and amphetamine. There are also numerous synthetic phenethylamines, including the 2-C family, NBOMes, and other NPS. They exert their effects by influencing the serotonergic and dopaminergic systems.
3. **Deliriants:** various plants, particularly *Datura stramonium*, contain tropane alkaloids, anticholinergic compounds such as atropine, hyoscyamine, and scopolamine, and are classified as deliriants. They cause intense and realistic hallucinations which can last for days and carry a high risk of toxicity.

4. Dissociatives: phencyclidine (PCP or 'angel dust') and ketamine are dissociative anesthetics and are also liable to abuse due to their hallucinogenic qualities. These drugs influence GABA and glutamate activity, which at high doses may cause the user to experience out-of-body sensations.

Hallucinogens and Dissociative Anesthetics and Menopause

In recent years, there has been a resurgence of interest in the potential therapeutic use of many hallucinogens and dissociatives. For example, psilocybin has been investigated as a treatment for a variety of mental health disorders with promising results. Likewise, ketamine is showing great potential in the treatment of depression.

These findings have been publicized although the drugs are not yet widely available for medical use. Patients considering self-medicating should be reminded of the importance of using these substances in a safe and supportive environment, preferably as part of an ongoing therapy program. Medical screening is also recommended for older patients to ensure that no complications occur as a result of comorbidities or polypharmacy.

There are also a growing number of ayahuasca retreats and ketamine clinics opening in locations around the world. Patients should perform due diligence before attending these centers to ensure they are legitimate and have sufficient safety measures in place.

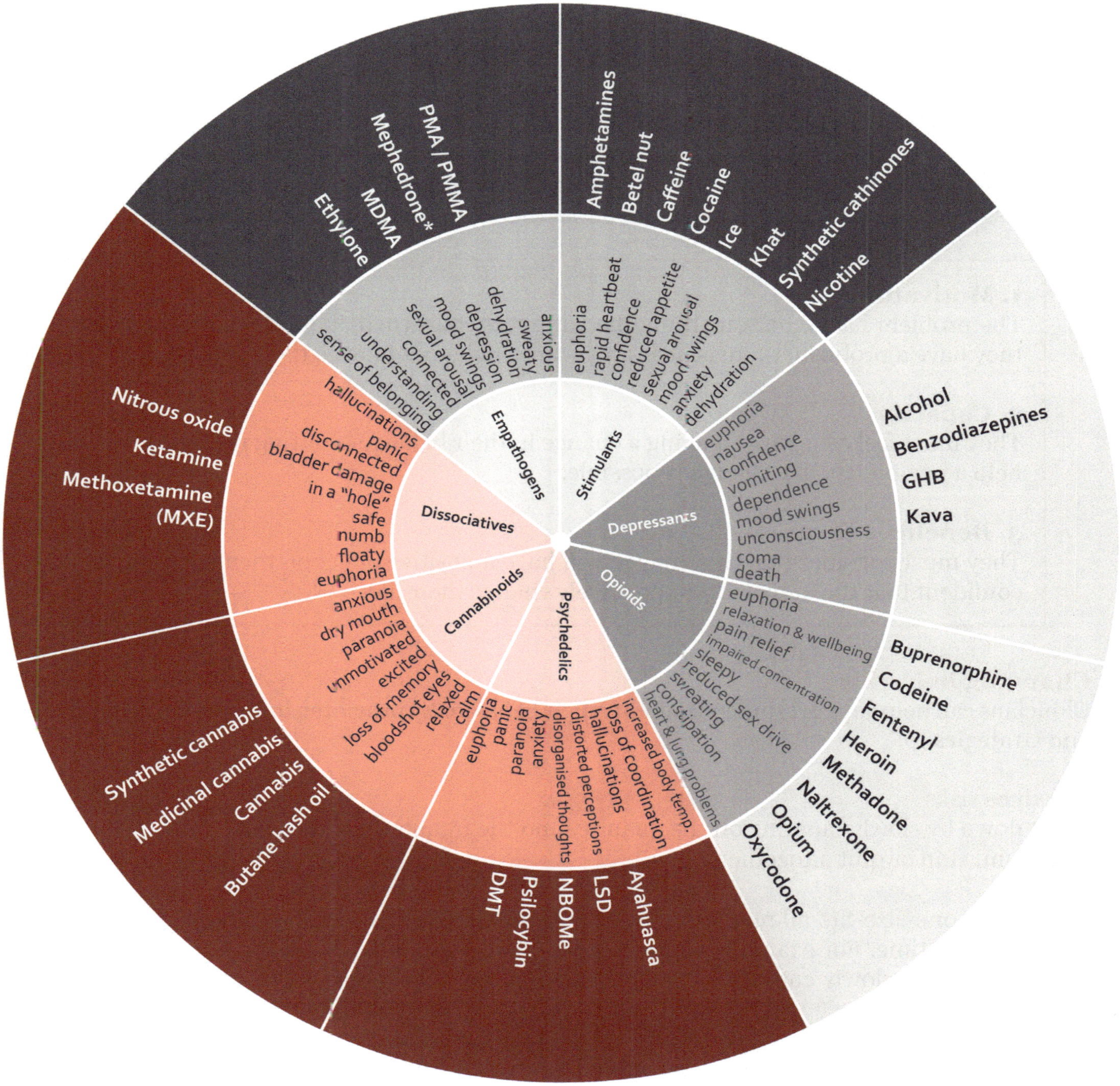

Figure 5.5: Drug wheel[22]

[22] Image Source: The Drugs Wheel by Mark Adley based on a work at www.thedrugswheel.com

Motivating Behavioral Change

One of the principal aims of any brief intervention is to assess the person's readiness for changing their drinking or drug use. It is important to identify what your patient wants and their expectation of your role in providing support for this. You can help them to identify their readiness for changing their behavior and assist them in setting realistically achievable goals.

1. Motivation
The problem has to be something the patient is concerned about. If they do not think they have a problem, there is little scope to be able to influence their behavior.

2. Capacity
They must feel capable of making a change in their behavior. Setting realistic goals can help a person feel like change is possible.

3. Benefit
They must consider that this change will have a positive effect on them. They must be confident that the outcome will positively change their life.

Changing Behavior

Clinicians can help support someone modify their behavior by providing information, treatment, and strategies to:

- Reduce risks
- Cut down by slowly tapering off the quantity and the frequency of drug use
- Abstain, stop or quit altogether

There is no one-size-fits-all method. There are those that respond well to tapering or reducing their use over time. For example, someone may choose to smoke one less cigarette a day over a period of time, slowly cutting down. Or those that go 'cold turkey,' choosing to stop using a substance altogether.

It is important to note that people are more likely to do well if they have someone to support them. Find out who else can help, for example, a close friend, spouse, partner, or family member. Considerations for treatment include: what the client wants, severity of problems and losses due to drug use, and safety of the patient, for example, other health risks.

Drug Use Assessment

These are the key questions to ask when conducting a drug use assessment:

- ☐ Drug of choice
- ☐ Desired effect - what purpose does it serve?
- ☐ Dosage
- ☐ Frequency of use
- ☐ Duration of use
- ☐ Date and time of last use
- ☐ Route of administration
- ☐ Previous seven day's consumption
- ☐ Typical week's consumption
- ☐ Periods of abstinence and how they were achieved
- ☐ Previous withdrawal syndromes
- ☐ Identified relapse triggers
- ☐ Readiness and motivation to change

Summary

How drug use, misuse, and dependence affect menopause is a largely understudied area. However, it appears that the majority of recreational substances will have some degree of negative impact. While some drugs do have therapeutic potential, they should be used responsibly, in moderation, and preferably with medical supervision to reduce the risk of adverse outcomes.

As clinicians, we have the opportunity to educate our patients about the potential consequences of their drug use and support them should they wish to stop. Therefore, it is essential to provide a comfortable and non-judgmental environment so that patients feel able to discuss their drug use openly and honestly.

References

Allen, SS., Hatsukami, DK., Blade, T., (2004). Transdermal nicotine use in postmenopausal women: Does the treatment efficacy differ in women using and not using hormone replacement therapy? Oxford Academic, Nicotine & Tobacco Research: Nicotine & Tobacco Research, Volume 6, Issue 5, October 2004, (pp 777–788), https://doi.org/10.1080/14622200420000274239. https://academic.oup.com/ntr/article-abstract/6/5/777/1021513

Raval, AP., (2011). Nicotine Addiction Causes Unique Detrimental Effects on Women's Brains. Taylor & Francis Online, Journal of Addictive Diseases: Volume 30, 2011 – Issue 2 (pp 149-158) https://doi.org/10.1080/10550887.2011.554782 https://www.tandfonline.com/doi/abs/10.1080/10550887.2011.554782

Tansavatdi, K., McClain, B., Herrington, DM., (2004). The effects of smoking on estradiol metabolism. NIH, National Library of Medicine, National Center for Biotechnology Information: Minerva Ginecol. 2004 Feb;56(1). (pp 105-14). https://pubmed.ncbi.nlm.nih.gov/14973414/

Tankó, LB., Christiansen, C., (2004). An update on the antiestrogenic effect of smoking: a literature review with implications for researchers and practitioners, NIH, National Library of Medicine, National Center for Biotechnology Information: Menopause. Jan-Feb 2004;11(1):(pp 104-9). doi: 10.1097/01.GME.0000079740.18541.DB.
https://pubmed.ncbi.nlm.nih.gov/14716190/

Copeland, AL., Peltier, MR., Geiselman, PJ, (2016). Severity of Menopausal Symptoms and Nicotine Dependence amongst Postmenopausal Women Smokers, Cambridge University Press: Published online by Cambridge University Press: 21 June 2016
https://www.cambridge.org/core/journals/journal-of-smoking-cessation/article/abs/severity-of-menopausal-symptoms-and-nicotine-dependence-amongst-postmenopausal-women-smokers/D4267F3D169CBC466D7AC93491721A39

Faubion, SS., Sood, R., Thielen, JM., et al. (2015). Caffeine and menopausal symptoms: what is the association? NIH, National Library of Medicine, National Center for Biotechnology Information: Menopause. 2015 Feb;22(2): (pp 155-8). doi: 10.1097/GME.0000000000000301.
https://pubmed.ncbi.nlm.nih.gov/25051286/

Bouchard, C., (2015). Coffee or caffeine intake and effects on menopausal symptoms, unsolved issue, Menopause, The Journal of The North American Menopause Society: Menopause: February 2015 - Volume 22 - Issue 2 - (pp 129-130) doi: 10.1097/GME.0000000000000412.
https://journals.lww.com/menopausejournal/Citation/2015/02000/Coffee_or_caffeine_intake_and_effects_on.3.aspx

Rhee, JJ., Qin, F-F., Hedlin, HK., et al. (2015). Coffee and caffeine consumption and the risk of hypertension in postmenopausal women, Oxford Academic, The American Journal of Clinical Nutrition: The American Journal of Clinical Nutrition, Volume 103, Issue 1, January 2016, (pp 210–217), https://doi.org/10.3945/ajcn.115.120147.
https://academic.oup.com/ajcn/article/103/1/210/4569306

Waer, FB., Laatar, R., Jouira, G., et al. (2021). Functional and cognitive responses to caffeine intake in middle-aged women are dose depending, Elsevier: Behavioral Brain Research, Volume 397, 15 January 2021, 112956.
https://www.sciencedirect.com/science/article/abs/pii/S0166432820306550

Cappelletti, S., Daria, P., Sani, G., et al. (2015). Caffeine: Cognitive and Physical Performance Enhancer or Psychoactive Drug, NCBI, PMC, US National Library of Medicine, National Institutes of Health, Current Neuropharmacology: Curr Neuropharmacol. 2015 Jan; 13(1): (pp 71–88). Published online 2015 Jan. doi: 10.2174/1570159X13666141210215655. https://www.ncbi.nlm.nih.gov/pmc/articles/PMC4462044/

Mount Sinai Health System, (2017), Researchers reveal connection between female estrogen cycle, addictive potential of cocaine, Science Daily.
https://www.sciencedaily.com/releases/2017/01/170110154428.htm

Ramôa, CP., Doyle, SE., Naim, DW., et al. (2013). Estradiol as a Mechanism for Sex Differences in the Development of an Addicted Phenotype following Extended Access Cocaine Self-Administration, NCBI, PMC, US National Library of Medicine, National Institutes of Health: Neuropsychopharmacology. 2013 Aug; 38(9): (pp 1698–1705). Published online 2013 Mar 27. Prepublished online 2013 Mar 12. doi: 10.1038/npp.2013.68
https://www.ncbi.nlm.nih.gov/pmc/articles/PMC3717535/

Calipari, ES., Juarez,B., Morel, C., et al (2017). Dopaminergic dynamics underlying sex-specific cocaine reward, Nature Communications: Article number: 13877 (2017)
https://www.nature.com/articles/ncomms13877

Quiñones-Jenab, V., Perrotti, LI., Ho, A., et al (2000). Cocaine affects progesterone plasma levels in female rats, NIH, National Library of Medicine, National Center for Biotechnology Information: Pharmacol Biochem Behav. 2000 Jun;66(2) (pp 449-53). doi: 10.1016/s0091-3057(00)00213-6.
https://pubmed.ncbi.nlm.nih.gov/10880704/

Reece, AS., Norman, A., Hulse, GK., (2017). Acceleration of cardiovascular-biological age by amphetamine exposure is a power function of chronological age, NCBI, PMC, US National Library of Medicine, National Institutes of Health: Heart Asia. 2017; 9(1):(pp 30–38). Published online 2017 Jan 10. doi: 10.1136/heartasia-2016-010832
https://www.ncbi.nlm.nih.gov/pmc/articles/PMC5307374/

CDC Centers for Disease Control and Prevention. (Sourced January 2021). Alcohol Use and Your Health: CDC, Alcohol & Public Health, Alcohol Basics
https://www.cdc.gov/alcohol/fact-sheets/alcohol-use.htm

Milic, J., Glisic, M., Voortman, T., et al. (2018). Menopause, ageing, and alcohol use disorders in women, Elsevier: Maturitas, Volume 111, May 2018, (pp 100-109).
https://www.sciencedirect.com/science/article/abs/pii/S037851221731-027

Taneri, PE., Kiefte-de-Jong, JC., Bramer, WM., et al, (2016). Association of alcohol consumption with the onset of natural menopause: a systematic review and meta-analysis, Oxford Academic: Human Reproduction Update, Volume 22, Issue 4, July/August 2016, (pp 516–528).
https://doi.org/10.1093/humupd/dmw013
https://academic.oup.com/humupd/article/22/4/516/2573866?login=true

Proserpio, P., Marra, S., Campana, C., et al (2020). Insomnia and menopause: a narrative review on mechanisms and treatments, NIH, National Library of Medicine, National Center for Biotechnology Information: Climacteric. 2020 Dec;23(6):539-549. doi: 10.1080/13697137.2020.1799973. Epub 2020 Sep 3.
https://pubmed.ncbi.nlm.nih.gov/32880197/

Gibson, CJ., Li, Y., Huang, AJ., et al, (2019). Menopausal Symptoms and Higher Risk Opioid Prescribing in a National Sample of Women Veterans with Chronic Pain, NCBI, PMC, US National Library of Medicine, National Institutes of Health: J Gen Intern Med. 2019 Oct; 34(10): (pp 2159–2166). Published online 2019 Aug 14. doi: 10.1007/s11606-019-05242-w
https://www.ncbi.nlm.nih.gov/pmc/articles/PMC6816610/

Smith, YR., Stohler, CS., Michols,TE., et al. (2006). Pronociceptive and Antinociceptive Effects of Estradiol through Endogenous Opioid Neurotransmission in Women, NCBI, PMC, US National Library of Medicine, National Institutes of Health: J Neurosci. 2006 May 24; 26(21): (pp 5777–5785). doi: 10.1523/JNEUROSCI.5223-05.2006
https://www.ncbi.nlm.nih.gov/pmc/articles/PMC1808228/

Katz, N., Mazer, NA., (2009), The Impact of Opioids on the Endocrine System, 2009 Lippincott Williams & Wilkins.
https://pubmed.ncbi.nlm.nih.gov/19333165/

Garcia-Romeu, A., Kersgaard, B., Addy, PH., (2016). Clinical Applications of Hallucinogens: A Review, NCBI, PMC, US National Library of Medicine, National Institutes of Health, HHS Publix Access, Author manuscript: Exp Clin Psychopharmacol. Author manuscript; available in PMC 2017 Aug 1. Published in final edited form as: Exp Clin Psychopharmacol. 2016 Aug; 24(4): (pp 229–268). doi: 10.1037/pha0000084
https://www.ncbi.nlm.nih.gov/pmc/articles/PMC5001686/

Daniel, J., Haberman, M., (2017). Clinical potential of psilocybin as a treatment for mental health conditions, NCBI, PMC, US National Library of Medicine, National Institutes of Health, The Mental Health Clinic: Ment Health Clin. 2017 Jan; 7(1): (pp 24–28). Published online 2018 Mar 23. doi: 10.9740/mhc.2017.01.024
https://www.ncbi.nlm.nih.gov/pmc/articles/PMC6007659/

Serafini, G., Howland, RH., Rovedi, F., et al. (2014). The Role of Ketamine in Treatment-Resistant Depression: A Systematic Review, NCBI, PMC, US National Library of Medicine, National Institutes of Health, Current Neuropharmacacology: Curr Neuropharmacol. 2014 Sep 12(5): (pp 444–461). Published online 2014 Sep. doi:10.2174/1570159X12666140619204251
https://www.ncbi.nlm.nih.gov/pmc/articles/PMC4243034/

SECTION 6 - Diet and Nutrition

7 Tips for Good Food Choices

Michael Pollan is the author of several bestselling books including The Omnivore's Dilemma, In Defense of Food, and Food Rules. His best advice is:

1. Don't eat anything your great grandmother wouldn't recognize as food.

2. Don't eat anything with more than five ingredients, or ingredients you can't pronounce.

3. Stay out of the middle of the supermarket; shop on the perimeter of the store. Real food tends to be on the outer edge of the store near the loading docks, where it can be replaced with fresh foods when it goes bad.

4. Don't eat anything that won't eventually rot (with the exception of honey).

5. If it came from a plant, eat it. If it was made in a plant, don't.

6. Enjoy meals with the people you love. Families traditionally ate together, around a table and not a TV, at regular meal times. It's a good tradition.

7. It is not just what you eat but how you eat. (See Chapter 7.1. Yangsheng: The Art of Self Care).

Pollan, M, (2006). The Omnivore's Dilemma: A Natural History of Four Meals. The Penguin Press : New York, USA.

Pollan, M, (2008). In Defense of Food: An Eater's Manifesto. The Penguin Press : New York, USA.

Pollan, M, (2009). Food Rules: An Eater's Manual. The Penguin Press : New York, USA.

6.1 Digestion, Absorption, and Elimination

Nutrition is a critical factor when it comes to transitioning smoothly through menopause. It also has a significant impact on health and wellbeing in the years to come, with good nutrition allowing women to optimize their quality of life well into middle age and beyond.

Eating a healthy, balanced diet should preferably begin in one's 30s or even earlier. And while most of us are aware of the fundamentals of good nutrition, it is essential to assess each patient's individual needs and advise them accordingly.

Furthermore, there are additional aspects to consider in menopausal patients. As well as looking at what our patients eat, we must also assess how well they are able to digest, absorb, and eliminate these foods.

Much of the information in this chapter, and the following two, is based on the teachings of Susan Kath, a naturopathic nutritionist with a special interest in supporting cognitive health and reversing cognitive decline.

Factors Influencing Digestion, Absorption, and Elimination

Bone and Muscle Mass

Older women are likely to have reduced bone mass (osteopenia) and muscle mass (sarcopenia). Therefore, their nutritional requirements will differ from younger women.

Basal Metabolic Rate

Muscle mass is one of the most significant factors influencing basal metabolic rate. Therefore, the sarcopenia that naturally occurs with aging can slow one's metabolism and thus reduce energy requirements.

Metabolic Dysregulation

Metabolic dysregulation can occur as a result of hypothyroidism, reduced glucose tolerance or insulin resistance, and metabolic syndrome. Menopause is also associated with changes in lipid metabolism which can increase the risk of cardiovascular disease. While the focus during menopause is often on estrogen, balancing all of a woman's hormones will allow them to function optimally.

Absorption of Nutrients

Postmenopausal women have a reduced ability to absorb certain nutrients such as calcium. Furthermore, certain substances may either enhance or inhibit the absorption of others. For example, vitamin C enhances iron absorption while caffeine interferes with it.

Sleep Quality

Menopausal women often suffer from reduced sleep quantity and quality. Short sleep durations are associated with increases in the hormone ghrelin, an appetite stimulator, and decreases in the hormone leptin, an appetite suppressant. These changes may contribute to increased calorie intake and weight gain.

Energy and Fatigue

Reduced energy is a common issue among menopausal women and is often seen as a normal part of the aging process. It may be related to lack of sleep, chronic illness, poorly regulated blood sugar, circulatory disorders, mitochondrial dysfunction, or general lack of nutrition.

Stressors and Stress Resistance

The primary stress hormone, cortisol, increases glucose in the bloodstream and curbs functions that would be nonessential in a fight or flight situation, such as suppressing the immune, digestive, and reproductive systems and slowing growth processes. Therefore, raised cortisol levels are detrimental over long periods as in cases of chronic stress. Additionally, adrenaline increases heart rate, elevates blood pressure, and boosts short-term energy supplies.

Environmental Toxin Exposure

Exposure to toxins, including xenoestrogens, mold, water or tick-borne disease, polychlorinated biphenyls (PCBs), phthalates, parabens, pesticides, and chlorine, coupled with reduced liver function will impact a woman's nutritional needs.

Genetics

Genetic testing can help to identify areas where nutritional supplementation may be beneficial. Single nuclear polymorphisms (SNPs) can influence nutrient absorption and metabolism as well as hormonal balance and detoxification.

Methylation

Methylation plays a key role in gene expression, and its dysregulation can contribute to a range of chronic conditions (see Chapter 2.4 Genetics and Epigenetics for more detail).

Some of the key nutrients for regulating methylation include methionine (an essential amino acid), vitamins B2, B6, and B12, folate, choline, betaine, magnesium, zinc, plant polyphenols (including catechin, epicatechin, and epigallocatechin gallate found in green tea), genistein, flavonoids (including quercetin, fisetin, myricetin), and the supplement S-adenosylmethionine (SAMe).

Chronic Health Issues

Chronic health issues, including inflammatory conditions and viral overload, can alter nutritional requirements and the ability to digest and absorb nutrients.

Other critical factors to consider include gut health, hormonal balance, and vitamin and micronutrient intake, which we will discuss in more detail in the following sections.

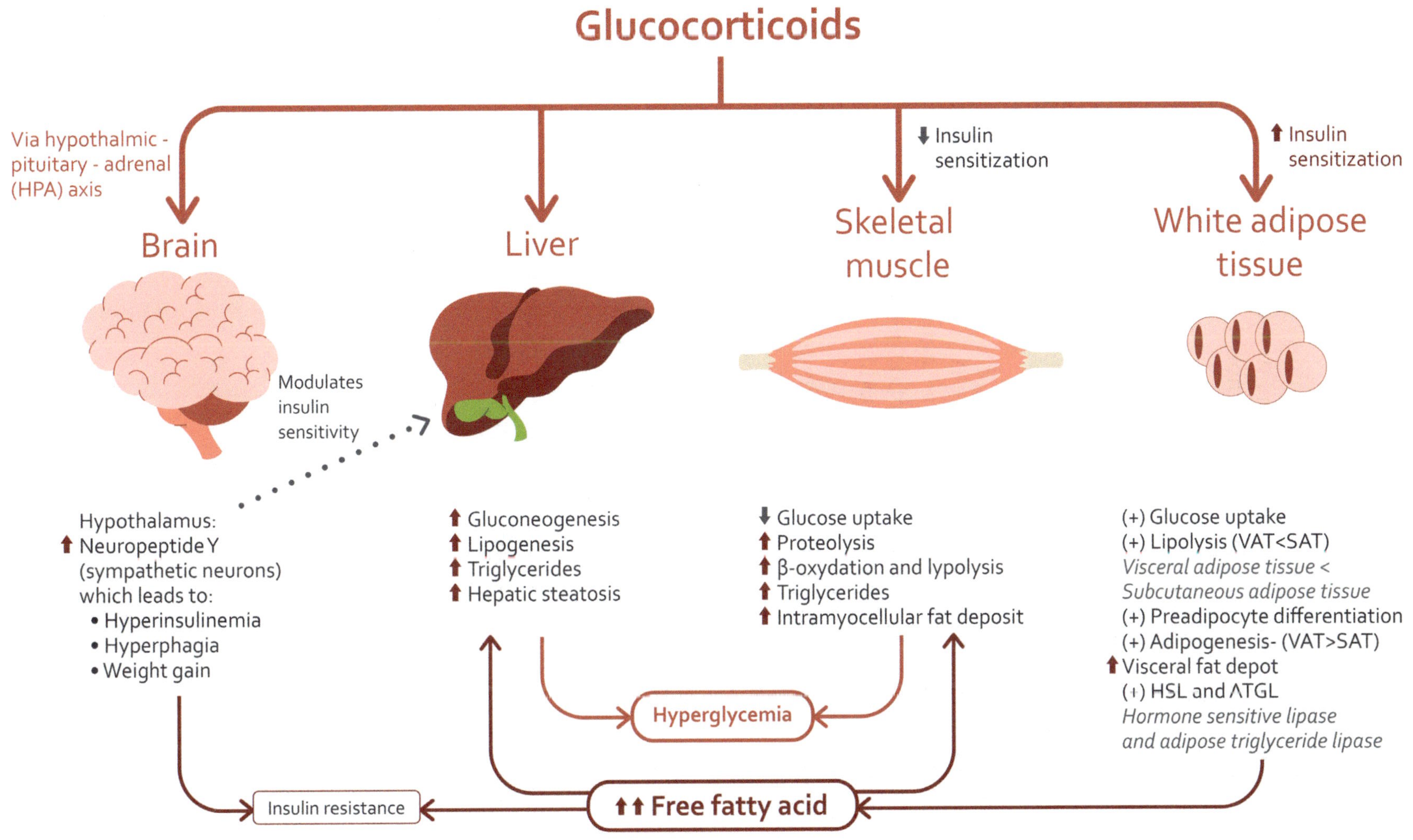

Figure 6.1a: Mechanisms of glucocorticoid-induced insulin resistance.[23]

Source: Courtesy of the U.S. National Library of Medicine.

[23] Geer, EB., Islam, J., Buettner, C., (2014) Mechanisms of Glucocorticoid-Induced Insulin Resistance, NIH National Library of Medicine, HHS Public Access: Endocrinol Metab Clin North Am. Author manuscript; available in PMC 2015 Mar 1. Published in final edited form as: Endocrinol Metab Clin North Am. 2014 Mar; 43(1): 75–102. doi: 10.1016/j.ecl.2013.10.005. https://www.ncbi.nlm.nih.gov/pmc/articles/PMC3942672/

Gut Health

The gut controls a large proportion of hormone synthesis and regulation. Gut health relies heavily on the microbiota, the population of microorganisms that inhabit the digestive tract. Having greater diversity within the microbiota is considered more beneficial for health.

Advantages of a Healthy Gut Microbiota

- Clearing excess hormones.
- Clearing xenoestrogens and other toxins.
- Lowering triglycerides and excess cholesterol, thus reducing the risk of cardiovascular disease.
- Regulating body weight by influencing insulin sensitivity and blood sugar.
- Enhancing immunity.
- Anticarcinogenic effects.
- Improving mood and emotional stability via gamma-aminobutyric acid (GABA) and serotonin production, as well as communication with the brain via the vagus nerve.
- Controlling harmful microorganisms e.g. parasites, fungi, and yeast.
- Breaking down fiber to release additional nutrients from food.
- Improving mineral absorption and balance.
- Synthesis of micronutrients e.g. fatty acids, B vitamins, and vitamin K2, which ensures calcium deposits in bones and not in the arteries.

Dysbiosis

When the microbiota becomes imbalanced, the resulting condition is known as dysbiosis. Some common examples include small intestinal bacterial overgrowth (SIBO) and irritable bowel syndrome (IBS), which can cause symptoms such as changes in bowel patterns, abdominal pain and bloating.

In some cases, dysbiosis affects the oestrobolome, the portion of the microbiota responsible for estrogen metabolism. The result is excess estrogen re-entering the bloodstream rather than being excreted. Complications include:

- Obesity
- Estrogen-receptor positive cancers
- Uterine hyperplasia
- Endometriosis
- Fibroids
- Premenstrual syndrome
- Menorrhagia
- Cardiovascular disease
- Cancer
- Cognitive issues
- Metabolic syndrome

Improving Gut Health

It is possible to significantly improve gut health by switching from a standard westernized diet to one that is rich in plant-based fiber and polyphenols from brightly colored fruit and vegetables.

Alcohol, non-steroidal anti-inflammatory drugs (NSAIDs), some antibiotics, oral contraceptives, stress, and high-sugar, high-fat diets all have a negative impact on gut health and should be minimized or avoided altogether.

Prebiotics

Prebiotics increase the diversity of the microbiota, including firmicutes and bifidogenic strains. These microorganisms ferment carbohydrates to produce butyrate, a short-chain fatty acid that plays a role in energy metabolism, gut barrier function, and reducing inflammation.

Sources of Prebiotics

Vegetables, fruit, grains, fructooligosaccharides (FOS), inulin, galactooligosaccharides (GOS), partially hydrolysed guar gum (PHGG), resistant starch, soluble fiber, and polyphenols.[24]

Probiotics

Probiotics contain live cultures of beneficial microorganisms and can help to maintain a healthy microbiota. Fermented foods are rich in probiotics and they are also available as supplements. However, care should be taken with probiotic drinks as they may have a high sugar content. Furthermore, many commercial fermented foods are pasteurized and will, therefore, have little impact on gut health. Patients should focus on fresh products such as yogurt or kefir rather than those stored in jars with a long shelf-life. Those with a desire to do so could also ferment their own probiotic foods at home.

Sources of Probiotics

Live yogurt, kefir, beet kvass, sauerkraut, kimchi, and kombucha.

Bone broth

Bone broth is rich in collagen and other beneficial substances that improve gut barrier integrity to prevent the leakage of pro-inflammatory compounds, including lipopolysaccharides and endotoxins.

---

[24] It is necessary to exercise caution when recommending high-fiber diets to patients with dysbiosis or digestive disorders such as irritable bowel syndrome. Patients should switch from low-fiber to higher-fiber diets gradually and under the supervision of a qualified nutritionist or dietician.

Cholesterol

Hormone synthesis requires an adequate intake of cholesterol since this molecule is the basis for all steroid hormones, including estrogen and progesterone. It is also essential for healthy cell membranes and synthesizing vitamin D from sunlight. (See Chapter 2.2 Female Reproductive Hormones, figure 2.2a Sex hormone biosynthesis pathway, page 23.).

Cholesterol is derived from animal food sources and plant-based fats but is also synthesized endogenously by the liver. It is circulated in the bloodstream in two forms:

1. High-Density Lipoprotein (HDL) Cholesterol
HDL cholesterol is often referred to as "good cholesterol." It picks up excess cholesterol in the blood and carries it back to the liver where it is broken down and removed from the body.

2. Low-Density Lipoprotein (LDL) Cholesterol
High levels of LDL cholesterol may eventually build up in the blood vessels causing atherosclerosis and narrowing of the arteries, thus raising the risk of cardiovascular disease. For this reason, LDL cholesterol is often referred to as "bad cholesterol."

However, the total LDL shown on a standard blood test may not reliably indicate the absolute risk of cardiovascular disease. This is because several other factors have a more significant impact, including having a higher number of particles of smaller size, and whether they are oxidized.

Furthermore, APOE genetic status affects how the body utilizes cholesterol and subsequently its overall levels. People who have the APOE4 genotype have a predisposition to higher cholesterol levels. Therefore, it is necessary to consider genetics and monitor whether dietary modifications to reduce saturated fat and cholesterol intake improve a patient's cholesterol levels.

Care should be taken with dietary cholesterol since many high-cholesterol foods are also high in saturated fats, a major contributing factor to cardiovascular disease (see below). Therefore, it is preferable to select sources that are lower in saturated fats.

Low-Fat Sources of Cholesterol

Avocado, fish, and chicken.

High-Fat Sources of Cholesterol

Beef, cheese, and butter.

Improving Hormonal Clearance

Enhancing Liver Function

The liver plays an essential role in the clearance of excess hormones via the pathways of sulfation and glucuronidation. These processes can be enhanced by several foods, including grapefruit, cruciferous vegetables, and nutrients like vitamins B6, B12, folate, molybdenum, and the amino acids cysteine (poultry, eggs, beef, whole grains) and methionine (eggs, cod, chicken, beef, pork, milk, rice).

Liver function can be supported by eating more bitter foods (e.g. endive, radicchio, dandelion, rocket, watercress, etc.) which help to reduce fatty liver, improve bile flow, and clear estrogens and toxins.

Glutathione Synthesis

It is also helpful to improve glutathione synthesis. Glutathione is the body's master antioxidant. It is composed of the amino acids cysteine, glycine, and glutamate. Adequate intake of methionine from protein is required to produce homocysteine that is then synthesized into cysteine, the rate-limiting amino acid involved in the production of glutathione. This occurs via the transsulfuration pathway.

Glutathione synthesis also requires adequate intake of several other nutrients, including B vitamins and betaine. Notably, the intermediary molecule, homocysteine, can damage endothelial cells and increase the risk of cardiovascular disease. Adequate intake of B vitamins, vitamin C, and vitamin E may offer some protection.

Calcium-D-Glucarate

Calcium-D-glucarate plays a vital role in estrogen metabolism. It is the calcium salt of glucaric acid, which is present in a variety of foods. Calcium-D-glucarate is also available as a supplement.

Sources of Glucaric Acid

Oranges, apples, grapefruit, and cruciferous vegetables.

Increase Elimination

There are two major types of elimination: excretion and biotransformation.

Excretion

Excretion is the removal of substances from the body, mainly by urine or feces. Therefore, maintaining regular bowel movements and urination is essential, and adequate fiber and water intake is key. Eating plenty of fiber is also associated with a lower risk of heart disease, stroke, type 2 diabetes, and bowel cancer.

Sources of Fiber

Breakfast cereals: wholewheat cereal biscuits, shredded wholegrain pillows, and porridge oats.

Starchy carbohydrates: potatoes, bread, cereals, rice, and pasta.

Pulses: baked beans, red, green, yellow and brown lentils, chickpeas (chana or garbanzo beans), garden peas, black-eyed peas, runner beans, broad beans (fava beans), kidney beans, butter beans (Lima beans), haricot beans, cannellini beans, flageolet beans, pinto beans, and borlotti beans.

Other Excretion Pathways

Other elimination pathways include excretion into bile, sweat, saliva, milk (via lactation), or other body fluids. Volatile substances, such as gaseous anesthetics, alcohol, and some drugs, are excreted via the lungs into expired air.

Biotransformation

Biotransformation is the process by which a substance is chemically converted by the body to a metabolite. The enzymes involved in the biotransformation of drugs are primarily located in the liver and other tissues such as the kidneys, lungs, small intestine, and skin.

Engaging in physical exercise and practices such as skin brushing, saunas, and breathing can help to eliminate toxins via the skin and lungs, thus taking some of the strain off the liver and allowing for better hormone clearance. It is also essential to reduce one's exposure to toxins, including xenoestrogens, pesticides, heavy metals, etc. to reduce the burden on the body and detoxify effectively. This is especially important if there are multiple inherited genetic polymorphisms on genes involved in detoxification processes.

Hormonal Imbalances

Some common hormonal imbalances are listed in table 6.1a on page 281.

Imbalance	Symptoms	Advice
Estrogen dominance (estrogen is relatively high in comparison to progesterone)	PMS Menstrual irregularities Low libido Fatigue Fibroids Endometriosis Fibrocystic breasts	Natural aromatase inhibitors (e.g. lignans) Reduce adipose tissue Reduce alcohol intake Check for gut dysbiosis Remove endocrine disruptors and toxins Check for exposure to molds and biotoxins
DHT (dihydrotestosterone)	Insulin resistance PCOS Hair loss Hirsutism Obesity Breast cancer	Increase protein intake Reduce sodium intake Licorice Reduce alpha-reductase activity (with zinc, nettle, saw palmetto, green tea)

Table 6.1a: Hormone imbalances.

Summary

Menopause can alter a person's nutritional requirements significantly. Numerous factors including altered metabolism, gut health, and hormonal status can have an impact. Therefore, menopausal patients should consider consulting a professional such as a naturopathic nutritionist to determine their individual needs and design an appropriate eating plan.

References

Kath, S., (2019). Nutrition, Food supplements and Lifestyle for Optimising Midlife and Beyond. Treating Women Academy: Online Menopause Masterclass.
https://www.treatingwomen.com/store/5tpUJ3Fk

Agostini, D., Zeppa, SD., Lucertini, F., et al. (2018). Muscle and Bone Health in Postmenopausal Women: Role of Protein and Vitamin D Supplementation Combined with Exercise Training, PMC US National Library of Medicine, National Institutes of Health, Nutrients MDPI: Nutrients. 2018 Aug; 10(8) (pp 1103). Published online 2018 Aug 16. doi: 10.3390/nu10081103.
https://www.ncbi.nlm.nih.gov/pmc/articles/PMC6116194/

Taheri, S., Lin, L., Austin, D., et al. (2004). Short Sleep Duration Is Associated with Reduced Leptin, Elevated Ghrelin, and Increased Body Mass Index, PMC US National Library of Medicine, National Institutes of Health, PLOS Medicine: PLoS Med. 2004 Dec; 1(3): e62. Published online 2004 Dec 7. doi: 10.1371/journal.pmed.0010062.
https://www.ncbi.nlm.nih.gov/pmc/articles/PMC535701/

Azzolino, D., Arosio, B., Marzetti, E., et al. (2020). Nutritional Status as a Mediator of Fatigue and Its Underlying Mechanisms in Older People, PMC US National Library of Medicine, National Institutes of Health, Nutrients MDPI: Nutrients. 2020 Feb; 12(2): 444. Published online 2020 Feb 10. doi: 10.3390/nu12020444.
https://www.ncbi.nlm.nih.gov/pmc/articles/PMC7071235/

Ko, S-H., Kim, H-S., (2020). Menopause-Associated Lipid Metabolic Disorders and Foods Beneficial for Postmenopausal Women, PMC US National Library of Medicine, National Institutes of Health, Nutrients MDPI: Nutrients. 2020 Jan; 12(1): 202. Published online 2020 Jan 13. doi: 10.3390/nu12010202.
https://www.ncbi.nlm.nih.gov/pmc/articles/PMC7019719/

Kampa, A., Daimon, M., Murakami, H., et al. (2016). Association between Higher Serum Cortisol Levels and Decreased Insulin Secretion in a General Population, PMC US National Library of Medicine, National Institutes of Health, PLOS One: PLoS One. 2016; 11(11): e0166077. Published online 2016 Nov 18. doi: 10.1371/journal.pone.0166077.
https://www.ncbi.nlm.nih.gov/pmc/articles/PMC5115704/

Wellwood, C., Rardin, S., (2014). Adrenal and Thyroid Supplementation Outperforms Nutritional Supplementation and Medications for Autoimmune Thyroiditis, PMC US National Library of Medicine, National Institutes of Health, IMCJ, Integrative Medicine: A Clinician's Journal: Integr Med (Encinitas). 2014 Jun; 13(3): (pp 41–47).
https://www.ncbi.nlm.nih.gov/pmc/articles/PMC4684134/

Jin, Z., Liu, Y., (2018). DNA methylation in human diseases, Elsevier, Genes & Diseases: Genes Dis. 2018 Mar; 5(1): 1–8. Published online 2018 Jan 31. doi: 10.1016/j.gendis.2018.01.002.
https://www.ncbi.nlm.nih.gov/pmc/articles/PMC6147084/

Kadayifci, FZ., Zheng, S., Pan, Y-X., (2018). Molecular Mechanisms Underlying the Link between Diet and DNA Methylation, PMC US National Library of Medicine, National Institutes of Health, MDPI, International Journal of Molecular Sciences: Int J Mol Sci. 2018 Dec; 19(12): 4055. Published online 2018 Dec 14. doi: 10.3390/ijms19124055.
https://www.ncbi.nlm.nih.gov/pmc/articles/PMC6320837/

Kwa, M., Plottel, CS., Blaser, MJ., et al. (2016). The Intestinal Microbiome and Estrogen Receptor–Positive Female Breast Cancer, PMC US National Library of Medicine, National Institutes of Health, JNCI, Journal of the National Cancer Institute: J Natl Cancer Inst. 2016 Aug; 108(8): djw029. Published online 2016 Apr 22.
doi: 10.1093/jnci/djw029 https://www.ncbi.nlm.nih.gov/pmc/articles/PMC5017946/

Donohoe, Dr.., Garge, N., Zhang, X., et al. (2011). The Microbiome and Butyrate Regulate Energy Metabolism and Autophagy in the Mammalian Colon, PMC US National Library of Medicine, National Institutes of Health, HHS Public Access, Author Manuscript: Cell Metab. Author manuscript; available in PMC 2012 May 4. Published in final edited form as: Cell Metab. 2011 May 4; 13(5): (pp 517–526). doi: 10.1016/j.cmet.2011.02.018.
https://www.ncbi.nlm.nih.gov/pmc/articles/PMC3099420/

Liu, H., Wang, J., He, T., et al. (2018). Butyrate: A Double-Edged Sword for Health? Oxford Academic: Advances in Nutrition, Volume 9, Issue 1, January 2018, (pp 21–29), https://doi.org/10.1093/advances/nmx009.
https://academic.oup.com/advances/article/9/1/21/4849000

Soliman, GA., (2018). Dietary Cholesterol and the Lack of Evidence in Cardiovascular Disease,PMC US National Library of Medicine, National Institutes of Health, MDPI, Nutrients: Nutrients. 2018 Jun; 10(6): (pp 780). Published online 2018 Jun 16. doi: 10.3390/nu10060780.
https://www.ncbi.nlm.nih.gov/pmc/articles/PMC6024687/

National Library of Medicine, National Center for Biotechnology Information. (2002). Calcium-D-glucarate: PMID: 12197785.
https://pubmed.ncbi.nlm.nih.gov/12197785/

Lu, SC., (2013). Glutathione Synthesis, PMC US National Library of Medicine, National Institutes of Health, HHS Public Access, Author Manuscript: Biochim Biophys Acta. Author manuscript; available in PMC 2014 May 1. Published in final edited form as: Biochim Biophys Acta. 2013 May; 1830(5): (pp 3143–3153). Published online 2012 Sep 17. doi:10.1016/j.bbagen.2012.09.008.
https://www.ncbi.nlm.nih.gov/pmc/articles/PMC3549305/

Lee, SR., Lee, S-Y., Kim, S-Y., et al. (2017). Hydroxylation and sulfation of sex steroid hormones in inflammatory liver, PMC US National Library of Medicine, National Institutes of Health, The Journal of Biomedical Research: J Biomed Res. 2017; 31(5): (pp 437–444).. doi: 10.7555/JBR.31.20170031.
https://www.ncbi.nlm.nih.gov/pmc/articles/PMC5706436/

Nimni, ME., Han, B., Cordoba, F., (2007). Are we getting enough sulfur in our diet? PMC US National Library of Medicine, National Institutes of Health, Nutrition & Metabolism: Nutr Metab (Lond). 2007; 4: 24. Published online 2007 Nov 6. doi: 10.1186/1743-7075-4-24.
https://www.ncbi.nlm.nih.gov/pmc/articles/PMC2198910/

Larsson, SC., Håkansson, N., Wolk, A., (2015). Dietary Cysteine and Other Amino Acids and Stroke Incidence in Women, Unit of Nutritional Epidemiology, Institute of Environmental Medicine, Karolinska Institutet, Stockholm, Sweden: URL: http://www.clinicaltrials.gov. Unique identifier: NCT01127698. (Stroke. 2015;46:922-926.
DOI: 10.1161/STROKEAHA.114.008022.)
https://www.ahajournals.org/doi/pdf/10.1161/STROKEAHA.114.008022.

Kohlmeier, M., (2003). Methionine, Science Direct:
https://www.sciencedirect.com/topics/agricultural-and-biological-sciences/methionine

Perna, AF., Ingrosso, D., Lombardi, C., et al. (2003). Possible mechanisms of homocysteine toxicity, Kidney International ISN: Homocysteine| Volume 63, Supplement 84, S137-S140, May 01, 2003
https://www.kidney-international.org/article/S0085-2538(15)49237-3/fulltext

6.2 Vitamins, Minerals, and Micronutrients

Vitamins, minerals, and various other micronutrients are organic compounds that are essential for cellular function and maintaining health. While it is important to consume enough micronutrients at every stage of life, menopause can increase the necessity for specific vitamins and minerals. Many other micronutrients may also be beneficial for menopausal and post-menopausal patients, potentially reducing symptom severity and decreasing the risk of chronic disease.

Essential Micronutrients for Menopause

Some of the most crucial micronutrients during menopause are discussed in detail below. A further summary of all the essential micronutrients and their sources can be found in table 6.2a.

Vitamin A

Vitamin A is necessary for the conversion of pregnenolone to progesterone or DHEA. It is present in its active form, retinol, in animal sources. However, in plant sources, it is available as carotenoids, which must be converted to retinol in the body. Therefore, vegans or those eating a largely plant-based diet may require supplementation.

B Vitamins

There are eight B vitamins, collectively called B complex vitamins. They are thiamine (B1), riboflavin (B2), niacin (B3), pantothenic acid (B5), pyridoxine (B6), biotin (B7), folate (B9), and cobalamin (B12). Though each of these vitamins has unique functions, they generally help the body produce energy and synthesize important molecules within the cells. Aside from B12, the body cannot store these vitamins for long periods, so it is necessary to replenish them regularly through food.

In terms of hormonal balance, vitamin B3 is necessary for the conversion of pregnenolone to progesterone or DHEA, and vitamin B5 supports adrenal health. Meanwhile, vitamins B6, B12, and B9 improve methylation, a process that alters the expression of DNA, potentially offering protection against certain cancers.

Vitamin D

Vitamin D is a prohormone and, along with vitamin K and calcium, is involved in hormone signaling. It also aids the absorption of calcium and, thus, supports bone health.

The primary source of vitamin D is sunlight on the skin. Therefore, many people living in regions with limited sunlight may require supplementation, especially during winter. There are also several dietary sources, like oily fish, liver, and egg yolks.

Vitamin K

There are two forms of vitamin K; K1 (phylloquinone) and K2 (menaquinone). Vitamin K1 is found in several dietary sources, primarily leafy green vegetables. Vitamin K2 is found in fermented dairy products. As well as being available from dietary sources, some vitamin K is synthesized by gut bacteria, further emphasising the importance of a healthy microbiota.

Vitamin K works synergistically with vitamin D to support bone and cardiovascular health. It also appears to play a role in metabolism by regulating insulin secretion and signaling.

Choline

Choline is a source of methyl groups necessary for many steps in metabolism. It is essential for the signaling function of cell membranes and deficiency can lead to liver and muscular dysfunction as well as nonalcoholic fatty liver disease (NAFLD or hepatosteatosis).

Choline is required for synthesizing acetylcholine, the primary neurotransmitter of the parasympathetic nervous system. Its functions include regulating smooth muscle control of the lungs, blood vessels, and heart. It is also important for memory and learning and is deficient in cases of dementia and Alzheimer's disease.

Postmenopausal women have higher choline requirements due to their decreased estrogen levels. Furthermore, certain genetic mutations, such as PEMT, may reduce de novo choline synthesis, increasing reliance on dietary intake.

Sources of Choline

Meat (especially beef liver), poultry, fish, dairy products, hard boiled eggs, shiitake mushrooms, baked red potatoes (flesh and skin), Brussels sprouts, broccoli, cauliflower, green peas, cabbage, beans (soybeans, kidney beans, green beans), peanuts, sunflower seeds, whole grains.

Spinach, beets, wheat, and shellfish are also good sources of the choline metabolite, *betaine*.

Beneficial Micronutrients

Micronutrient	Benefits	Sources
Alkylresorcinols (phenolic lipids)	May reduce the risk of diabetes, cardiovascular disease, and several cancers	• Wholegrains • Wheat • Rye
Allicin	Antimicrobial – may reduce the risk of ulcers and reduce blood cholesterol	• Garlic • Onions • Leeks • Chives
Carotenoids (including beta-carotene, lycopene, lutein, etc.)	Antioxidant effects – may reduce the risk of cancer and other chronic diseases	• Apricots • Cantaloupe • Carrots • Pumpkin • Sweet potato • Tomatoes • Broccoli • Spinach
Capsaicin	Anticoagulant and anti-inflammatory – may reduce the risk of fatal blood clots	Hot peppers
Curcumin[25]	Antioxidant, anti-inflammatory, and anticoagulant – may suppress carcinogen activating enzymes	Turmeric
Flavonoids (including flavones, isoflavones, flavanols, catechins)	Antioxidant effects – neutralize reactive oxygen species and carcinogens, may inhibit cells proliferation	• Black and green tea • Wine • Whole wheat • Soy beans Fruit, vegetables, and herbs, especially: • Celery • Citrus fruit • Olives • Onions • Oregano • Berries • Purple grapes
Genistein and daidzein	Phytoestrogens – weakly mimic or modulate estrogen activity. May reduce the risk of some cancers and osteoporosis and inhibit GI cell proliferation	• Soy beans • Soy milk • Soy flour • Tofu • Textured vegetable protein • Other legumes and legume products

[25] Curcumin is fat-soluble and should be consumed with a healthy fat to facilitate absorption. Piperine (found in black pepper) also significantly enhances its bioavailability.

Micronutrient	Benefits	Sources
Indoles	May stimulate the production of enzymes that inhibit DNA damage and estrogen activity due to carcinogens	Cruciferous vegetables, including: • Broccoli • Brussels sprouts • Cabbage • Cauliflower • Mustard greens • Kale • Horseradish
Isothiocyanates	Antioxidant – may inhibit carcinogen-activating enzymes	Cruciferous vegetables
Monoterpenes (e.g., limonene)	May stimulate the production of enzymes that detoxify carcinogens and inhibit cell proliferation	Citrus peel and citrus peel oil
Phenolic acids	May increase the water-solubility of carcinogens and improve excretion	• Coffee • Oats • Potatoes • Soy beans Fruit, especially: • Apples • Cherries • Grapes • Blueberries • Oranges • Prunes • Pears
Resveratrol	Antioxidant and anti-inflammatory – may suppress cancer cell growth, reduce LDL cholesterol oxidation, and prevent clot formation	• Red wine • Grapes • Raspberries • Peanuts
Saponins	May interfere with DNA replication and prevent cancer cell proliferation, support immune response	• Soy beans • Potatoes • Green vegetables • Alfalfa and other sprouts • Tomatoes
Tannins	Antioxidant, may inhibit carcinogen activation and cancer progression	• Black-eyed peas • Grapes • Lentils • Wine • Tea

Table 6.2a: Sources of micronutrients.[26]

[26] Ko, S-H., Kim, H-S., (2020). Menopause-Associated Lipid Metabolic Disorders and Foods Beneficial for Postmenopausal Women, PMC US National Library of Medicine, National Institutes of Health, Nutrients MDPI: Nutrients. 2020 Jan; 12(1): 202. Published online 2020 Jan 13. doi: 10.3390/nu12010202. https://www.ncbi.nlm.nih.gov/pmc/articles/PMC7019719/

Minerals

Mineral	Functions	Sources
Calcium	Maintains healthy bones and teeth Regulates muscle contractions, including the heart Plays a role in blood clotting	• Dairy products • Cereals • Nuts • Seeds • Pulses • Leafy greens
Iron	A component of hemoglobin	• Liver • Offal • Red meat • Beans • Nuts • Dried fruit • Fortified cereals
Magnesium	Regulates sodium and potassium levels Aids absorption and metabolism of other nutrients Supports parathyroid glands for bone health	Widespread in foods, especially: • Wholemeal bread • Spinach • Nuts
Manganese	Aids in production and activation of certain enzymes	• Whole grain cereals • Nuts • Bread • Green vegetables, including peas
Molybdenum	Aids in production and activation of certain enzymes	• Legumes • Whole grains • Nuts • Beef liver
Phosphorus	Maintains healthy bones and teeth Releases energy from food	• Red meat • Dairy products • Fish • Poultry • Bread • Brown rice • Oats
Potassium	Controls fluid balance within the body to maintain blood pressure Assists heart muscle function	• Bananas • Nuts • Seeds • Parsnips• Beef • Fish • Pulses • Poultry • Broccoli • Brussels sprouts
Zinc	Supports cell and enzyme production Processes carbohydrates, fats, and protein Supports wound healing	• Meat • Shellfish • Bread • Dairy products • Cereals

Table 6.2b: Sources of minerals.[27]

[27] Minerals from plant-based sources are often bound by phytic acid which decreases their bioavailability significantly. The phytic acid content of foods can be reduced by milling, soaking, germinating, and fermenting. Therefore, these processes are recommended to facilitate more efficient nutrient absorption.
Table source: https://www.nhs.uk/conditions/vitamins-and-minerals/

Water-Soluble Vitamins

Vitamin	Functions	Sources
B1	Breaks down and releases energy from food	• Peas • Bananas • Oranges • Nuts • Whole grain bread • Fortified cereals • Liver
B2	Maintains eye, skin, and nervous system health Releases energy from food	• Milk • Eggs • Mushrooms • Fortified cereals • Plain yogurt
B3	Maintains skin and nervous system health Releases energy from food	• Meat • Fish • Eggs • Wheat flour
B5	Releases energy from food	• Chicken • Mushrooms • Kidneys • Eggs • Avocado • Fortified cereals • Beef • Liver
B6	Aids the body's storage of protein and carbohydrates A component of hemoglobin	• Pork • Poultry • Peanuts • Some fish • Soya beans • Wheatgerm • Bananas • Oats • Fortified cereals • Milk
B7	Aids synthesis of fatty acids	Produced by intestinal microbiota, only found in very low levels in food
B9	Aids production of red blood cells Reduces risk of birth defects, such as spina bifida	• Broccoli • Leafy greens • Brussels sprouts • Peas • Chickpeas • Kidney beans • Liver • Fortified cereals
B12	Aids production of red blood cells Supports nervous system function Releases energy from food Assists the body in utising folate (B9)	• Meat • Fish • Milk • Eggs • Cheese • Fortified cereals
C	Aids iron absorption Aids collagen production to maintain healthy skin, blood vessels, cartilage, and bone Aids wound healing Antioxidant	• Citrus fruit • Peppers • Strawberries • Potatoes • Blackberries • Broccoli • Blackcurrants • Brussels sprouts

Table 6.2c: Water-soluble vitamins.[28]

[28] As these nutrients are water-soluble, cooking methods such as boiling can significantly reduce their concentration in food. Lightly steaming or stir-frying helps to preserve water-soluble nutrients and is the recommended method for cooking vegetables.

Fat-Soluble Vitamins

Vitamin	Functions	Sources
A	Supports immune function Improves eye health, especially night vision Maintains the health of skin and mucous membranes	• Liver • Oily fish • Egg yolks • Squashes • Dairy products • Sweet potatoes • Carrots • Mangoes • Papaya • Maize • Dark leafy greens
D	Aids calcium absorption Maintains healthy bones and teeth Supports nervous system function	• Sunlight • Meat • Oily fish • Egg yolk • Butter • Cereals • Fortified spreads
E	Maintains the health of cell walls Antioxidant	• Vegetable oils • Lettuce • Nuts • Seeds • Leafy greens • Wheatgerm
K	Aids blood clotting Supports bone health	• Leafy greens • Vegetable oils • Cereals • Cheese • Liver • Fermented dairy products

Table 6.2d: Fat-soluble vitamins.[29]

Long-term overconsumption of fat-soluble vitamins can be toxic and even fatal. Although hypervitaminosis is rare and unlikely to occur from normal dietary intake, anyone taking supplements should ensure they do not exceed the maximum dosage. It is also essential to keep in mind that supplements such as multivitamins and fish oils both contain fat-soluble vitamins and should not be taken together.

Summary

Adequate intake of vitamins, minerals, and other micronutrients is essential throughout life and the demand for certain micronutrients may increase during and after menopause. Ideally, patients should meet these nutritional needs by consuming a varied diet rather than taking supplements. However, supplements may be appropriate for some individuals with specific micronutrient deficiencies or medical conditions. In these cases, supplements should be taken with guidance from a doctor, nutritionist or qualified dietician.

[29] As these vitamins are fat-soluble, it is necessary to consume them with some dietary fat to aid absorption.

References

Kath, S., (2019). Nutrition, Food Supplements and Lifestyle for Optimising Midlife and Beyond. Treating Women Academy: Online Menopause Masterclass.
https://www.treatingwomen.com/store/5tpUJ3Fk

NIH, National Institutes of Health, Office of Dietary Supplements. (2021). Molybdenum Fact Sheet for Health Professionals.
https://ods.od.nih.gov/factsheets/Molybdenum-HealthProfessional

Albahrani, AA., Greaves, RF., (2016). Fat-Soluble Vitamins: Clinical Indications and Current Challenges for Chromatographic Measurement, PMC US National Library of Medicine, National Institutes of Health, AACB, The Clinical Biochemist Reviews: Clin Biochem Rev. 2016 Feb; 37(1):(pp 27–47).
https://www.ncbi.nlm.nih.gov/pmc/articles/PMC4810759/

Marcinowska-Suchowiersk,. E., Kupisz-Urbaska, M., Łukaszkiewicz, J., et al. (2018). Vitamin D Toxicity–A Clinical Perspective, PMC US National Library of Medicine, National Institutes of Health, Frontiers in Endocrinology: Front Endocrinol (Lausanne). 2018; 9: 550. Published online 2018 Sep 20. doi: 10.3389/fendo.2018.00550.
https://www.ncbi.nlm.nih.gov/pmc/articles/PMC6158375/

Kennedy, DO., (2016). B Vitamins and the Brain: Mechanisms, Dose and Efficacy—A Review, PMC US National Library of Medicine, National Institutes of Health, Nutrients MDPI: Nutrients. 2016 Feb; 8(2): 68. Published online 2016 Jan 28. doi: 10.3390/nu8020068
https://www.ncbi.nlm.nih.gov/pmc/articles/PMC4772032/

Gilbert, C., (2013). What is vitamin A and why do we need it? PMC US National Library of Medicine, National Institutes of Health, Community Eye Health Journal: Community Eye Health. 2013; 26(84): 65.
https://www.ncbi.nlm.nih.gov/pmc/articles/PMC3936685/

Gupta, RK., Gangoliya, SS., Singh, NK., (2015). Reduction of phytic acid and enhancement of bioavailable micronutrients in food grains, PMC US National Library of Medicine, National Institutes of Health, Springer: J Food Sci Technol. 2015 Feb; 52(2): (pp 676–684). Published online 2013 Apr 24. doi: 10.1007/s13197-013-0978-y.
https://www.ncbi.nlm.nih.gov/pmc/articles/PMC4325021/

Ko, S-H., Kim, H-S., (2020). Menopause-Associated Lipid Metabolic Disorders and Foods Beneficial for Postmenopausal Women, PMC US National Library of Medicine, National Institutes of Health, Nutrients MDPI: Nutrients. 2020 Jan; 12(1): 202. Published online 2020 Jan 13. doi: 10.3390/nu12010202.
https://www.ncbi.nlm.nih.gov/pmc/articles/PMC7019719/

van Ballegooijen, AJ,. Pilz, S., Tomaschitz, A., et al. (2017). The Synergistic Interplay between Vitamins D and K for Bone and Cardiovascular Health: A Narrative Review, PMC US National Library of Medicine, National Institutes of Health, International Journal of Endocrinology: Int J Endocrinol. 2017; 2017: 7454376. Published online 2017 Sep 12. doi: 10.1155/2017/7454376.
https://www.ncbi.nlm.nih.gov/pmc/articles/PMC5613455/

Fischer, LM., da Costa, K-A., Kwock, L., et al. (2010). Dietary choline requirements of women: effects of estrogen and genetic variation, PMC US National Library of Medicine, National Institutes of Health, The American Journal of Clinical Nutrition: Am J Clin Nutr. 2010 Nov; 92(5): (pp 1113–1119). Published online 2010 Sep 22. doi: 10.3945/ajcn.2010.30064.
https://www.ncbi.nlm.nih.gov/pmc/articles/PMC2954445/

NIH, National Institutes of Health, Office of Dietary Supplements, (2021). Choline, Fact Sheet for Health Professionals.
https://ods.od.nih.gov/factsheets/Choline-HealthProfessional/

6.3 Diet, Lifestyle, and Disease Prevention

Menopause increases the risk of many chronic diseases, including cardiovascular disease, diabetes, osteoporosis, Alzheimer's disease, and cancer. In many cases, modifiable factors including diet and other lifestyle choices can either increase or decrease the risk significantly.

Eating a healthy, balanced diet should preferably begin in a woman's 30s or even earlier in order to maximize the benefits.

Body Weight

Hormone loss and imbalance, slowing metabolism, reduced activity, gut dysbiosis, chronic HPA overstimulation, stress, and mitochondrial dysfunction can all lead to weight gain following menopause.

Being overweight or obese is associated with a plethora of diseases, including chronic inflammation, cardiovascular disease, diabetes, and cancer. However, being underweight is also far from ideal as estrogen is produced in adipose tissue post-menopause.

The best way to maintain a healthy body weight is to balance one's calorie intake and output. Daily calorie requirements depend upon basal metabolic rate (BMR) and physical activity levels. Unfortunately, calculating BMR is not a simple equation and depends on numerous factors, including age, height, weight, and body mass composition. As a general guideline, women should aim to consume 2000 calories per day for weight maintenance, and fewer for weight loss.

Some other ways to aid weight loss and maintain a healthy body mass index are discussed in the following paragraphs.

Weight loss

Diet

It is important to adjust portion size and calorie intake according to physical activity levels. Calorie intake can be limited by avoiding high-calorie, high-fat foods that have a low nutritional value and increasing consumption of fiber and protein, which increase satiety.

Plant-based foods are a good source of low-calorie nutrition, although fruit should be limited due to its sugar content. Eating 6–8 portions of vegetables, 1–2 portions of starchy vegetables, and 1–2 pieces of whole fruit daily is ideal. A small quantity of raw or dry-roasted nuts and seeds can be added to meals or eaten as snacks.

Protein intake should be increased to 30–40g per meal, with a focus on lean protein, such as chicken, fish, legumes, and whole grains. Whole grains are also a good source of carbohydrates and provide a steadier supply of energy than their processed counterparts.

Consumption of stimulants, including caffeine and sugar, should be reduced, as should alcohol intake.

Fasting

Intermittent fasting for 14–18 hours per day induces ketogenesis to help burn fat as an energy source. However, it is not appropriate for everyone and should only be undertaken with professional supervision.

Physical Activity

Increased physical activity burns excess calories and is one of the best ways to maintain a healthy weight. As well as aerobic exercise, which increases the heart rate, menopausal women should aim to increase their muscle mass. Not only will this help to combat the effects of sarcopenia and prevent falls, but increased muscle mass will raise basal metabolic rate and daily calorie requirements.

Stress and Sleep

Both chronic stress and sleep deprivation can result in hormonal dysregulation and interrupt metabolic processes. Therefore, stress management and good sleep hygiene have critical roles to play in maintaining a healthy weight.

Weight Gain

Being underweight poses a number of risks to post-menopausal women, including nutritional deficiencies, anemia, and an increased risk of osteoporosis. However, gaining weight is not as simple as consuming more calories. It is important to increase energy intake from healthy sources and avoid those high in sugar and unhealthy fats.

Furthermore, being underweight can be a symptom of serious medical conditions, including cancer. This is especially true if unexpected or sudden weight loss occurs. Therefore, underweight individuals should undergo clinical investigations to determine the cause and begin a weight gain diet under the supervision of a professional nutritionist.

Heart Health

Menopause increases the risk of heart disease due to the loss of estrogen and its protective effects on the cardiovascular system. As well as maintaining a healthy weight as detailed above, some further dietary and lifestyle measures which may help include the following:

Reduce "Bad" Fats and Increase "Good" Fats

Fats may be classified as "good" or "bad" depending on their overall impact on the body. For example, trans fats and saturated fats increase the risk of heart disease and should be kept to a minimum. Meanwhile, mono and polyunsaturated fats, including omega-3 fatty acids, may offer some protection against cardiovascular disease (see below).

All types of fat are high in energy. A gram of fat, whether saturated or unsaturated, provides twice as much energy as carbohydrates and proteins.

"Good" Fats Examples

Monounsaturated Fats (MUFAs)

MUFAs protect the heart by maintaining HDL and reducing LDL cholesterol levels.

Sources of MUFAs

Extra virgin olive oil, macadamia oil, almonds, Brazil nuts, peanuts, and avocados.
Note: Canola oil is rich in MUFAs. However, it also contains polyunsaturated fatty acids (PUFAs), which oxidize due to heat applied during processing. Oxidized polyunsaturated fatty acids are associated with oxidative stress and inflammation.

Polyunsaturated Fats (PUFAs)

PUFAs include omega-3 and omega-6 fatty acids, which cannot be made by the body and are therefore essential in small amounts in the diet. They help to lower LDL cholesterol levels, thus benefiting cardiovascular health.

Omega-3 and 6

Omega-3 fatty acids are also involved in hormone signaling and play a crucial role in menopausal health. They could assist in the management of menopausal symptoms as well as offering protection against osteoporosis, breast cancer, and cardiovascular disease.

Most adults get enough omega-6 in their diet but are advised to consume more omega-3 by eating at least two portions of fish a week, including one portion of oily fish. Vegetable sources of omega-3 fats are not thought to have the same benefits on heart health as those found in fish.

A 1:1-4 ratio of omega-3 to omega-6 fats is considered optimal for good health. Excess omega-6 (common in processed vegetable oils, takeaways, and restaurant-prepared foods) are pro-inflammatory, increasing the risk of chronic diseases, especially when these oils are oxidized by exposure to high temperatures.

Sources of Omega-3

Oily fish[30] (kippers, herring, trout, sardines, salmon, mackerel), soybeans (roasted), walnuts, chia seeds, flaxseeds, and hemp seeds.

Sources of Omega-6

Vegetable oils such as rapeseed (canola), corn, and sunflower oil, walnuts, sesame seeds, sunflower seeds, and sacha inchi seeds.

"Bad" Fats Examples

Trans Fats

Trans fats increase disease risk, even when eaten in small quantities. They are primarily found in processed foods made with trans fat from partially hydrogenated oil. Hydrogenation is when liquid vegetable oil turns into a semi-solid or solid. Manufacturers use hydrogenated oils to improve the texture, flavor, and shelf life of packaged foods. Partially hydrogenated oils contain trans fatty acids which raise LDL cholesterol and lower HDL cholesterol.

Sources of Trans Fat

Fried foods (e.g. donuts) and baked goods, including commercial cakes, pie crusts, pastries, biscuits, frozen pizza, cookies, crackers, stick margarine, vegetable shortening, and other spreads.

Saturated Fats

While not as harmful as trans fats, in comparison to unsaturated fats, saturated fats may negatively impact health and are best consumed in moderation. However, saturated fats are more stable and less likely to oxidize to pro-inflammatory compounds than polyunsaturated fats.

Medium-chain saturated fats, such as coconut oil, may be beneficial on certain dietary protocols, providing an alternative fuel source to carbohydrates.

Sources of Saturated Fats

Fatty cuts of meat, animal products, including sausages, pies, butter, ghee, lard, cheese (especially hard cheese like cheddar), cream, sour cream, ice cream, most packet savoury snacks like cheese crackers and microwave popcorn, chocolate confectionery, biscuits, cakes, pastries, palm oil, coconut oil, and coconut cream.

Control Blood Sugar and Insulin

High blood sugar can damage the blood vessels over sustained periods, leading to cardiovascular disease and circulatory disorders. Therefore, it is essential to keep the blood sugar at healthy levels by eating a low glycemic index diet, minimizing refined sugars and carbohydrates, and keeping stress levels to a minimum. Equally, it is important to support insulin function by maintaining a healthy body weight as detailed above.

---

[30] It is best to avoid or minimize large oily fish such as bill fish and tuna due to higher levels of mercury and other toxins.

Control Blood Pressure

High blood pressure is a major risk factor for cardiovascular events, including heart attacks and strokes. Since it is usually asymptomatic, it is important to monitor the blood pressure regularly.

Factors that influence blood pressure include diet, activity levels, body weight, and conditions such as diabetes. One of the most important dietary factors is salt, which should be kept to a minimum (<6g daily). The best way to do this is by avoiding salty snacks, packaged and processed foods, and cooking from scratch. Beware of hidden salt in products such as cheese, bread, and cereals. Rather than seasoning food with salt, use herbs, spices, and black pepper instead.

DASH Eating Plan

The Dietary Approaches to Stop Hypertension (DASH) Eating Plan was specially formulated to help hypertensive patients reduce blood pressure through diet.

A typical serving guide for a patient following the DASH diet is as follows[31] :

1. **Vegetables:** about five servings per day
2. **Fruits:** about five servings per day
3. **Carbohydrates:** about seven servings per day
4. **Low-fat dairy products:** about two servings per day
5. **Lean meat products:** about two or fewer servings per day
6. **Nuts and seeds:** 2-3 times per week

Manage Chronic Inflammation

Chronic inflammation is strongly linked with cardiovascular disease and a host of other serious conditions. Stress is a major contributing factor to chronic, low-grade inflammation and should be kept to a minimum (see Chapter 5.2 Stress, Trauma and Resistance). Smoking is another significant cause of inflammation and one of the most substantial risk factors for cardiovascular disease.

Diet and gut health also play a role as many foods have either pro-inflammatory or anti-inflammatory properties. The microbiome is responsible for metabolizing these dietary components and maintaining gut integrity to prevent pro-inflammatory metabolites from entering the bloodstream. Diets that are reported to have positive effects on inflammation include vegetarian diets and the Mediterranean diet.

---

[31] Challa. HJ., Ameer. MA., Uppaluri. KR., (2021). DASH Diet To Stop Hypertension, StatPearls [Internet], Treasure Island (FL): StatPearls Publishing; 2021 Jan-. https://www.ncbi.nlm.nih.gov/books/NBK482514/

Pro-Inflammatory Foods	Anti-Inflammatory Foods
Refined flours Gluten Trans fats Saturated fats Dairy products Red meat Processed meat Fried foods Alcohol	• Omega-3 PUFAs • MUFAs • Phytochemicals • Flavonoids, especially anthocyanins (blueberries, strawberries, etc.) • Vitamin D • Fruit with enzymatic proteins, such as papain and bromelain (papaya, mango, pineapple) • Ginger • Turmeric with black pepper • Green tea • Legumes

Table 6.3a: Pro- and anti-inflammatory foods.

Bone Health

Women should aim to optimize bone health starting from their 20s in order to reduce the risk of osteoporosis.

Nutrients

Calcium is one of the most important nutrients for building bone and vitamin D aids its absorption. Dairy products are one of the best sources of calcium, although not everyone can tolerate them. People with lactose intolerance and vegans may require supplementation. From a TCEAM perspective, people with Spleen deficiencies or excessive dampness should also avoid excessive dairy consumption, although low or non-fat dairy products may be better tolerated.

Other important nutrients for bone health include vitamin K2, phosphorus, and magnesium. Plant based sources of calcium include wombok (Chinese cabbage, which is very well absorbed and almost equivalent to dairy), buttered dark leafy greens and cruciferous vegetables, soy products and other legumes, almonds, sesame seeds (tahini), and seaweeds (wakame).

Exercise

Undertaking regular physical activity to maintain flexibility, balance, and strength is critical for bone health. Weight-bearing exercise, such as strength or resistance training, helps to build bone mass. It is important to consider both the upper and lower body, with weight-lifting for the upper body and activities like brisk walking, jogging, jumping, or skipping for the lower. Practices such as tai chi and yoga can help to improve balance and reduce the risk of falls.

Manage Mood

Depression and anxiety are independent risk factors for dementia. Therefore, it is essential to manage one's mood in order to maintain brain health and prevent cognitive decline post-menopause. One key way to do this is by improving stress resilience (see Chapter 5.2, Stress, Trauma, and Stress Resistance). Removing stimulants and depressants, including alcohol and caffeine, may also help to stabilize mood and emotional balance.

Other beneficial activities include relaxation techniques such as meditation, mindfulness, breathing exercises, acupuncture, massage, connecting with others, or engaging in therapy if necessary, to resolve challenging emotions.

Gut Health

It is necessary to optimize gut health and integrity to boost nutrient absorption, regulate the gut-brain axis, and eliminate bacterial overgrowth, which can lead to brain fog. There also appears to be an association between gut inflammation, dysbiosis, and mood disorders.

Blood Sugar

Poorly regulated blood sugar can have a negative impact on mood. Glycotoxicity also has a severe negative impact on brain health. Therefore, improving blood sugar regulation with cinnamon and chromium may help, as may the ability to utilize both glucose and ketones as a source of energy by consuming both healthy fats and carbohydrates.

Inflammation

Chronic inflammation is associated with depression as well as other chronic health conditions, which may have a negative impact on mood. Eating an anti-inflammatory diet may help to ameliorate some of these issues (see Table 6.3a).

Diet

Adequate intake of protein, especially the amino acids phenylalanine, tyrosine, and tryptophan, is critical for neurotransmitter synthesis.

Other key nutrients include vitamins B3, B6, folate, B9, B12, and C, magnesium, manganese, iron, copper, and zinc. Carbohydrates aid the transport of amino acids across the blood-brain barrier.

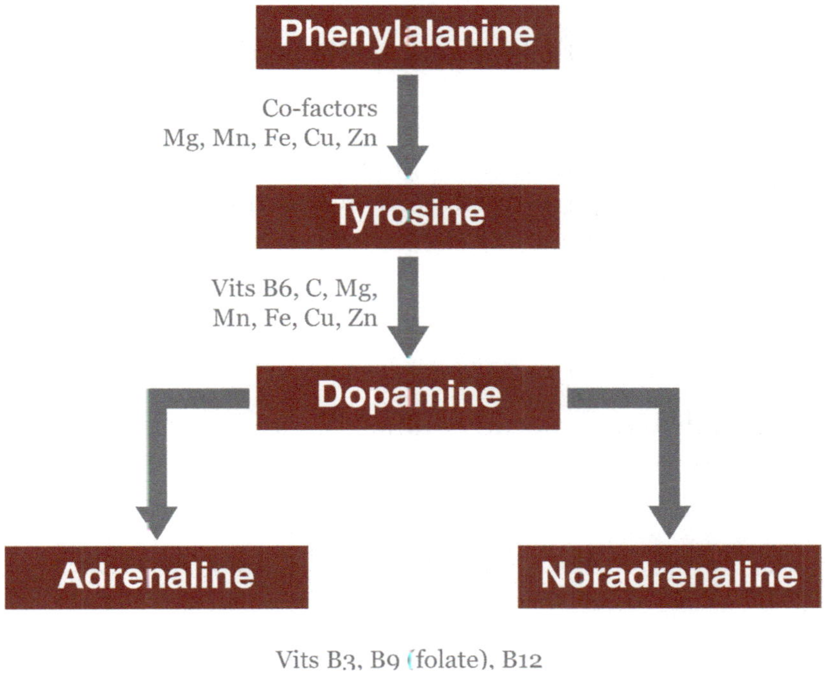

Figure 6.3a: Nutrients to neurotransmitters. [32]

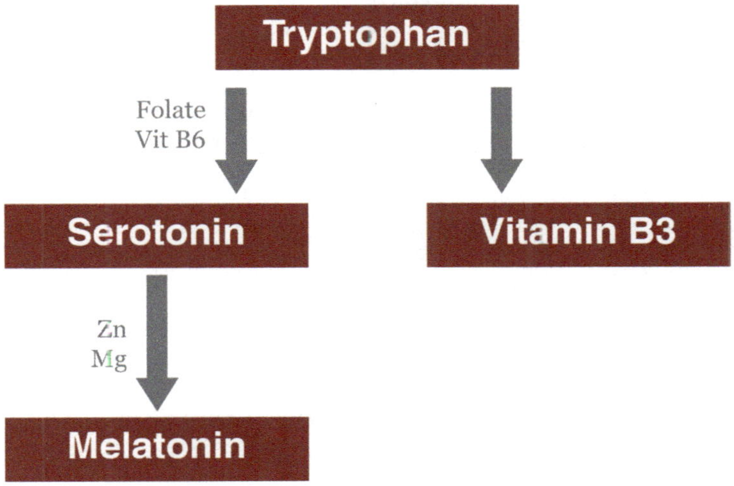

Figure 6.3b: Nutrients to neurotransmitters.

[32] Kath, S., (2019). Nutrition, Food supplements and Lifestyle for Optimising Midlife and Beyond. Treating Women Academy: Online Menopause Masterclass. https://www.treatingwomen.com/store/5tpUJ3Fk

Neurotrophic Factors
Neurotrophic factors are molecules that influence cell function within the nervous system. They include:

- Healthy fats: omega-3 (EPA, DHA), extra virgin olive oil, phospholipids, and cholesterol
- Choline: aids the synthesis of neurotransmitters acetylcholine and phosphatidylcholine
- Vitamin D: aids methylation and neurotransmitter production
- Antioxidants and phytonutrients
- Beta-hydroxybutyrate supports ketone production

Toxins
Toxins such as heavy metals have a negative impact on brain function. Therefore, it is crucial to reduce toxic load by avoiding exposure to environmental toxins as well as improving the body's detoxification and clearance functions (see Chapter 6.1, Digestion, Absorption, and Elimination).

Sleep
Sleep promotes healthy functioning within the glymphatic system, a macroscopic system that helps to clear waste products such as soluble proteins and metabolites from the brain. Dysfunction in this system has been implicated in the development of neurodegenerative disorders, traumatic brain injury, and strokes. (See Chapter 5.3, Sleep, Energy, and Fatigue).

Exercise
Exercise has numerous benefits for brain health, including increasing brain-derived neurotrophic factor (BDNF), releasing endorphins, enhancing mood, improving circulation, promoting better sleep, and increasing energy.

Mental Stimulation
It is important to stay mentally active in order to maintain brain health. Helpful activities include games and social activities, computer use, and craft activities.

Cancer Prevention

Prevent Obesity

Obesity is one of the most significant risk factors for many different types of cancer, including endometrial, esophageal adenocarcinoma, colorectal, postmenopausal breast, and renal cancers, among others. Possible mechanisms include dysregulation of insulin, insulin-like growth factor-I, sex steroids, and adipokines, chronic inflammation, oxidative stress, crosstalk between cancerous cells and adipose tissue, migrating adipose stromal cells, obesity-induced hypoxia, genetics, and immune dysfunction.

Decrease HCAs and PAHs

Heterocyclic amines (HCAs) and polycyclic aromatic hydrocarbons (PAHs) are chemicals formed when muscle meat, including beef, pork, fish, or poultry, is cooked using high-temperature methods, such as pan-frying or grilling directly over an open flame. In laboratory experiments, HCAs and PAHs have been found to be mutagenic, causing changes in DNA that may increase the risk of cancer.

In order to decrease HCA and PAH consumption, food should be marinated before grilling to avoid charring. High-temperature cooking methods, such as pan-frying or grilling directly over an open flame should also be avoided. Cruciferous vegetables appear to combat some of the detrimental effects of HCAs and PAHs and should be consumed liberally.

Alcohol and Smoking

Both alcohol consumption and smoking are risk factors for cancer. Alcohol may increase the risk of breast cancer by promoting the aromatization of androgens to estrogens. However, the same process could potentially offer some protection against cardiovascular disease and osteoporosis. Therefore, while excessive alcohol use is harmful, moderate consumption could provide some benefits.

Smoking should be avoided completely.

Symptom/Risk	Advice
Hot Flashes	• Eat more cooling foods (salad, above-ground vegetables, cold soups) • Lignans (flax seeds, whole grains, legumes, fruit, vegetables) • Isoflavones (soy, daidzein, genistein) • Pomegranate • Adzuki, alfalfa, mung beans, celery seed, parsley • Herbal teas: alfalfa, calendula, fennel, licorice, raspberry leaf, red clover, sage • Replace lost electrolytes and magnesium (coconut water, sea vegetables) • Avoid aggravating factors (alcohol, caffeine, spicy food) • Reduce "bad" fats • Avoid insulin resistance (eat a low-GI diet) • Reduce stress • Reframe attitude: think of hot flashes as a "power surge" or "trip to tropics" • Address hormone imbalances • Supplements (consult a professional) e.g. soy isoflavones, flaxseed, maca, *Panax ginseng*, pine bark, red clover, white mulberry, tribulus
Weight Gain	• Address hormonal imbalances and gut dysbiosis • Reduce stress • Increase physical activity • Intermittent fasting if appropriate • Increase fiber and prebiotics • Increase protein, "good" fats, "smart carbs" • Adjust portion size according to activity levels • Increase muscle mass to improve metabolism • Increase plant foods (6–8 portions daily) • "Eat the rainbow" • Decrease stimulant intake (caffeine, sugar) • Decrease alcohol intake • Avoid nutrient-poor, high-calorie foods • Avoid pro-inflammatory foods

Symptom/Risk	Advice
Brain Health	• Manage mood (relaxation techniques, exercise, etc.) • Remove stimulants and depressants • Improve blood sugar control (cinnamon, chromium) • Increase nutrients for neurotransmitter synthesis (magnesium, manganese, iron, copper, zinc, calcium, B2, B3, B9 (folate)) • Optimize gut health • Reduce stress • Improve sleep • Ensure good social/emotional support network • Increase healthy fats, omega 3, choline, vitamin D, antioxidants, phytonutrients, ketones
Fatigue and Energy	• Improve hormesis (fasting, high-intensity interval training, sauna, cold showers) • Reduce stress • Improve sleep (melatonin, B3, avoid stimulants) • Key nutrients: B6, B12, magnesium, methionine, SAMe • Support mitochondrial health (B3, B6, B9, vitamin C, CoQ10, vitamin K1, B7 (biotin), magnesium, manganese) • Increase antioxidants to combat oxidative stress (alpha-lipoic acid, organ meat, spinach, cruciferous veg, red meat, beets) • Increase phytochemicals (curcumin, resveratrol, green tea)
Vaginal Dryness, Atrophy, and Low Libido	• Improve circulation and blood flow • Increase healthy fats (omega 3, olive oil) • Increase zinc, vitamin D, magnesium, potassium • Increase nitrate-rich foods • Prebiotics and probiotics • Use natural lubrication (coconut, avocado, olive, jojoba oil) • Stay sexually active • Topical estrogen cream if indicated

Symptom/Risk	Advice
Diabetes	• Control blood sugar and insulin • Eat more "smart carbs" and "good" fats • Maintain healthy weight
Cardiovascular Disease	• Control blood pressure, oxidized LDL particles, triglycerides • Manage chronic inflammation
Dementia/ Alzheimer's	• X-patterning activities (juggling, tai chi) • Check BDNF, glucotoxicity
Osteoporosis	• Maintain flexibility, balance, and strength • Calcium, magnesium, vitamin D, vitamin K2
Cancer	• Avoid obesity • Reduce alcohol intake/ quit smoking • Increase exercise • Reduce methoxy-estrone

Table 6.3b: Menopause symptoms and risk factors.

Summary

Modifiable diet and lifestyle factors play a critical role in a person's risk of developing numerous chronic conditions. As clinicians, we are uniquely placed to offer our patients guidance on how to adopt a healthier lifestyle and maintain their wellbeing for years to come. However, it is essential to make these suggestions in a manner that is easy for the patient to accept and follow. This might involve prioritizing certain aspects to offer manageable changes rather than suggesting many significant changes at once.

References

Kath, S., (2019). Nutrition, Food Supplements and Lifestyle for Optimising Midlife and Beyond. Treating Women Academy: Online Menopause Masterclass.
https://www.treatingwomen.com/store/5tpUJ3Fk

NIH, National Library of Medicine. (2020). Facts about polyunsaturated fats, Medline Plus: Home > Medical Encyclopedia > Facts about polyunsaturated fats.
https://medlineplus.gov/ency/patientinstructions/000747.htm

Saldeen. P., Saldee, T., (2004). Women and omega-3 Fatty acids, NIH National Library of Medicine, National Center for Biotechnology Information: Obstet Gynecol Surv. 2004 Oct;59(10):(pp 722-30); quiz 745-6.
doi: 10.1097/01.ogx.0000140038.70473.96. https://pubmed.ncbi.nlm.nih.gov/15385858/

Awada, M., Soulage, CO., Meynier, A., et al. (2012). Dietary oxidized n-3 PUFA induce oxidative stress and inflammation: role of intestinal absorption of 4-HHE and reactivity in intestinal cells, PMC US National Library of Medicine, National Institutes of Health, JLR, Journal of Lipid Research: J Lipid Res. 2012 Oct; 53(10): (pp 2069–2080).
doi: 10.1194/jlr.M026179.
https://www.ncbi.nlm.nih.gov/pmc/articles/PMC3435540/

Bustamante, MF., Agustín-Perez, M., Cedola, F., et al. (2020). Design of an anti-inflammatory diet (ITIS diet) for patients with rheumatoid arthritis, PMC US National Library of Medicine, National Institutes of Health, Elsevier, Contemporary Clinical Trials Communications: Contemp Clin Trials Commun. 2020 Mar; 17: 100524.. Published online 2020 Jan 21.
doi: 10.1016/j.conctc.2020.100524.
https://www.ncbi.nlm.nih.gov/pmc/articles/PMC6997513/

Liu, Y-Z., Wang, Y-X., Jiang, C-L., (2-17). Inflammation: The Common Pathway of Stress-Related Diseases, PMC US National Library of Medicine, National Institutes of Health, Frontiers in Human Neuroscience: Front Hum Neurosci. 2017; 11: 316. Published online 2017 Jun 20. doi: 10.3389/fnhum.2017.00316.
https://www.ncbi.nlm.nih.gov/pmc/articles/PMC5476783/

Bishehsari, F., Magno, E., Swanson, G., et al. (2017). Alcohol and Gut-Derived Inflammation, PMC US National Library of Medicine, National Institutes of Health, Alcohol Research, Current Reviews: Alcohol Res. 2017; 38(2): (pp 163–171).
https://www.ncbi.nlm.nih.gov/pmc/articles/PMC5513683/

PLOS Medicine, (2005). Smoking and Inflammation, PMC US National Library of Medicine, National Institutes of Health: PLoS Med. 2005 Jun; 2(6): e198. Published online 2005 Jun 28. doi: 10.1371/journal.pmed.0020198,
https://www.ncbi.nlm.nih.gov/pmc/articles/PMC1160597/

Office of the Surgeon General (US). (2004). Bone Health and Osteoporosis: A Report of the Surgeon General. Office of the Surgeon General (US). Rockville (MD): Office of the Surgeon General (US); 2004.
https://www.ncbi.nlm.nih.gov/books/NBK45523/

Clapp, M., Aurora, N., Herrera, L., et al. (2017). Gut microbiota's effect on mental health: The gut-brain axis, PMC US National Library of Medicine, National Institutes of Health, Clinics and Practice, an Open Access Journal by MDPI: Clin Pract. 2017 Sep 15; 7(4): 987. Published online 2017 Sep 15. doi: 10.4081/cp.2017.987.
https://www.ncbi.nlm.nih.gov/pmc/articles/PMC5641835/

Jessen, NA., Munk, ASF., Lundgaard, I., et al. (2015). The Glymphatic System – A Beginner's Guide, PMC US National Library of Medicine, National Institutes of Health, HHS Public Access, Author Manuscript: Neurochem Res. Author manuscript; available in PMC 2016 Dec 1. Published in final edited form as: Neurochem Res. 2015 Dec; 40(12): (pp 2583–2599). Published online 2015 May 7. doi: 10.1007/s11064-015-1581-6.
https://www.ncbi.nlm.nih.gov/pmc/articles/PMC4636982/

Krell-Roesch, J. Vemuri, P., Pink, A., et al. (2017). Association Between Mentally Stimulating Activities in Late Life and the Outcome of Incident Mild Cognitive Impairment, With an Analysis of the APOE 4 Genotype, Jama Network: JAMA Neurol. 2017;74(3): (pp 332-338). doi:10.1001/jamaneuro.2016.3822.
https://jamanetwork.com/journals/jamaneurology/fullarticle/2598835

De Pergola, G,. Silvestris, F., (2013). Obesity as a Major Risk Factor for Cancer, PMC US National Library of Medicine, National Institutes of Health, Journal of Obesity: J Obes. 2013; 2013: 291546. Published online 2013 Aug 29.
doi: 10.1155/2013/291546 https://www.ncbi.nlm.nih.gov/pmc/articles/PMC3773450/

Al-Sader, H., Abdul-Jabar, H., Allawi. Z., (2009). Alcohol and Breast Cancer: The Mechanisms Explained, PMC US National Library of Medicine, National Institutes of Health, Journal of Clinical Medicine Research: J Clin Med Res. 2009 Aug; 1(3): (pp 125–131). Published online 2009 Jul 3. doi: 10.4021/jocmr2009.07.1246.
https://www.ncbi.nlm.nih.gov/pmc/articles/PMC3318874/

6.4 Herbs and Botanicals

Many women would prefer to avoid taking MHT and opt for alternative treatments instead. The following herbs and botanical extracts are all popular examples.

Unfortunately, although some women experience benefits while taking these products, the clinical evidence relating to most of them is sparse. Another major issue with herbal remedies is that many people assume they are safe. However, they can and do cause adverse effects and, in some cases, serious drug interactions. Therefore, they should only be used under the supervision of a qualified herbalist.

Below are some of the most commonly used herbal remedies for menopausal symptoms. An exhaustive list is beyond the scope of this publication as there are so many options available.

Soy Isoflavones

Isoflavones are a type of flavonoid found in legumes, especially soybeans. They possess a similar chemical structure to estradiol and, for this reason, are sometimes classified as phytoestrogens (plant estrogens). Soy products make up a large proportion of Asian diets and it has been hypothesized that this is one reason why Asian women typically experience milder menopausal symptoms than Westerners, although this is currently unproven.

Active compounds

There are many types of isoflavones present in soybeans. The most well-researched are genistein and daidzein. However, it is interesting to note that these compounds only exist in their inactive forms in soy and are converted by intestinal bacteria to biologically active substances.

Proposed mechanisms

It appears that soy isoflavones act as selective estrogen receptor modulators. Studies suggest that they have an agonistic effect in the absence of estradiol and an antagonistic effect in its presence. This means that they could potentially stimulate these receptors and produce estrogen-like effects in post-menopausal individuals.

Efficacy

The evidence surrounding soy isoflavones for menopausal symptoms is mixed. However, they do appear to have a positive effect on lipid profiles, reducing LDL cholesterol and triglycerides while increasing HDL cholesterol. They have also shown some promise for improving bone health and protecting breast tissue.

Adverse effects

There may be some risks associated with soy isoflavones due to their effects on estrogen receptors. Therefore, they should be avoided by those with a history or family history of breast cancer, other estrogen-receptor positive cancers, or estrogen-sensitive conditions.

Red Clover (*Trifolium pratense*)

Red clover is native to Europe, Central Asia, and North Africa. Its flowers were traditionally used as an anti-spasmodic and anti-cancer treatment, and have only been promoted as a remedy for menopausal symptoms more recently. Like soy, red clover contains isoflavones and is, therefore, often considered a phytoestrogen.

Active compounds

Genistein, daidzein, formononetin, and biochanin A.

Proposed mechanisms

As well as its estrogenic effects, red clover appears to influence mu and delta opioid receptors, which play a role in temperature regulation, mood, and hormone production.

Efficacy

The evidence that red clover relieves menopausal symptoms, such as hot flashes, is mixed. There is limited evidence surrounding its benefits for bone health and lipid profiles.

Adverse effects

Reported side effects include mild headaches, muscular pain, and nausea. Due to its estrogenic effects, it should be avoided by women with estrogen-sensitive conditions.

Chaste Tree/Chaste Berry (*Vitex agnus-castus*)

The chaste tree is native to the Mediterranean region and its berries have been used medicinally since ancient Greek times. It has phytoestrogenic properties and is often employed as a natural remedy for female reproductive issues, infertility, PMS, and hyperprolactinemia. In recent years, its potential as a treatment for menopausal symptoms has also been explored.

Active compounds

Flavonoids, flavones, flavonols (3-methyl kaempferol, luteolin, apigenin, casticin), terpenoids, neolignans, and phenolic compounds.

Proposed mechanisms

Vitex agnus-castus (VAC) acts upon dopamine receptors in the pituitary gland, especially the region responsible for LH secretion. It also has an affinity for mu and delta opioid receptors, which play a role in regulating mood, appetite, and HPA activity.

Efficacy

There is limited evidence that VAC could reduce vasomotor symptoms and anxiety in menopausal women, as well as potentially enhancing mood.

Adverse effects

Side effects include mild gastrointestinal upsets, rash, and itching. VAC can interact with antidepressants and should not be taken by those with a history or family history of breast cancer.

Maca Root (*Lepidium meyenii*)

Maca is a member of the mustard family and has been consumed as a root vegetable in the mountains of Peru for centuries. It reportedly has a wealth of benefits and has traditionally been used to increase energy, maintain health, and promote hormonal balance. Several studies have investigated its usefulness as a treatment for menopausal symptoms.

Active Compounds

Plant sterols (campesterol, stigmasterol, beta-sitosterol), polyunsaturated fatty acids and their amides (macaenes, macamides), amino acids, and aromatic glucosinolates.

Proposed Mechanisms

Maca appears to modulate the production of several hormones (including estrogen and FSH) and other compounds without direct estrogenic or androgenic activity. It has been suggested that it affects hormonal processes via the HPO axis, although further study is required.

Efficacy

There is some evidence that maca alleviates vasomotor symptoms and reduces anxiety, depression, and sexual dysfunction. It may also improve bone mineral density markers in early post-menopausal women.

Adverse Effects

None reported, although further research into the herb's safety has been recommended. Due to its possible estrogenic effects, it should be avoided by patients with estrogen-sensitive conditions.

Black Cohosh (*Cimicifuga racemosa*)

Black cohosh is native to Canada and the eastern United States. Its rhizomes were traditionally used by Native Americans as a remedy for menstrual irregularities. However, in recent years, it has been promoted as a treatment for menopausal symptoms, including hot flashes. It has also been promoted as increasing bone mineral density.

Active compounds

Triterpene glycosides (actein, cimicifugoside), fatty acids, resins, caffeic acids, isoferulic acids, and isoflavones.

Proposed mechanisms

It was previously thought that the isoflavones found in black cohosh directly stimulated estrogen receptors. However, it now seems more likely that the herb has more centrally-acting effects, including the stimulation of dopaminergic receptors. Black cohosh also appears to reduce circulating LH levels, particularly through the activity of its triterpene glycosides.

Efficacy

There is insufficient evidence to confirm the efficacy of black cohosh for menopausal symptoms or increasing bone mineral density. Some studies suggest it may have increased efficacy in combination with other herbs and botanicals.

Adverse effects

Reported side effects include breast pain and enlargement, infections, vaginal bleeding, gastrointestinal disturbances, and musculoskeletal complaints. There have also been isolated cases of hepatitis, hepatic failure, facial odema, and cutaneous vasculitis. However, it is not possible to confirm whether all of these adverse reactions were directly related to black cohosh.

Ginseng (*Panax ginseng*)

Ginseng is one of the best known herbal remedies and a staple of traditional Chinese medicine, where it is known as Ren Shen. Although it is most widely used as a general tonic and adaptogen, it has also been investigated as a treatment for menopausal symptoms. *Panax ginseng* is usually known as Asian or Korean ginseng and should not be confused with *Panax quinquefolius* (American ginseng), although the two do have somewhat similar properties.

Active Compounds

Triterpene saponins (ginsenosides).

Proposed Mechanisms

Ginsenosides appear to exhibit estrogenic activity without binding directly to estrogen receptors. However, further study into these compounds' effects on the hormone is needed as the mechanism is still not fully understood.

Efficacy

Studies into ginseng's impact on menopausal symptoms have yielded mixed results. Some suggest improvements in several areas, including sexual arousal, depression, and general health. However, evidence regarding the herb's efficacy in treating hot flashes is less consistent. Ginseng may also provide some benefits for cardiovascular health and play a role in reducing the risk of metabolic disorder.

Adverse Effects

Ginseng can have anticoagulant effects and may cause vaginal bleeding. Patients with estrogen-sensitive conditions should not take ginseng due to its potentially estrogenic effects.

Dong Quai (*Angelica sinensis*)

Dong quai (Dang Gui) is commonly used in Chinese herbal medicine, most often in combination with other herbs. Sometimes known as 'female ginseng,' its primary indications include enriching the Blood and promoting circulation in the treatment of menstrual disorders. However, it has also been promoted as a remedy for menopausal symptoms, including headaches and fatigue.

Active compounds

Polysaccharides, Z-ligustilide, ferulic acid, and furocoumarins.

Proposed mechanisms

Dong quai has been shown to have weak estrogenic effects. It also displays immunostimulatory, anti-inflammatory, antioxidant, vasodilatory, and anti-atherosclerotic properties.

Efficacy

There is insufficient evidence regarding the efficacy of dong quai for menopausal symptoms as a single herb. However, it may be effective in combination with other ingredients. It may also offer some protection against atherosclerosis and strokes.

Adverse effects

Possible drug interactions (including blood thinners, such as warfarin), photosensitivity, possible carcinogenic effects. Due to its estrogenic effects, dong quai may not be appropriate for women with estrogen-receptor positive cancers.

Evening Primrose Oil (*Oenothera biennis*)

Evening primrose is a wildflower native to North America but is now found in many different regions worldwide. The flower's seeds produce an oil that is rich in fatty acids and has many purported therapeutic benefits. Evening primrose oil (EPO) has been extensively researched for women's health issues, primarily breast pain and PMS. It has also been investigated as a remedy for menopausal symptoms, such as hot flashes.

Active compounds

Omega-6 fatty acids (linolenic acid, gamma-linolenic acid), phenolic acids, and flavonoids.

Proposed mechanisms

Little information is available regarding how EPO might benefit menopausal symptoms. In general, its fatty acids act as precursors for series 1 prostaglandins, which have anti-inflammatory effects. They may also counteract the high prolactin levels that are seen in some women with PMS.

Efficacy

There is insufficient evidence to confirm that EPO effectively reduces hot flash frequency, although some studies suggest it may reduce their severity. It might also help to alleviate psychological symptoms such as irritability and depression.

Adverse effects

Some patients may experience bloating, nausea, or headaches while taking EPO. It may interact with medications, including anticoagulant and antiplatelet drugs, and should be used with caution in epilepsy.

St. John's Wort (*Hypericum perforatum*)

St. John's wort is native to Europe but now grows throughout many temperate regions of the world. It has been used medicinally since ancient Greek times, with wide-ranging indications, including wound healing, inducing diuresis, and alleviating menstrual disorders. Nowadays, it is most recognized as a remedy for depression and is one of the most widely studied herbs for this condition. It is sometimes used in combination with black cohosh to relieve vasomotor symptoms, irritability, mood swings, and insomnia associated with menopause.

Active compounds

Hypericin, hyperforin, and flavonoids (rutin, quercetin, kaempferol).

Proposed mechanisms

St. John's wort's antidepressant properties appear to stem from its active constituents hypericin and hyperforin. Hypericin increases blood flow and mildly inhibits monoaminoxidase (MAO) A and B, the enzymes responsible for metabolizing amine neurotransmitters. Meanwhile, hyperforin inhibits the reuptake of several neurotransmitters, including serotonin, dopamine, noradrenaline, GABA, and L-glutamate.

Efficacy

Numerous studies suggest that St. John's wort has antidepressant, antioxidant, neuroprotective, and possible anti-inflammatory properties. Although the evidence relating to St. John's wort for menopausal symptoms is more limited, it does show some promise, especially in combination with black cohosh.

Adverse effects

Common side effects include dry mouth, gastrointestinal upsets, allergic reaction, lethargy, dizziness, confusion, and restlessness. St. John's wort is also known to interact with many pharmaceuticals, including anticoagulants, digoxin, cyclosporine, proteases inhibitors, and oral contraceptives.

Valerian (*Valeriana officinalis*)

Valerian has been a popular herbal remedy for decades. Its root extract has purported sedative, hypnotic, antidepressant, and anxiolytic properties. It appears to improve sleep without imparting a hangover effect, making it one of the most common herbal remedies for stress and sleep disorders.

Active compounds

Terpenoids (bornyl acetate, valepotriates, valerenic acid), and hydroxy pinoresinol.

Proposed mechanisms

Valerenic acid appears to inhibit the breakdown of GABA, the primary inhibitory neurotransmitter, to induce sedation. The active compound hydroxypinoresinol has also shown an affinity for benzodiazepine receptors.

Efficacy

Studies suggest that valerian could help to improve sleep quality, although none have focused specifically on menopausal women.

Adverse effects

Adverse reactions to valerian include sedation, dizziness, diarrhea, and withdrawal symptoms upon cessation. There have been several reports of liver toxicity, especially when using valerian alongside other herbal remedies, including black cohosh.

Ginkgo (*Ginkgo biloba*)

Ginkgo is a prehistoric tree that is native to China but now grows worldwide. In China, its edible nuts are considered a delicacy. However, it is ginkgo leaves that have the most therapeutic potential. In TCEAM, they are known as Bai Guo Ye and their indications include circulatory problems, asthma, tinnitus, vertigo, and cognitive dysfunction.

Ginkgo is one of the best-researched herbal remedies and the German Commission E has approved it for cerebral insufficiency, peripheral vascular disease, vertigo, and tinnitus. It may, therefore, be a popular choice for post-menopausal women experiencing cognitive decline.

Active compounds

Terpenoids, flavonoids, flavonol glycosides (quercetin, catechin), and proanthocyanidins.

Proposed mechanisms

Ginkgo leaf extract increases cerebral blood flow, improves brain cells' ability to take up glucose, and enhances nerve transmission. It also displays antioxidant, neuroprotective, and vasorelaxant activity.

Efficacy

There is a reasonable amount of clinical evidence suggesting that ginkgo improves cognition while enhancing mood and emotional function.

Adverse effects

Possible side effects include headache, palpitations, gastrointestinal upsets, constipation, and allergic skin reactions. Ginkgo should be used with caution in patients with bleeding disorders or those taking anticoagulant, anti-platelet, or non-steroidal anti-inflammatory drugs.

Turmeric (*Curcuma longa*)

Turmeric is a member of the ginger family. It is native to the Indian subcontinent where it is an important culinary and medicinal spice. In TCEAM, it is known as Yu Jin and its indications include promoting qi and Blood circulation, clearing Heart-heat, and relieving depression. The plant's rhizome is best known for its potent anti-inflammatory properties, which could offer some level of protection against numerous age-related diseases. It has also been investigated as a treatment for anxiety and depression.

Active compounds

Turmeric contains over 100 chemical compounds but the best studied of these is curcumin. It also contains d-alpha-phellandrene, d-sabinene, cinol, borneol, zingiberene, and various sesquiterpenes.

Proposed mechanisms

Turmeric is best known for its anti-inflammatory effects. It is also antioxidant, antimicrobial, and has anticarcinogenic properties, including inhibiting cell proliferation and inducing apoptosis.

Efficacy

There is plenty of evidence for turmeric's efficacy as an anti-inflammatory herb. However, curcumin alone has poor bioavailability. Its absorption can be enhanced by consuming it together with a small quantity of healthy fat and some black pepper, which contains the bioenhancer, piperine.

Adverse effects

Side effects are rare but may include diarrhea, headache, and rash.

CBD (*Cannabidiol*)

CBD is just one of the many active compounds produced by *Cannabis sativa* plants, including hemp. Although its discovery was relatively recent, it has quickly become one of the most popular natural remedies available. Unlike the cannabinoid delta-9-tetrahydrocannabinol (THC), CBD does not have intoxicating effects. However, research has shown that it has powerful anti-inflammatory, antioxidant, and neuroprotective effects and may benefit a wide variety of physical and psychological symptoms.

Active compounds

CBD products fall into three categories: isolates, broad-spectrum, and full-spectrum. Broad and full-spectrum CBD products contain a variety of other cannabinoids, terpenoids, and flavonoids in addition to CBD.

Proposed mechanisms

CBD appears to work primarily by enhancing the functionality of the body's endogenous cannabinoid system. It inhibits the enzyme FAAH, which breaks down anandamide, a fatty acid that acts as a neurotransmitter among its many other functions. Early research also suggests that CBD influences several receptor types outside of the endogenous cannabinoid system, including 5HT1A receptors, TRPV1 receptors, and PPAR-gamma receptors.

Efficacy

There is evidence that CBD possesses anti-inflammatory, antioxidant, neuroprotective, and anti-tumor effects. It appears to benefit a range of conditions, including epilepsy, anxiety, sleep disorders, and pain. However, it has poor bioavailability when taken orally, calling into question the usefulness of many commercial products.

Adverse effects

Side effects are uncommon but include dry mouth, gastrointestinal upsets, and drowsiness. Long-term use of high doses may affect liver function and there is a high potential for drug interactions.

Summary

Herbal remedies are becoming increasingly popular due to their cost-effectiveness and ease of access, being widely available over the counter and online. They also reduce reliance on a gynecologist or medical doctor for prescriptions and may be perceived as safer alternatives to MHT due to their natural origin.

However, these remedies are not necessarily safe or suitable for everyone, and patients should always seek medical advice before beginning any new treatment, especially if their symptoms are severe.

It should also be noted that the supplements market is poorly regulated and care should be taken to choose products that are well-manufactured, efficacious, and free from contaminants. The best brands are very transparent regarding their ingredients and processing methods and provide up-to-date laboratory reports confirming each product's precise contents.

References

Ang, Q., Ge, X., Tian, X., et al. (2013). Soy isoflavone: The multipurpose phytochemical (Review), PMC US National Library of Medicine, National Institutes of Health, Biomedical Reports: Biomed Rep. 2013 Sep; 1(5): (pp 697–701). Published online 2013 Jun 3. doi: 10.3892/br.2013.129
https://www.ncbi.nlm.nih.gov/pmc/articles/PMC3916987/

Pabich, M., Materska, M., (2019). Biological Effect of Soy Isoflavones in the Prevention of Civilization Diseases, PMC US National Library of Medicine, National Institutes of Health, Nutrients: Nutrients. 2019 Jul; 11(7): 1660. Published online 2019 Jul 20. doi: 10.3390/nu11071660
https://www.ncbi.nlm.nih.gov/pmc/articles/PMC6683102/

Naseri, R., Farnia, V., Yazdchi, K., et al. (2019). Comparison of Vitex agnus-castus Extracts with Placebo in Reducing Menopausal Symptoms: A Randomized Double-Blind Study, PMC US National Library of Medicine, National Institutes of Health, KJFM, Korean Journal of Family Medicine: Korean J Fam Med. 2019 Nov; 40(6): (pp 362–367). Published online 2019 May 9. doi: 10.4082/kjfm.18.0067
https://www.ncbi.nlm.nih.gov/pmc/articles/PMC6887765/

Webster, DE., He, Y., Chen, S-N., et al. (2012). Opioidergic mechanisms underlying the actions of Vitex agnus-castus L,PMC US National Library of Medicine, National Institutes of Health. HHS Public Access, Author Manuscript: Biochem Pharmacol. Author manuscript; available in PMC 2012 Jan 1. Published in final edited form as: Biochem Pharmacol. 2011 Jan 1; 81(1): (pp 170–177). Published online 2010 Sep 18. doi: 10.1016/j.bcp.2010.09.013.
https://www.ncbi.nlm.nih.gov/pmc/articles/PMC2993511/

Chen, S-N., Friesen, JB., Webster, D., et al, (2012). Phytoconstituents from Vitex agnus-castus fruits, PMC US National Library of Medicine, National Institutes of Health, HHS Public Access, Author Manuscript: Fitoterapia. Author manuscript; available in PMC 2012 Jun 1. Published in final edited form as: Fitoterapia. 2011 Jun; 82(4): (pp 528–533). Published online 2010 Dec 13. doi: 10.1016/j.fitote.2010.12.003
https://www.ncbi.nlm.nih.gov/pmc/articles/PMC3081944/

Meissner, HO., Mscisz, A., Reich-Bilinska, H., et al. (2006). Hormone-Balancing Effect of Pre-Gelatinized Organic Maca (Lepidium peruvianum Chacon): (II) Physiological and Symptomatic Responses of Early-Postmenopausal Women to Standardized doses of Maca in Double Blind, Randomized, Placebo-Controlled, Multi-Centre Clinical Study, PMC US National Library of Medicine, National Institutes of Health, IJBS, International Journal of Biomedical Science: Int J Biomed Sci. 2006 Dec; 2(4): (pp 360–374).
https://www.ncbi.nlm.nih.gov/pmc/articles/PMC3614647/

Meissner, HO., Mscisz, A., Reich-Bilinska, H., et al. (2006). Hormone-Balancing Effect of Pre-Gelatinized Organic Maca (Lepidium peruvianum Chacon): (III) Clinical responses of early-postmenopausal women to Maca in double blind, randomized, Placebo-controlled, crossover configuration, outpatient study,PMC US National Library of Medicine, National Institutes of Health, IJBS, International Journal of Biomedical Science: Int J Biomed Sci. 2006 Dec; 2(4): (pp 375–394).
https://www.ncbi.nlm.nih.gov/pmc/articles/PMC3614644/

Lee, MS., Shin, B-CS., Lim, H-J., et al. (2011). Maca (Lepidium meyenii) for treatment of menopausal symptoms: A systematic review, NIH National Library of Medicine, National Center for Biotechnology Information: Maturitas, 2011 Nov;70(3):(pp 227-33). doi: 10.1016/j.maturitas.2011.07.017. Epub 2011 Aug 15.
https://pubmed.ncbi.nlm.nih.gov/21840656/

Brooks, NA., Wilcox, G., Walker, ZK., et al. (2008). Beneficial effects of Lepidium meyenii (Maca) on psychological symptoms and measures of sexual dysfunction in postmenopausal women are not related to estrogen or androgen content, NIH National Library of Medicine, National Center for Biotechnology Information: Randomized Controlled Trial Menopause. Nov-Dec 2008;15(6):(pp 1157-62). doi: 10.1097/gme.0b013e3181732953.
https://pubmed.ncbi.nlm.nih.gov/18784609/

Stojanovska, L., Law, C., Lai, B., et al. (2015). Maca reduces blood pressure and depression, in a pilot study in postmenopausal women, NIH National Library of Medicine, National Center for Biotechnology Information: Randomized Controlled Trial Climacteric 2015 Feb;18(1): (pp 69-78). doi: 10.3109/13697137.2014.929649. Epub 2014 Aug 7.
https://pubmed.ncbi.nlm.nih.gov/24931003/

Leach, MJ., Moore, V., (2012). Black cohosh (Cimicifuga spp.) for menopausal symptoms, PMC US National Library of Medicine, National Institutes of Health, Cochrane Library: Cochrane Database Syst Rev. 2012 Sep; 2012(9): CD007244. Published online 2012 Sep 12. doi: 10.1002/14651858.CD007244.pub2.
https://www.ncbi.nlm.nih.gov/pmc/articles/PMC6599854/

Kim, M-S., Lim, H-J., Yang, HJ., et al. (2013). Ginseng for managing menopause symptoms: a systematic review of randomized clinical trials, PMC US National Library of Medicine, National Institutes of Health, Elsevier: J Ginseng Res. 2013 Mar; 37(1): (pp 30–36). doi: 10.5142/jgr.2013.37.30.
https://www.ncbi.nlm.nih.gov/pmc/articles/PMC3659624/

Lee, HW., Choi, J., Lee,YJ., et al. (2016). Ginseng for managing menopausal woman's health; A systematic review of double-blind, randomized, placebo-controlled trials, PMC US National Library of Medicine, National Institutes of Health, Medicine: Medicine (Baltimore). 2016 Sep; 95(38): e4914. Published online 2016 Sep 23. doi: 10.1097/MD.0000000000004914.
https://www.ncbi.nlm.nih.gov/pmc/articles/PMC5044908/

Yoon, SJ., Kim, SK., Lee, NA., et al. (2021). Effect of Korean Red Ginseng on metabolic syndrome, PMC US National Library of Medicine, National Institutes of Health, Elsevier: J Ginseng Res. 2021 May; 45(3): (pp 380–389). Published online 2020 Nov 12. doi: 10.1016/j.jgr.2020.11.002.
https://www.ncbi.nlm.nih.gov/pmc/articles/PMC8134847/

Wu, Y-C., Hsieh, C-L., (2011). Pharmacological effects of Radix Angelica Sinensis (Danggui) on cerebral infarction, PMC US National Library of Medicine, National Institutes of Health, Chinese Medicine BMC: Chin Med. 2011; 6: 32. Published online 2011 Aug 25. doi 10.1186/1749-8546-6-32.
https://www.ncbi.nlm.nih.gov/pmc/articles/PMC3174116/

Lau, CBS., Ho, TCY., Chan, TWL., et al. (2005). Use of dong quai (Angelica sinensis) to treat peri- or postmenopausal symptoms in women with breast cancer: is it appropriate? NIH, National Library of Medicine, National Center for Biotechnology Information: Menopause. Nov-Dec 2005;12(6): (pp 734-40). doi: 10.1097/01.gme.0000184419.65943.01. Epub 2005 Nov 8.
https://pubmed.ncbi.nlm.nih.gov/16278617/

Mahboubi, M., (2019). Evening Primrose (Oenothera biennis) Oil in Management of Female Ailments, PMC US National Library of Medicine, National Institutes of Health, JMM, Journal of Menopausal Medicine: J Menopausal Med. 2019 Aug; 25(2):(pp 74–82). Published online 2019 Aug 5. doi: 10.6118/jmm.18190.
https://www.ncbi.nlm.nih.gov/pmc/articles/PMC6718646/

Horrobin, DF., (1983). The role of essential fatty acids and prostaglandins in the premenstrual syndrome, PMC US National Library of Medicine, National Institutes of Health, NIH, National Center for Biotechnology Information: J Reprod Med. 1983 Jul;28(7): (pp 465-8).
https://pubmed.ncbi.nlm.nih.gov/6350579/

Timoszuk, M., Bielawska, K., Skrzydlewska, E., (2018). Evening Primrose (Oenothera biennis) Biological Activity Dependent on Chemical Composition, PMC US National Library of Medicine, National Institutes of Health, Antioxidants MDPI: Antioxidants (Basel). 2018 Aug; 7(8): 108. Published online 2018 Aug 14. doi: 10.3390/antiox7080108.
https://www.ncbi.nlm.nih.gov/pmc/articles/PMC6116039/

Klemow, KM., Bartlow, A., Crawford, J., et al. (2011). Chapter 11 Medical Attributes of St. John's Wort (Hypericum perforatum), NCBI, Herbal Medicine: Biomolecular and Clinical Aspects. 2nd edition: Benzie IFF, Wachtel-Galor S, editors. Boca Raton (FL): CRC Press/Taylor & Francis; 2011.
https://www.ncbi.nlm.nih.gov/books/NBK92750/

Al-Akoum, M., Maunsell, E., Verreault, R., et al. (2009). Effects of Hypericum perforatum (St. John's wort) on hot flashes and quality of life in perimenopausal women: a randomized pilot trial, NIH, National Library of Medicine, National Center for Biotechnology Information: Randomized Controlled Trial Menopause. Mar-Apr 2009;16(2): (pp 307-14). doi: 10.1097/gme.0b013e31818572a0.
https://pubmed.ncbi.nlm.nih.gov/19194342/

Bent, S., Padula, A., Moore, D., et al. (2006). Valerian for Sleep: A Systematic Review and Meta-Analysis, PMC US National Library of Medicine, National Institutes of Health, HHS Public Access, Author Manuscript: Am J Med. Author manuscript; available in PMC 2015 Apr 13. Published in final edited form as: Am J Med. 2006 Dec; 119(12): (pp 1005–1012). doi: 10.1016/j.amjmed.2006.02.026 https://www.ncbi.nlm.nih.gov/pmc/articles/PMC4394901/
LiverTox: Clinical and Research Information on Drug-Induced Liver Injury [Internet]. (2012). Valerian.
https://www.ncbi.nlm.nih.gov/books/NBK548255/

Houghton, PJ., (1999). The scientific basis for the reputed activity of Valerian, NIH, National Library of Medicine, National Center for Biotechnology Information: J Pharm Pharmacol. 1999 May;51(5): (pp 505-12).
doi: 10.1211/0022357991772772.
https://pubmed.ncbi.nlm.nih.gov/10411208/

Brondino, N., De Silvestri, A., Re, S., et al. (2013). A Systematic Review and Meta-Analysis of Ginkgo biloba in Neuropsychiatric Disorders: From Ancient Tradition to Modern-Day Medicine, PMC US National Library of Medicine, National Institutes of Health, Hindawi: Evid Based Complement Alternat Med. 2013; 2013: 915691. Published online 2013 May 28. doi: 10.1155/2013/915691
https://www.ncbi.nlm.nih.gov/pmc/articles/PMC3679686/

Nguyen, T., Alzahrani, T., (2021). Ginkgo Biloba, NCBI, StatPearls {Internet}: Treasure Island (FL): StatPearls Publishing; 2021 Jan-. https://www.ncbi.nlm.nih.gov/books/NBK541024/

Chen, S-N., Friesen, JB., Webster, D., et al (2012). Phytoconstituents from Vitex agnus-castus fruits, PMC US National Library of Medicine, National Institutes of Health, HHS Public Access, Author Manuscript: Fitoterapia. Author manuscript; available in PMC 2012 Jun 1. Published in final edited form as: Fitoterapia. 2011 Jun; 82(4): (pp 528–533). Published online 2010 Dec 13. doi: 10.1016/j.fitote.2010.12.003.
https://www.ncbi.nlm.nih.gov/pmc/articles/PMC3081944/

Prasad, S., Aggarwal, BB., (Sourced January 2021). Chapter 13: Turmeric, the Golden Spice, Herbal Medicine: PMC US National Library of Medicine, National Institutes of Health, Biomolecular and Clinical Aspects. 2nd edition: Benzie IFF, Wachtel-Galor S, editors. Boca Raton (FL): CRC Press/Taylor & Francis; 2011.
https://www.ncbi.nlm.nih.gov/books/NBK92752/

Hewlings, SJ., Kalman, DS. (2017). Curcumin: A Review of Its Effects on Human Health, Foods, PMC US National Library of Medicine, National Institutes of Health, MDPI: Foods. 2017 Oct; 6(10): 92. Published online 2017 Oct 22. doi: 10.3390/foods6100092. https://www.ncbi.nlm.nih.gov/pmc/articles/PMC5664031/

World Health Organization, (2018). CANNABIDIOL (CBD), Critical Review, Report
https://www.who.int/docs/default-source/controlled-substances/whocbdreportmay2018-2.pdf

Huestis, MA., Solimini, R., Pichini, S., et al. (2019). Cannabidiol Adverse Effects and Toxicity, PMC US National Library of Medicine, National Institutes of Health, Current Neuropharmacology: Curr Neuropharmacol. 2019 Oct; 17(10): (pp 974–989). Published online 2019 Oct. doi: 10.2174/1570159X17666190603171901.
https://www.ncbi.nlm.nih.gov/pmc/articles/PMC7052834/

Geller, SE., Studee, L., (2007). Botanical and Dietary Supplements for Menopausal Symptoms: What Works, What Doesn't, PMC US National Library of Medicine, National Institutes of Health, HHS Public Access, Author Manuscript: J Womens Health (Larchmt). Author manuscript; available in PMC 2007 Jan 8. Published in final edited form as: J Womens Health (Larchmt). 2005 Sep; 14(7): (pp 634–649). doi: 10.1089/jwh.2005.14.634.
https://www.ncbi.nlm.nih.gov/pmc/articles/PMC1764641/

Geller, SE., Studee, L., (2007). Contemporary Alternatives to Plant Estrogens for Menopause, PMC US National Library of Medicine, National Institutes of Health, HHS Public Access, Author Manuscript: Maturitas. Author manuscript; available in PMC 2007 Nov 1. Published in final edited form as: Maturitas. 2006 Nov 1; 55(Suppl 1): S3–13. Published online 2006 Aug 1. doi: 10.1016/j.maturitas.2006.06.012.
https://www.ncbi.nlm.nih.gov/pmc/articles/PMC1780040/

«Three parts medicine, seven parts nurturing health.
Skill in treating is not as good as skill in nurturing health.»

Chinese saying.

Source: Deadman, P., (2016). Live Well, Live Long: Teachings from the Chinese Nourishment of Life Tradition and Modern Research. The Journal of Chinese Medicine Ltd: Hove, England.

SECTION 7 - Self-care

7.1 Yangsheng: The Ancient Art of Self-Care

The practice of self-care is one of the most effective ways to stay healthy at any age. However, it is especially important as we grow older since the body becomes less adept at recovering from lifestyle-related physiological stress.

Daily activities have a far more significant impact in the long-term than treatment alone. Therefore, encouraging and empowering patients to take responsibility for their wellbeing can greatly improve outcomes in the vast majority of cases.

Broadly speaking, there are two primary ways to become and remain healthy:

1. Avoid harms: behaviors, foods, substances, or events that may cause physical or emotional damage (such as eating junk food, binge drinking, and being sedentary).

2. Actively make healthy choices: eating well, exercising regularly, connecting with friends and family, getting adequate rest, and moderate consumption of alcohol.

Chinese medicine extends this second principle and prescribes a universal self-care formula to cultivate health and longevity: *yangsheng*.

The character *yang* (养) translates as 'to support,' 'to cultivate,' or 'to nourish' and the character *sheng* (生) translates as 'life' or 'living.' Therefore, the most widely used translation of the term *yangsheng* is 'nourishment of life.'

As the name suggests, the aim of *yangsheng* is to promote a long and healthy life. It involves the regulation of one's diet, emotions, activity levels, and sleep, with a strong emphasis on moderation in all areas.

Chapter 1 of the *Su Wen* describes how, during a period referred to as 'high antiquity,' people had an average lifespan of 100 years[33] :

"Eating and drinking had their limit,
Activity and rest had their norm,
Not exhausting themselves thoughtlessly,
Body and spirit held together,
Having reached the natural span
They departed at 100 years of age."

[33] Larre, C., translated from French by Firebrace, P. (1994) The Way of Heaven Monkey Press. Cambridge, UK.

The following practices are all essential to the *yangsheng* tradition:

1. Cultivating the mind and managing the emotions
2. Regulating the diet, including how, when, and what we consume
3. Cultivating the body by balancing appropriate rest, activity, and exercise, including deep breathing
4. Getting enough good quality sleep
5. Having a healthy and fulfilling sex life
6. Making time for leisure activities, such as spending time in nature or enjoying music, dance, and art
7. Making appropriate lifestyle adaptations during pregnancy and following childbirth
8. Caring for children wisely
9. Accepting the aging process and managing it as well as possible

The Four Legs of a Chair

According to Peter Deadman, the author of Live Well Live Long: Teachings from the Chinese Nourishment of Life Tradition and Modern Research (2016), the first four of these principles are paramount to good health at every stage in life: mind and emotions, diet, exercise, and sleep. Analogous to the four legs of a chair, they all carry equal importance.

Homeostasis, the interdependent and optimal functioning of all systems of the human organism, is the chair. If one of these 'legs' is weak or broken the chair becomes unstable.

Cultivating the Mind and Emotions

It is considered healthy to express one's emotions at the appropriate time, at an appropriate level, and in a considerate way. Conversely, emotional extremes, outbursts, or getting 'stuck' in one emotion can have detrimental consequences. For example, so-called 'destructive anger' has been linked to an increased risk of coronary heart disease while chronic stress is known to compromize immunity and cause damage to various organs and tissues (see Chapter 5.2 Stress, Trauma and Stress Resistance).

Practices such as mindfulness and meditation, which allow the individual to observe their emotions without engaging in them, can be especially helpful here. Other beneficial activities include those which harmonize the body and mind. Tai chi, qi gong, meditation, and yoga are all good examples of activities with both physical and psychological benefits. Slow, deep breathing, in particular, can help to activate the parasympathetic branch of the central nervous system, which is associated with relaxation and rest.

It may also be helpful to cultivate a more positive mindset by focusing on emotions such as friendship, gratitude, kindness, and forgiveness. With regards to menopause, specifically, it can be helpful to reframe the experience as a positive one. Having a sense of optimism regarding menopause and what lies beyond can make the entire process much easier. It also allows menopause to become an opportunity to heal and grow (see Chapter 1.2, Your Role as a Clinician).

Diet and Eating Habits

There is a saying in Chinese that "medicine and food share a common origin." However, in the West, food is viewed more as fuel than medicine. For example, food is measured in calories and kilojoules, which are the units of energy needed to raise the temperature of one gram of water by 33.8°F. Therefore all foods are measured by the amount of energy they provide. Chinese medicine, on the other hand, views food as something that can heal or cause harm. Helping patients shift this mindset is a big part of midlife health management.

As well as eating foods that are nutritious, natural, and in season, it is essential to pay attention to the way these foods are eaten. Once again, balance is key here and it is important to eat well without becoming obsessive or following overly restrictive diets.

Yangsheng places importance on how and when a person eats, extending beyond the axiom "you are what you eat." Within this framework, the emphasis is on the person, timing, and their environment, not only the food being consumed.

How to Eat

Eating should be enjoyable and only done when in a calm state of mind. Using all of one's senses when eating can improve digestion by enhancing what is known as the 'cephalic phase.' This term is used to describe the impact of sufficiently smelling and tasting food on the release of pancreatic enzymes and gastric acid. This crucial phase of optimal digestion is undermined by eating on the go, not chewing food sufficiently, or engaging in other activities (such as driving, speaking on the phone, or watching TV) while eating. Therefore, meals should be eaten slowly while sitting down and paying full attention to their various tastes and textures.

How Much to Eat

As women enter midlife, they may benefit from a certain degree of calorie restriction. This can be achieved by only eating when hungry and stopping before one is completely full. However, it is crucial to ensure that the diet remains nutritionally complete to avoid deficiencies. Good advice for patients is to eat to 70% full, never over or under-eating.

When to Eat

Timing is another key factor and food eaten in the first half of the day, while the Spleen is functioning at its peak, will be digested more efficiently. Conversely, food eaten late in the evening can lead to stagnation and Stomach-heat, with symptoms such as abdominal discomfort and insomnia. Eating too late in the evening can also reduce one's appetite the following morning, making it difficult to eat a good breakfast.

What to Eat

Modern advances in refrigeration, preservation, and food transport mean that we can now import foods outside of their natural season from anywhere in the world. While, at first, this may seem great in terms of taste and variety, it is not so beneficial for our health.

Imported foods, such as fruits, are often picked before they have ripened fully, and artificially engineered to appear ripe. They may look juicy and appealing on the shelf, but these foods are often not what they seem. Worse still, many people now eat large amounts of highly processed foods that are low in nutrition and high in fat, sugar, salt, and hidden additives.

Most importantly, consuming food that is fresh and grown locally means only eating in accordance with the season. Seasonal foods ripen fully and naturally and are packed with nutrition, unlike those which have traveled from halfway across the world with their nutrients engineered out.

Another advantage of eating local, seasonal food is that it will meet the body's changing requirements at different times of year. For example, many people find that they are instinctively drawn towards energy-rich comfort food in the fall and winter (belonging to the earth element), whereas in spring and summer they prefer fresh, juicy fruit and vegetables (wood element).

Yangsheng also places emphasis on a balance of the five tastes; sour, bitter, sweet, acrid (pungent), and salty. These correspond to the five elements and their principal yin organs: the Liver, Heart, Spleen, Lungs, and Kidneys. Meals require a balance of the five tastes and avoidance of over-consuming any one in excess.

Furthermore, food preparation is categorized into five temperature groups, or natures; heating, warming, neutral, cooling, and cold. All foods are also seen as having distinct properties depending on the location, season, and climate in which they are grown. This allows food to be used as a medicine, with cooling foods such as cucumbers and watermelon being useful in hot diseases, and warming foods such as ginger and garlic being useful for the symptoms of cold.

Individuals should also eat according to their own constitution. For instance, damp, moistening foods such as dairy, wheat, avocados, and bananas could be helpful for people with dry conditions such as dry skin or constipation. However, if they are eaten by someone with a damp constitution and symptoms such as fatigue, heavy limbs, and loose stools, these foods could make matters much worse.

Yangsheng takes the view that the diet should be tailored to suit one's constitutional strengths with avoidance of foods that are likely to cause illnesses. Depending on where an individual's primary imbalances lie, certain foods could either alleviate or exacerbate the symptoms of their condition. Therefore, what is considered healthy for one person could be extremely harmful to another (see Chapter 3.6, Five Elements, Five Phases).

In terms of the make-up of meals, rich, fatty, and strongly flavored foods should be combined with those that are bland and easy to digest. However, the correct balance will vary depending on an individual's energy requirements and constitution. For example, during adolescence and pregnancy, individuals will require more rich, energy-dense foods to support healthy growth and development.

On the other hand, those who are convalescing or have weak digestion will benefit from eating more bland foods. Likewise, those who are extremely physically active will require more energy-dense foods than those who live a more sedentary lifestyle. Menopausal women require smaller quantities of highly nutritious food and should avoid spicy, processed foods, and refined sugar.

Exercise, Physical Activity, and Breathing

Physical activity is crucial throughout life but becomes even more so leading up to menopause. Weight gain is common during the menopausal transition, which contributes to the risk of developing chronic health conditions such as diabetes, cardiovascular disease, arthritis, and some forms of cancer. Regular exercise can also help to combat mood disorders such as depression and anxiety.

However, exercising to the point of exhaustion is counterproductive. From a TCEAM perspective, excessive sweating means fluid loss, which can contribute to yin deficiency and the leakage of qi through the pores. In biomedical terms, over-exercising increases circulating cortisol levels, a contributing factor to sleep problems and blood glucose dysregulation.

It is, therefore, appropriate to balance high-intensity workouts with gentler activities, such as tai chi, qi gong, and yoga. Muscle-strengthening exercise is also essential during midlife to combat the effects of sarcopenia (muscle loss).

> **Breathing and Free Flow**
> "Free flow is the smooth and unobstructed circulation of qi, Blood and fluid through the healthy body and essentially means that all bodily processes are working at their optimum state."[34]

---

[34] Deadman, P., (2016). Live Well, Live Long: Teachings from the Chinese Nourishment of Life Tradition and Modern Research. The Journal of Chinese Medicine Ltd : Hove, England.

How to Breathe Exercise by Peter Deadman[35]

The lungs can expand in all three dimensions... upwards/downwards, sideways, and forwards/backwards. Because of constraint from the rib cage, however, the greatest possible area of expansion is downwards.

When we deepen our breathing, the diaphragm descends, pushing down the abdominal contents and allowing air to fill the lower lobes of the lung which are rich in blood vessels and so able to absorb oxygen efficiently.

Breathing is unusual among our visceral (body organ) processes in that it can be both unconsciously maintained (like the beating of the heart), and consciously controlled. For most of the day we are unaware of breathing in the same way that we are unaware of our digestive process. Unlike digestion, however, we can choose to control breathing, and in both the Chinese tradition and in modern stress and anxiety management training, the emphasis is on slow and deep abdominal (diaphragmatic) breathing, rather than breathing into the chest walls.

The conventional way of learning this breathing is to sit in a chair – relaxed but upright, so that the abdomen is not restricted. One hand can be placed on the chest, and the other on the abdomen below the navel. As we inhale, the hand resting on the chest should barely move, while the hand on the abdomen will move outwards as the abdomen expands like a balloon on inhalation and sinks back on exhalation.

Inhalation should always be through the nose (if possible), while exhalation can be from the nose or mouth. The art is to allow the breathing to become smooth and relaxed of its own accord, and never to try to make it so. Forcing the breath by trying to inhale or exhale too deeply, or holding it for extended periods, risks causing mental agitation and disturbance, rather than calm.

When we allow the breath to sink, rather than forcing it, while maintaining a calm and centered attention, the breath will begin to slow down naturally. As we practise and gain experience, we can start to feel the breath filling the whole pelvic region, not just the front of the abdomen where we practised resting the hand, but also the sides, the lower back and the pelvic floor. Like all worthwhile skills, this requires patience to develop but in time the experience will be deeply rewarding.

Breathing in this way can slow the heartbeat, lower or stabilize blood pressure, and help in the relief of anxiety.

[35] Deadman, P., (2016). Live Well, Live Long: Teachings from the Chinese Nourishment of Life Tradition and Modern Research. The Journal of Chinese Medicine Ltd : Hove, England.

Tai Chi and Qi Gong

Tai chi (or taiji) and qi gong are often considered forms of moving meditation and combine smooth, flowing movements with deep and controlled breathing. The principles underlying the two practices are similar and they provide similar benefits, including improved balance and strength as well as mental relaxation.

Qi gong is older than tai chi and it tends to involve simpler movements and is easier to learn. Meanwhile, tai chi is usually more choreographed with particular movements carried out in a fixed sequence. Furthermore, there are many different forms of tai chi and qi gong, each with subtle differences in the way that they are performed.

Sleep

Good sleep is one of the most important ways to maintain good health. Unfortunately, getting a good night's sleep can be difficult during menopause due to symptoms such as night sweats and insomnia. Generally speaking, women are more prone to insomnia throughout life as they are more likely to be Blood deficient than men. These issues often worsen with age due to declining yin.

Fortunately, these issues can be combated to some degree by maintaining good sleep hygiene. Regularity is key, and those suffering from sleep problems should aim to go to bed and get up at the same time each day, even at weekends. One can prepare the body for sleep by dimming the lights in the evening and avoiding electronic screens to promote melatonin production. Overly stimulating activities should also be avoided during the evening, including talking too much and overeating. Caffeine should not be consumed after mid-afternoon, or even earlier for sensitive individuals.

Keeping the bedroom cool is a good way to reduce night sweats, although it is advisable to sleep under light bed clothes rather than uncovered. According to Chinese traditions, the best position for sleep is on one side with the knees bent.

Soaking the feet in hot water before bed can help to draw yang downwards and promote restful sleep. See Chapter 7.3 for a selection of foot soak recipes.

The remaining *yangsheng* principles are:

Healthy and Fulfilling Sex Life

Another form of physical activity which is often referred to in *yangsheng* traditions is sexual activity. The consensus is that excessive sexual activity in men leads to loss of *jing* and, therefore, contributes to the aging process.

However, for women there is an alternative school of thought that suggests that maintaining a healthy level of sexual activity during menopause and midlife could help to counter symptoms such as vaginal dryness and atrophy. We explore this further in Chapter 5.4, Sexual Activity.

Enjoying Nature, Music, Dance, and Art

Living in Harmony With Nature and the Seasons

Living in harmony with the seasons is another critical element of *yangsheng*, and it is necessary to make adjustments to one's lifestyle throughout the year to maintain health and prevent disease. This particular aspect of *yangsheng* is especially difficult to adhere to in modern society, as the majority of people have to start and finish work at the same time each day regardless of changing daylight hours and temperatures.

However, it is possible to modify one's lifestyle in a way that makes transitioning through the seasons easier, even if the circumstances are less than ideal. For example, by eating seasonal foods and engaging in the proper levels of physical activity, one can move through the seasons smoothly and reduce the likelihood of becoming unwell.

Moving harmoniously with the seasons means moving harmoniously with yin and yang, and maintaining the proper balance between the two. The idea of balance and avoiding extremes lies right at the core of the *yangsheng* tradition.

Spring

Spring is a time of awakening and invigoration as yang begins to take over from yin. It is a time to reintroduce movement and vitality after the stillness of the winter months. Spring is associated with the Liver and, therefore, the muscles and tendons. It is appropriate to increase one's physical activity during this season, with an emphasis on improving suppleness and flexibility. It is also the right time to eat more leafy green vegetables, herbs, shoots, and sour-tasting foods.

Summer

Summer is the season of maturity, with yang reaching its zenith during the warmer months. The days are longer, allowing for increased outdoor activity, although it is essential to avoid overexposure to the sun. Equally, the use of air-conditioners and electric fans is viewed as extremely damaging to one's health. It can result in disharmony between yin and yang, which may manifest as illness during the fall and winter months. Cooling the body should be primarily done by eating appropriate foods, such as watermelon, cucumbers, gourds, and so on.

Fall

Throughout the fall months, yang begins to decline as yin increases. The days become shorter and colder, and it is appropriate to spend more time indoors. If it is necessary to perform outdoor activities, one should wear enough clothing to keep warm. Fall is also associated with dryness and it is necessary to moisten and nourish the Lungs to avoid symptoms such as coughing and sore throats. Appropriate foods for protecting the Lungs during fall include pears, radishes, mushrooms, and tofu.

Winter

Winter is the season of maximum yin. It is a time for stillness, reflection, and conserving one's resources. Exerting too much energy during the winter can be injurious to the Kidneys, as can failing to stay sufficiently warm. Ideally, all activity should be done during the daylight hours, although in modern life this is rarely feasible. It is best to eat energy-rich foods such as root vegetables, as well as those that nourish the Kidneys, including black rice, soy sauce, and sea vegetables.

Other examples of connecting with nature and the seasons include gardening, walking and hiking, camping, and outdoor activities. Exploring forests, oceans, and mountains - even the local park - provides an opportunity to be at one with nature.

The Moon Cycle

Women who are grieving the loss of their menstrual cycle may choose to align themselves with the moon in order to continue experiencing a natural energetic ebb and flow. Traditionally, the waxing moon has been associated with the pre-ovulation phase and increasing *yin*. Meanwhile, the waning moon represents the post-ovulation phase and increasing *yang*. Women may simply choose to observe these changes or adjust their activities accordingly.

Music, Dance, and Art

Given that menopause is fundamentally about change, many women find it a time to explore creativity and try new things. For some women, the freeing up of time and resources with children growing up and becoming less dependent or moving out of the family home means they have more time and energy for their own pursuits. Encouraging them to take up the *yangsheng* practice of nourishing one's creativity and artistic expression can harmonize the free flow of Blood and qi, boost confidence, and be an outlet for social connectivity and learning new skills.

Lifestyle During Pregnancy and Following Childbirth

Based on the philosophy of Confucianism and Daoism with ancestral worship at the core, conception is the fusion of yin and yang (man and woman) and continuation of family heredity (in modern terms the genetic line). *Yangsheng* places a huge emphasis on pregnancy and childbirth with a set of guidelines to protect health and wellbeing during the pregnancy and in the months and even years following childbirth. We discuss this in greater detail in Chapter 3.3 Gates of Life.

Caring for Children Wisely

Children are essential to the future wellbeing of our planet and society. Therefore, ensuring their wellbeing is beneficial, even for those who do not have children of their own. Chinese medicine has viewed pediatrics as a speciality area for centuries.

According to the famous physician Sun Simiao[36]:

> *"There is no Dao [literally 'path', but here in the sense of 'skill' or 'practice'] among the common people that is greater than the Dao of nurturing the young."*

There are many excellent textbooks on the subject of caring for children with TCEAM, and it is beyond the scope of this book to elaborate on the specialty of pediatrics.

Managing the Aging Process

With the exception of premature death, growing old is inevitable and as yet, cannot be prevented. However, we do have some control over how we age.

While genetics and unavoidable environmental factors do play a role, one's lifestyle and attitude can significantly influence the aging process. By incorporating *yangsheng* practices into our daily lives, we can potentially extend our active years and minimize the risk of chronic disease.

Summary

Although *yangsheng* is an ancient practice, it is still very much applicable today. By educating our patients and encouraging them to adopt these healthy habits and daily rituals, we can help them to improve their overall health and enhance the outcomes of treatment.

If a woman begins preparing for menopause well in advance, she can reduce the severity of many issues. By eating well, exercising sufficiently, and practicing *yangsheng* techniques, it is possible to remain healthy both during and after menopause.

---

[36] Deadman, P., (2016). Live Well, Live Long: Teachings from the Chinese Nourishment of Life Tradition and Modern Research. The Journal of Chinese Medicine Ltd : Hove, England.

References

Larre, C., translated from French by Firebrace, P. (1994) The Way of Heaven. Monkey Press. Cambridge, UK.
Deadman, P., (2006). Live Well Live Long: Teachings from the Chinese Nourishment of Life Tradition. The Journal of Chinese Medicine Ltd: Hove, England.

Deadman, P., (2019). Teachings from the Chinese Nourishment of Life Traditions. Treating Women Academy: Online Menopause Masterclass.
https://www.treatingwomen.com/store/5tpUJ3Fk

Davidson, KW., Mostofsky, E., (2010). Anger Expression and Risk of Coronary Heart Disease: Evidence From the Nova Scotia Health Survey, PMC US National Library of Medicine, National Institutes of Health, HHS Public Access, Author manuscript: Am Heart J. Author manuscript; available in PMC 2011 Feb 1. Published in final edited form as: Am Heart J. 2010 Feb; 159(2): (pp 199–206). doi: 10.1016/j.ahj.2009.11.007.
https://www.ncbi.nlm.nih.gov/pmc/articles/PMC2831051

Mariotti, A., (2015). The effects of chronic stress on health: new insights into the molecular mechanisms of brain–body communication, PMC US National Library of Medicine, National Institutes of Health, Future Science OA: Future Sci OA. 2015 Nov; 1(3): FSO23. Published online 2015 Nov 1. doi: 10.4155/fso.15.21.
https://www.ncbi.nlm.nih.gov/pmc/articles/PMC5137920

Katschinski, M., (2000). Nutritional implications of cephalic phase gastrointestinal responses, NIH, National Library of Medicine, National Center for Biotechnology Information: Appetite. 2000 Apr;34(2): (pp 189-96).
doi: 10.1006/appe.1999.0280.
https://www.ncbi.nlm.nih.gov/pubmed/10744909

Hill, EE., Zack, E., Battaglini, C., et al. (2008). Exercise and circulating cortisol levels: the intensity threshold effect, NIH, National Library of Medicine, National Center for Biotechnology Information: J Endocrinol Invest. 2008 Jul;31(7): (pp 587-91). doi: 10.1007/BF03345606..
https://www.ncbi.nlm.nih.gov/pubmed/18787373

7.2 Teas and Infusions

Tea is an integral part of the *yangsheng* tradition. It has been drunk in China since approximately 2700 BC. However, it was not popularized until the 8th century when Lu Yu wrote the Tea Classic, or *Cha Jing*.

Portuguese and Dutch traders brought tea back to Europe during the 16th century and it rapidly spread across the globe. It is now the most commonly drunk beverage in the world, with the only exception being water.

Not only is tea enjoyable to drink, but it also has a range of potential benefits for human health. These benefits derive from a range of compounds such as catechins that are present in varying levels in different types of tea.

Although all tea comes from the same plant, *Camellia sinensis*, the beverage can possess a broad range of characteristics depending on how it is processed.

After tea leaves are harvested, they begin to oxidize. This process can be halted by exposing the leaves to heat, a technique known as *shaqing* (literally 'kill green').

White and green teas undergo *shaqing* soon after harvesting, meaning that they do not become highly oxidized. On the other hand, oolong, red, and black teas are allowed to oxidize for much longer periods, sometimes with the additional process of fermentation.

Generally speaking, the less oxidation a tea undergoes, the more catechins it will retain. Meanwhile, as tea leaves become more oxidized, their caffeine content increases. It is for this reason that white and green teas are considered the most beneficial to health.

Teas and TCEAM

In TCEAM terms, tea leaves are classified as bitter in flavor and cool in nature. However, white and green teas are the most cooling, while red and black teas are warmer in nature.

In China, it is a commonly held belief that green tea is most appropriate for summer use, while red and black teas should be enjoyed in winter. However, the most appropriate tea for any individual will also depend on their constitutional type and symptomatology.

Tea has the ability to enter the Heart, Lung, and Stomach channels. Its traditional uses include promoting digestion, resolving phlegm, relieving thirst, refreshing the mind, inducing diuresis, and removing toxicity.

Green tea also possesses a number of benefits from a biomedical perspective. Numerous studies have shed light on its potential as a preventative measure against various chronic diseases. However, in order to derive any benefits, it is necessary to consume several cups each day.

Compound	Properties	Description
Caffeine	Stimulates the central nervous system. Increases alertness and energy. Acts as a diuretic. Increases production of stomach acid. May interfere with iron and calcium absorption. Increases heart rate and blood pressure.	Caffeine is an alkaloid compound, specifically, a methylxanthine. It acts as a central nervous system stimulant to impart a sense of alertness and energy, while also increasing heart rate and blood pressure. Caffeine also acts as a diuretic and increases stomach acid production. It can interfere with iron and calcium absorption, meaning that it should not be consumed at mealtimes.
Catechins	A type of plant polyphenol. Powerful antioxidant effects. Responsible for many of tea's health benefits.	Catechins are a type of plant polyphenol and possess powerful antioxidant properties. These are the compounds that are responsible for many of tea's potential benefits. Some of the most abundant catechins in tea are ECGC, EGC, and EC.
L-Theanine	Has a direct influence on mental function. Increases alpha brain waves. Induces relaxation without drowsiness.	L-theanine is an amino acid and it has a direct effect on mental function. Research has shown that it increases alpha-brain waves to induce a sense of calm and relaxation.
Theobromine	May possess antitumoral, anti-inflammatory, and cardioprotective effects. May improve respiratory health/relieve cough.	Like caffeine, theobromine is a methylxanthine compound. It may possess antitumoral, anti-inflammatory, and cardioprotective effects. It could also improve respiratory health to relieve symptoms such as coughing.
Theophylline	Found in low levels in black tea. Bronchodilator. Anti-inflammatory effects.	Another methylxanthine compound, theophylline is found in low levels in black tea. It acts as a bronchodilator and may also possess anti-inflammatory effects.

Table 7.2a: Properties of compounds found in tea.

Benefits of Tea

Stimulant Effects

Caffeine enhances acetylcholine activity and inhibits adenosine binding, giving it a stimulating effect on the central nervous system. This is perhaps one of the best-known properties of tea and other caffeine-containing beverages such as coffee.

Relaxant Effects

L-theanine has a calming effect, helping to balance out the stimulating effects of caffeine. For this reason, tea does not cause a 'wired' or jittery sensation in the same way that coffee can.

The act of drinking tea can be relaxing in itself when seen as an act of self-care or mindfulness. This practice can include listening to the kettle boil, watching the color change as the water pours over the tea leaves, and feeling the warmth of the cup in the hands. Most importantly though, the aroma and flavor of the tea should be truly savoured. Therefore, it is best to drink tea whilst sitting down and away from the computer or any other distractions.

Role in Weight Management

Various studies have shown tea to influence fat metabolism and promote weight loss, with these effects mainly attributed to the catechin EGCG (epigallocatechin gallate). Furthermore, tea is virtually calorie-free when drunk without milk or sugar, making it a healthier substitute for high-fat, high-sugar beverages.

Role in Diabetes Management

By helping women to maintain a healthy weight, tea may help in the prevention of diabetes and metabolic syndrome. Studies also suggest that catechins, including EGCG could play a role in reducing blood glucose and regulating insulin levels.

Cardioprotective Properties

Studies have shown that both black and green tea have potential cardioprotective properties, reducing the risk of hypertension, heart disease, and stroke. Again, many of these benefits are attributed to catechins such as EGCG.

Neuroprotective Properties

Although this area has not been studied rigorously, tea may also offer some neuroprotective benefits, reducing the risk of Alzheimer's and Parkinson's diseases. Once again, this is primarily due to the antioxidant properties of EGCG, although L-theanine may also play a role.

Bone Health Maintenance

There appears to be a positive correlation between tea drinking and bone mineral density, suggesting that tea could offer some protection against osteopenia and osteoporosis. Yet again, ECGC is the primary compound of interest here.

Anticarcinogenic Properties

Finally, tea has displayed anticarcinogenic properties, although the evidence is somewhat inconsistent. It appears to inhibit tumorigenesis in the digestive tract and green tea, specifically, has been linked with a reduced risk of developing breast cancer.

Nutritional Properties

Tea contains a range of essential minerals, including calcium, magnesium, chromium, manganese, iron, copper, zinc, molybdenum, selenium, sodium, phosphorus, cobalt, strontium, nickel, potassium, fluorine, and aluminium.

It also contains trace amounts of vitamins B, C, and E as well as lipids (linoleic and alpha-linolenic acids), and sterols (stigmasterol).

Other Benefits of Tea

Tea also has several other significant advantages as a tool for improving wellbeing.

It is widely available and financially accessible, unlike some other medications, herbs, and supplements, which are costly and sometimes hard to find. Furthermore, it is safe with a low risk of side effects, drug interactions, and no overdose or addiction profile.

It can be used at home, in the office, or even on the go. In China, it is common practice to carry a small tea flask containing an individual's prefered beverage. However, if this is not practical, it is easy to keep a few teabags or a supply of loose leaf tea in one's handbag or car so that it is always on hand.

Finally, there is the social aspect of meeting with friends and family to enjoy tea. This age-old ritual can provide a chance to connect with loved ones while enjoying a comforting brew. This may be especially beneficial for older women as they might feel less inclined to visit bars and nightclubs as their primary source of social interaction.

Precautions

Tea contains caffeine which should not be consumed in excess. The side effects of excessive caffeine consumption include increased heart rate, anxiety, and insomnia, all of which could potentially exacerbate menopausal symptoms. From a TCEAM perspective, tea opens the surface and is useful for that purpose. However, it can initiate perspiration and may aggravate menopausal sweats.

Furthermore, the tannins in tea can impair iron absorption when consumed concurrently. Although this does not appear to significantly alter long-term iron status, it may be best to avoid drinking tea (or other tannin-containing beverages, such as coffee) at mealtimes.

Herbal and Flower Infusions

Herbal 'teas' (more accurately *infusions*) are becoming more popular in the West, leading to an increased need for awareness regarding how they affect the body. Although not as strong as herbal decoctions, drinking the same herbal tea regularly may influence symptoms. Some herbal teas are more suitable for menopausal women than others and when matched appropriately can lead to enhanced treatment outcomes.

Herb	Traditional Uses	Modern Research
Ginger*	Colds Nausea Arthritis Migraines Hypertension	Antioxidant Anti-inflammatory Anti-nausea effects Possible anticarcinogenic activity
Peppermint	Colds Headaches Digestive issues	Antimicrobial Antiviral Antioxidant Antitumor activity Antispasmodic to relax gastrointestinal tissue Possible analgesic effects
Chamomile	Promotes calm and relaxation Sleep aid	Anti-inflammatory Antioxidant Mild astringent May affect estrogen receptors (more evidence needed) Possible benefits for osteoporosis Topical application may relieve vaginitis
Roselle (Hibiscus)	Improve cardiovascular health	Antioxidant Lowers blood pressure Lowers LDL cholesterol without affecting HDL Diuretic
Chinese Hawthorn	Aids digestion of fatty foods	Reduces LDL cholesterol while raising HDL May support fat loss

* Ginger opens the pores and can promote sweating.

Herb	Traditional Uses	Modern Research
Schisandra	Astringing Lung and Large Intestine Securing essence Replenishing qi Nourishing Kidney Promote body fluid production Calming Heart and promoting tranquilization	Hepatoprotective Anti-inflammatory Antioxidant Anticancer activity Modulates immune system Adaptogenic Benefits cardiovascular system Antimicrobial Cosmetic properties
Goji Berry	Nourish Kidney and Liver yin Supplement Blood and essence (*jing*) Benefit eyesight	Antioxidant Anti-inflammatory Maintains eye health Lowers LDL cholesterol and triglycerides while raising HDL Hypoglycemic effects Anticancer effects Modulates immune system Neuroprotective effects (reduces glutamate toxicity) Benefits cardiovascular system
Ginseng[37]	Reinforce original qi Tonify *zang* organs Promote body fluid production Promote tranquilization Improve intellect Nourish Blood	Modulates immune system Anti-cancer properties Hypoglycemic effects Neuroprotective effects
American Ginseng	Tonify qi Nourish yin Clear heat Promote generation of body fluids	Neuroprotective effects Anxiolytic Antioxidant Anti-cancer effects Hypoglycemic effects May aid weight management May help to prevent premature ovarian failure

Table 7.2b: Herbal and flower infusions.

[37] Ginseng is a warming herb and overuse can cause headaches, insomnia, and increased blood pressure. It is unsuitable for patients with Liver yang rising or existing hypertension.

Chinese Medicinal Teas

Chinese medicinal teas are milder and usually better-tasting than prescribed, multi-ingredient formulas. They usually contain one or two ingredients and can be drunk throughout the day as an adjunct to prescribed herbs, acupuncture, or other treatments.

However, it is still necessary to exercise caution and ensure that the ingredients are suitable for the patient's constitution and not contraindicated for any reason. The following recipes have been reproduced with permission from Honora Lee Wolfe's 1998 book, Managing Menopause Naturally with Chinese Medicine.

<table>
<tr><th colspan="2">Tea 1. Liver Depression / Qi Stagnation</th></tr>
<tr><th>Ingredients</th><th>Instructions</th></tr>
<tr><td>Fresh plums 100-150g

Water 320ml

Green tea 2g

Honey 25g</td><td>Boil the fresh plums in the water for 3 minutes.

Add the green tea and honey and steep for 10 minutes.

Take one dose in the morning and evening.</td></tr>
<tr><th colspan="2">Usage</th></tr>
<tr><td colspan="2">Long-term Liver qi stagnation can lead to depressive heat, which can affect the other organs and bowels. Plums soften the stools, dispel dampness, and harmonize the Liver to increase defecation, thus clearing heat from the yangming (Stomach and Large Intestine). Meanwhile, green tea reduces the impact of Liver qi stagnation on breast tissue and cools the Stomach.</td></tr>
</table>

Table 7.2c: Tea 1 for Liver depression / qi stagnation.

Tea 2. Liver Depression / Qi Stagnation	
Ingredients	**Instructions**
Zhi Shi (Aurantii Fructus Immaturus) 25g Chen Pi (Citri Reticulatae Pericarpium) or orange peel 25g Green tea 2g	Boil the two citrus products together in water for several minutes. Add the green tea and steep for 10 minutes. Drink the tea as a beverage any time during the day.
Usage	
Zhi Shi and Chen Pi move qi (especially Stomach and Liver qi), dispel and dry dampness. This benefits patients whose Spleen qi is impaired by Liver qi stagnation, thus weakening its ability to transform and transport fluids. It is a mild and pleasant tasting tea which provides an excellent daily beverage to transform dampness, boost Spleen function, and relieve Liver depression.	

Table 7.2d: Tea 2 for Liver depression / qi stagnation.

Tea 3. Liver Depression / Qi Stagnation	
Ingredients	**Instructions**
Yu Jin (Curcumae Radix i.e. turmeric) 10g Gan Cao (Glycyrrhizae Radix i.e. licorice) 5g [38] Green tea 2g Water 1 liter	Boil the turmeric and licorice in a liter of water. Add the green tea with a little honey to taste. Drink this tea as a beverage throughout the day.
Usage	
Yu Jin is a powerful qi mover and in biomedical terms it has anti-inflammatory properties. Gan Cao harmonizes the Stomach.	

Table 7.2e: Tea 3 for Liver depression / qi stagnation.

[38] People with high blood pressure should consume licorice with caution.

Tea 1. Liver Depression / Depressive Heat	
Ingredients	**Instructions**
Green tea 30g Shan Zhi Zi (Gardeniae Fructus) 30g Water 4 cups	Boil the tea and Shan Zhi Zi together until the liquid is reduced by half. Strain and drink one cup of this tea in the morning and evening.
Usage	
Note: In addition, Jasmine tea purchased at Asian specialty food shops is a good background beverage for those with Liver depression with or without heat.	

Table 7.2f: Tea 1 for Liver depression / depressive heat.

Tea 2. Liver Depression / Depressive Heat	
Ingredients	**Instructions**
Ju Hua (Chrysanthemi Flos) 15g Green tea 2g	Steep together in boiling water for 10 minutes. Drink tea as a beverage during the day.
Usage	
Ju Hua cools the Liver and benefits the eyes. This recipe is beneficial as a daily beverage when Liver heat is causing red, itchy, or burning eyes. It can be drunk warm or at room temperature, or kept in the refrigerator during the heat of summer.	

Table 7.2g: Tea 2 for Liver depression / depressive heat.

Spleen Vacuity Fatigue and Lack of Strength	
Ingredients	**Instructions**
Ren Shen (Ginseng Radix) 8g Water 1 cup	Boil the ginseng in water and let steep for an hour or more.* Drink this as a tea throughout the day.
Usage	
Ren Shen is a warming herb that supports the Spleen. It may be beneficial for patients whose Spleen deficiency is predominant and Liver depression is less significant, especially if their primary symptom is fatigue. A course of this simple tea drunk once daily can greatly improve treatment outcomes.	

Table 7.2h: Tea for Spleen vacuity fatigue and lack of strength.

*Note: Asian specialty food stores often sell small porcelain ginseng cookers. These are lidded cups meant to be placed in a pan of water to create a small double-cooker. Basically, the longer you cook ginseng, the more you get out of it. As a substitute for ginseng, you can use double the amount of Dang Shen (Codonopsis Radix).

PRECAUTION: Do not advise ginseng if your patient suffers from hypertension or high blood pressure.

Tea 1. Spleen Qi and Heart-Blood Vacuity	
Ingredients	**Instructions**
Tai Zi Shen (Pseudostellariae Radix) 9g Fu Xiao Mai (Tritici Fructus Levis) 15g	Place the roots and seeds in a thermos and steep in boiling water for 20 minutes. Drink the tea throughout the day.
Usage	
This tea enriches yin, generates fluids, gently supplements Spleen and Lung qi, and supplements Heart qi to stop sweating. It makes a good background beverage for patients with fatigue, thirst, and hot flashes due to Heart and Spleen deficiency.	

Table 7.2i: Tea 1. for Spleen qi and Heart-Blood vacuity.

Tea 2. Spleen Qi and Heart-Blood Vacuity	
Ingredients	**Instructions**
Long Yan Rou (Longan Arillus) 5–10 pieces	Place the dried fruits in a double boiler or pressure cooker and steam thoroughly. Place them in a teacup and steep in boiling water for 10 minutes. Drink the resulting liquid as a tea.
Usage	
This tea effectively nourishes the Blood and can be effective as a daily beverage to calm the *shen* and improve sleep in patients who are excessively worried, pensive, or forgetful. However, it is also quite damp-forming and is contraindicated for patients with damp or phlegm conditions, or patients where Liver qi stagnation has transformed into depressive heat.	

Table 7.2j: Tea 2. for Spleen qi and Heart-Blood vacuity.

Tea 3. Spleen Qi and Heart-Blood Vacuity	
Ingredients	**Instructions**
Da Zao (Jujubae Fructus) 10 pieces Green tea 5g	Place the fruit in water and boil until completely cooked and soft. Use the resulting liquid to steep the green tea. Drink this tea at any time throughout the day.
Usage	
This tea can be used to calm the *shen*, nourish Blood, and relieve irritability, emotional instability, or restlessness. Da Zao can also be cooked into rice congee or soup and 3-4 pieces eaten daily. However, they are contraindicated in cases of damp heat or phlegm heat.	

Table 7.2k: Tea 3. for Spleen qi and Heart-Blood vacuity.

Tea 1. Insomnia due to Heart Yin and Blood Vacuity	
Ingredients	**Instructions**
Bai Zi Ren (Platycladi Semen) 15g	Grind the seeds into pieces. Boil with water for 10 minutes and add honey to taste. Drink either before or after dinner.
Usage	
Bai Zi Ren nourishes Heart Blood and moistens Kidney yin. This tea is excellent for insomnia, forgetfulness, and palpitations, providing the patient has good digestion. It is not indicated for patients prone to diarrhea due to dampness and phlegm. The tea should be trialed for a few days before prescribing it for longer periods.	

Table 7.2l: Tea 1. for insomnia due to Heart yin and Blood vacuity.

Tea 2. Insomnia due to Heart Yin and Blood Vacuity	
Ingredients	**Instructions**
Sang Shen (Fructus Mori) 15g	Boil the fruit in water, strain and drink one serving per day.
Usage	
This tea nourishes Blood and enriches both Heart and Kidney yin. It can be quite effective for patients with dizziness, tinnitus, insomnia, and premature graying of the hair. However, it should not be used for patients who are prone to diarrhea due to dampness and/or a cold Spleen.	

Table 7.2m: Tea 2. for insomnia due to Heart yin and Blood vacuity.

Tea 3. Insomnia due to Heart Yin and Blood Vacuity	
Ingredients	**Instructions**
Wu Wei Zi (Schisandrae Fructus) Gou Qi Zi (Lycii Fructus)	Grind equal parts of each fruit into powder. Use 5g of this powder steeped in boiling water for 10 minutes. Drink as a tea throughout the day.
Usage	
This combination nourishes the Heart and calms the *shen*, astringes Lung qi, and enriches Kidney yin. It is especially good for chronic thirst, lower back soreness and weakness, and blurred vision. However, Gou Qi Zi can be difficult to digest for those with deficient Spleen qi.	

Table 7.2n: Tea 3. for insomnia due to Heart yin and Blood vacuity.

Tea 4. Insomnia due to Heart Yin and Blood Vacuity	
Ingredients	**Instructions**
Suan Zao Ren (Ziziphi Spinosi Semen) 9 g	Pound the fruit into pieces, steep in boiling water for 10 minutes. Drink throughout the day.
Usage	
This tea can be invaluable for patients with intractable insomnia or irritability due to Liver yin deficiency. It nourishes Heart yin and Liver Blood and clears deficient Heart heat. A small amount of Huang Qi (Astragali Radix) can be added if causing diarrhea is a concern. Some texts suggest only drinking this tea in the afternoon and evening before bed.	

Table 7.2o Tea 4. for insomnia due to Heart yin and Blood vacuity.

Phlegm Obstruction with Liver Depression / Depressive Heat	
Ingredients	**Instructions**
Shi Chang Pu (Acori Tatarinowii Rhizoma) 6 g Mo Li Hua (Jasmini Flos)* 6 g Green tea* 10g * or jasmine tea bought at an Asian specialty food shop	Grind the ingredients into a coarse powder. Soak some of the powder in boiling water. Drink as a tea any time of the day.
Usage	
Shi Chang Pu opens the orifices and disperses phlegm, strengthens digestion, and calms the *shen*. Because it opens the orifices, it can also benefit hearing and improve cognitive function, including memory. This tea is slightly warming but gentle and with the addition of Mo Li Hua, is unlikely to aggravate heat conditions.	

Table 7.2p: Tea for phlegm obstruction with Liver depression / depressive heat.

Phlegm Obstruction Disturbing the Heart Spirit but Without Heat	
Ingredients	**Instructions**
Long Chi (Mastodi Dentis Fossilia) 10 g Shi Chang Pu (Acori Tatarinowii Rhizoma) 3 g	Boil the Long Chi in water for 10 minutes. Add the Shi Chang Pu and continue boiling for another 10 to 15 minutes. Strain and drink any time of the day. 1–2 doses per day. The doses given are for a one day's supply.
Usage	
Long Chi is a useful medicinal for strongly calming the *shen* in patients with red eyes and other signs of unrestrained Liver yang rising. It restrains Liver yang and wind, although it is rarely used alone and is primarily included in formulas for insomnia with disturbing dreams, possibly with palpitations, tinnitus, or dizziness. In combination with Shi Chang Pu, its effect on the *shen* is strengthened and balanced.	

Table 7.2q: Tea for phlegm obstruction disturbing the Heart spirit but without heat.

Fire Disturbing the Heart Spirit	
Ingredients	**Instructions**
Deng Xin Cao (Junci Medulla) 60g Dan Zhu Ye (Lophatheri Herba) 60g	Boil the herbs, strain and drink the tea warm at any time of the day, one serving per day.
Usage	
Fire disturbing the Heart spirit is characterized by restlessness and insomnia, vexation, agitation, and heart palpitations. There will be a red tongue tip and sores on the tip of the tongue. Deng Xin Cao is one of the most commonly used medicinals in the Chinese materia medica. It facilitates the removal of heat via urination. It is useful for patients with both Heart symptoms (e.g. insomnia, anxiety) and urinary symptoms, such as painful, frequent, or dribbling urination, especially in combination with Dan Zhu Ye. The patient may also be irritable. Some sources describe this syndrome as Heart fire with Kidney yin deficiency.	

Table 7.2r: Tea for fire disturbing the Heart spirit.

Tea 1. Menstrual or Uterine Bleeding Due to Spleen-Kidney Dual Vacuity	
Ingredients	**Instructions**
Lian Zi (Nelumbinis Semen i.e. lotus seeds) 5g Tea leaves 30g	Soak the tea leaves in boiling water. Strain and reserve the tea. Soak the lotus seeds in warm water for a few hours. Stew the seeds with a little sugar. Add the tea water and stir well. Once again, strain and drink the remaining liquid as a tea throughout the day.
Usage	
Lotus seeds are another effective medicinal for insomnia and irritability. They are sweet and neutral, benefiting the Spleen, Kidney, and Heart. They also stop bleeding due to the Spleen being unable to contain the blood. This is a mild tea that can be used to re-establish communication between the Heart and Kidney and stop bleeding. Patients should be monitored for side effects such as constipation and abdominal distension. Although it is less likely to occur when lotus seeds are taken in this way, it is still possible. A much more complex formula will be necessary for chronic or severe uterine bleeding to address any specific patterns of disharmony.	

Table 7.2s: Tea 1. Menstrual or uterine bleeding due to Spleen-Kidney dual vacuity.

Tea 2. Menstrual or Uterine Bleeding Due to Heat	
Ingredients	**Instructions**
Qing Hao (Artemisiae Annuae Herba) 6g Mu Dan Pi (Moutan Cortex) 6g Tea leaves 3g	Wash the herbs and place them along with the tea leaves in a teacup. Cover with boiling water and allow it to steep for 15 to 20 minutes. Strain, add a little sugar to taste and drink frequently throughout the day.
Usage	
Excessive menstruation or functional uterine bleeding due to heat forcing the blood to move franetically or recklessly outside its pathways. Qing Hao cools the Blood and is useful for cases of deficiency heat. It can be used for fevers and rashes but is a popular herb for treating pathologic uterine bleeding due to yin deficiency. It is less likely to damage Blood and yin while clearing heat than other hemostatic medicinals. It may cause diarrhea in individuals with severe Spleen deficiency, although this is rare.	

Table 7.2t: Tea 2. Menstrual or uterine bleeding due to heat.

Depression Alternating With Agitation	
Ingredients	**Instructions**
Xiao Mai (Tritici Semen) 30g Da Zao (Jujubae Fructus) 10 pieces Gan Cao (Glycyrrhizae Radix) 6g [39]	Stir-fry the Gan Cao, add the other ingredients then boil in water. Strain the liquid and drink this frequently as tea.
Usage	
Xiao Mai is ripe wheat grain and does not float (unlike Fu Xiao Mai, which does). It nourishes Heart qi to relieve irritability and restlessness. In combination with Da Zao and Gan Cao, it makes the famous Gan Mai Da Zao Tang (licorice, wheat, and jujube decoction) formula. The quantity above will make over two liters of tea, which is an excellent background beverage for patients with insomnia, restlessness, and possibly irritability.	

Table 7.2u: Tea for depression alternating with agitation.

[39] Gan Cao can be omitted for patients with high blood pressure.

Patient Advice

> It is advisable for patients suffering from menopausal symptoms such as hot flashes to avoid very warming teas such as ginger.
> Asking a patient for details regarding what types of tea they are drinking and how often may aid diagnosis.
> If someone has recently drunk a cup of tea (or coffee) it can affect tongue and pulse diagnosis.
> Advise patients to avoid adding milk, sugar, or sweeteners to tea to reduce calories, inflammation, and damp formation.

Summary

Tea and herbal infusions have numerous benefits during and after menopause in terms of both physical and mental health. However, while true teas from Camellia sinensis have an excellent safety profile, it is necessary to exercise a little more caution with other herbs.

While herbal teas are less potent than full-strength medicinal decoctions, drinking the same infusion for a prolonged period can have noticeable effects. Therefore, it is advisable for women planning on doing this to seek professional advice to ensure their chosen tea is suitable for them.

References

Saunders, NC., (2017). The Qi of Tea: The History and Use of Tea in Traditional Chinese Medicine. Kindle Edition.

Delimont, NM., Haub, MD., Lindshield, BL., (2017). The Impact of Tannin Consumption on Iron Bioavailability and Status: A Narrative Review, NIH, National Library of Medicine, National Center for Biotechnology Information: CDN Current Developments in Nutrition, Curr Dev Nutr. 2017 Feb; 1(2): 1–12. Published online 2017 Jan 19. doi: 10.3945/cdn.116.000042 - https://www.ncbi.nlm.nih.gov/pmc/articles/PMC5998341

Saunders, NC., (2019). The Qi of Tea for Midlife and Menopause. Treating Women Academy: Online Menopause Masterclass.- https://www.treatingwomen.com/store/5tpUJ3Fk

Wolfe, HL., (1998). Managing Menopause Naturally with Chinese Medicine. Blue Poppy Press ; Portland, Oregon, USA.

7.3 Foot Soaks

The traditional practice of soaking the feet has many potential benefits. From a TCEAM viewpoint, it draws yang downward, thus countering the flaring up of heat and aiding relaxation and sleep. Furthermore, there are many key acupuncture points on the foot, relating to various organs and body parts. Therefore, treating the feet can have a positive influence on a person's overall wellbeing.

From a biomedical perspective, soaking the feet in hot water improves microcirculation in the area. Therefore, it may play a role in the treatment of local conditions, such as diabetic peripheral neuropathy (although care must be taken to ensure the water is not too hot if a patient has altered sensations in their feet). Soaking also increases skin permeability, allowing herbs' medicinal compounds to enter the bloodstream without the need for oral consumption, which may be prefered in some cases.

Although it is generally a well-tolerated and enjoyable modality, there are a few general guidelines to follow to ensure the patient's safety. Therefore, practitioners wishing to recommend the practice should advise their patients as follows:

- In most cases, the ideal temperature for soaking is 98 - 107°F.
- Soak the feet for an appropriate length of time:
    - At temperatures between 98- 107°F, soak for 10-30 minutes.
    - At cooler temperatures 93-97°F, soak for 15-30 minutes.
    - At temperatures between 107-111°F or below 91°F, do not exceed 10 minutes.
- The dosage for external medicines is relatively large and unsuitable for oral use. Furthermore, toxic herbs should be used with extreme caution.
- Soaking the feet is unsuitable for patients with fever or bleeding. Use with extreme caution in patients with high blood pressure, or a history/high risk of strokes.
- Deficient patients should exercise caution. Stop the treatment immediately if dizziness or lightheadedness occurs to avoid fainting.
- Soaking the feet can increase calorie expenditure leading to blood glucose reductions. Therefore, people with diabetes and older adults should proceed with caution.
- Soaking the feet diverts blood away from the digestive organs and should not be performed immediately after eating.
- Avoid rubbing or scratching the skin, which can lead to epidermal damage and increase the risk of infections.
- Soaking the feet can induce sweating. Avoid exposure to wind and cold during and after the treatment.
- After soaking, thoroughly wash and dry the feet.

The following are a few suggestions based on recipes from the book 速效足疗图典 (Su Xiao Zu Liao Tu Dian) by Zhu Wenzeng. There are many other formulas that may be suitable and prescriptions should be determined on a case-by-case basis.

Goji Leaf, Chrysanthemum, Andrographis, and Ilex Formula	
Actions	
Nourish the Liver and Kidneys, calm the Liver, descend Liver fire.	
Ingredients	**Instructions**
Gou Qi Ye (Lycii Folium) 60g Ju Hua (Chrysanthemi Flos) 20g Chuan Xin Lian (Andrographis Herba) 15g Ku Ding Cha (Ilicis Folium) 3g	Place the ingredients in a pot and cover them with water. Simmer for 30 minutes before straining off the liquid and placing it in a foot bath. Soak the feet for 30 minutes, once per evening for 10 days.
Usage	
Suitable for menopause syndrome characterized by menstrual disorders, dizziness, vexation, irritability, bitter taste in the mouth.	

Table 7.3a: Foot soak recipe goji leaf, chrysanthemum, andrographis, and ilex formula for menopause syndrome.

Kumquat Leaf and Chuan Xiong Formula	
Actions	
Course the Liver, resolve depression, rectify qi, transform phlegm.	
Ingredients	**Instructions**
Jin Ju Ye (Fortunellae Folium) 50g Qing Pi (Citri Reticulatae Pericarpium Viride) 20g Chuan Xiong (Chuanxiong Rhizoma) 20g Chen Pi (Citri Reticulatae Pericarpium) 30g	Place the ingredients in a pot and cover them with water. Simmer for 30 minutes before straining off the liquid and placing it in a foot bath. Soak the feet for 30 minutes, once per evening for 10 days.
Usage	
Suitable for menopause syndrome characterized by chest, hypochondrium, or abdominal fullness, distension, or pain, and depression.	

Table 7.3b: Foot soak recipe kumquat leaf and chuan xiong formula for menopause syndrome.

Cassia, Sanguisorba, and Mulberry Twig Formula	
Actions	
Course the Liver, clear heat.	
Ingredients	**Instructions**
Jue Ming Zi (Cassiae Semen) 30g Di Yu (Sanguisorbae Radix) 30g Sang Zhi (Mori Ramulus) 30g	Place the ingredients in a pot and cover them with water. Soak for 5-10 minutes then simmer to make a decoction. Place in a foot bath and allow to cool to a suitable temperature. Soak the feet for 30 minutes, twice daily for 10 days. The above recipe is for a two-day, i.e., four-dose supply.
Usage	
Suitable for menopause syndrome characterized by vexation and irascibility. Unsuitable for patients with numbness of the hands and feet, dry mouth, dry throat, etc.	

Table 7.3c: Foot soak recipe cassia, sanguisorba, and mulberry twig formula for menopause syndrome.

Tulip and Silk Tree Flower Formula	
Actions	
Tranquillize and quiet the *shen*.	
Ingredients	**Instructions**
Yu Jin Xiang (Tulipae Gesnerianae Herba) 30g He Huan Hua (Albizziae Flos) 30g	Place the ingredients in a pot and cover them with water. Soak for 5-10 minutes then simmer to make a decoction. Place in a foot bath and allow to cool to a suitable temperature. Soak the feet for 30 minutes, twice daily for 10 days. The above recipe is for a two-day, i.e., four-dose supply.
Usage	
Suitable for menopause syndrome.	

Table 7.3d: Foot soak recipe tulip and silk tree flower formula for menopause syndrome.

Silk Tree Formula	
Actions	
Resolve depression, calm the *shen*.	
Ingredients	**Instructions**
He Huan Pi (Albizziae Cortex) 30g	Place the ingredients in a pot and cover them with water. Soak for 5-10 minutes then simmer to make a decoction. Place in a foot bath and allow to cool to a suitable temperature. Soak the feet for 15-30 minutes just before bed. The above recipe is for a two-day supply.
Usage	
Suitable for emotional strain leading to insomnia, characterized by anger and melancholy, vacuity vexation, restlessness, poor memory.	

Table 7.3e: Foot soak recipe silk tree formula for insomnia.

Lodestone and Polygala Formula	
Actions	
Nourish the Heart, calm the *shen*.	
Ingredients	**Instructions**
Ci Shi (Magnetitum) 15g Jing Jie (Schizonepetae Herba) 15g Ye Jiao Teng (Polygoni Multiflori Caulis) 15g Dan Shen (Salviae Miltiorrhizae Radix) 15g Du Huo (Angelicae Pubescentis Radix) 15g Yuan Zhi (Polygalae Radix) 15g	Place the ingredients in a pot and cover them with water. Soak for 5-10 minutes then simmer to make a decoction. Place in a foot bath and allow to cool to a suitable temperature. Soak the feet for 15-30 minutes just before bed. The above recipe is for a two-day supply.
Usage	
Suitable for insomnia characterized by excessive dreaming.	

Table 7.3f: Foot soak recipe lodestone and polygala formula for insomnia.

Coptis and Cinnamon Formula	
Actions	
Tranquillize and calm the *shen*.	
Ingredients	**Instructions**
Huang Lian (Coptidis Rhizoma) 15g Rou Gui (Cinnamomi Cortex) 15g	Place the ingredients in a pot and cover them with water. Soak for 5-10 minutes then simmer to make a decoction. Place in a foot bath and allow to cool to a suitable temperature. Soak the feet for 15-30 minutes just before bed. The above recipe is for a two-day supply.
Usage	
Suitable for insomnia characterized by excessive dreaming.	

Table 7.3g: Foot soak recipe coptis and cinnamon formula for insomnia.

Salvia and Eucommia Formula	
Actions	
Clear heat, calm the *shen*.	
Ingredients	**Instructions**
Dan Shen (Salviae Miltiorrhizae Radix) 15g Du Zhong (Eucommiae Cortex) 15g Mu Gua (Chanemolis Fructus) 15g Dang Gui (Angelicae Sinensis Radix) 15g Hong Hua (Carthami Flos) 10g Xiang Fu (Cyperi Rhizoma) 10g Mang Xiao (Natrii Sulfas) 10g Chen Pi (Citri Reticulatae Pericarpium) 10g Sang Zhi (Mori Ramulus) 10g	Place the ingredients in a pot and cover them with water. Simmer for 30 minutes, place in a footbath and first steam then soak the feet. Repeat every evening before bed for 15 days.
Usage	
Suitable for agitation.	

Table 7.3h: Foot soak recipe salvia and eucommia formula for agitation.

Mugwort, Cinnamon, and Dahurian Angelica Formula	
Actions	
Return fire to the source.	
Ingredients	**Instructions**
Ai Ye (Artemisiae Argyi Folium) 20g Rou Gui (Cinnamomi Cortex) 10g Bai Zhi (Angelicae Dahuricae Radix) 10g	Place the ingredients in a pot and cover with water. Simmer for 30 minutes and strain. Soak a clean piece of gauze in the liquid and use it to wash the feet for 10-20 minutes each day.
Usage	
Suitable for agitation due to vacuity heat floating upward.	

Table 7.3i: Foot soak recipe mugwort, cinnamon, and Dahurian angelica formula for agitation.

Summary

Soaking the feet is a very traditional treatment modality. It allows the patient to relax while the active components of herbal medicines absorb through their skin.

Although it is generally well-tolerated, certain precautions must be taken to ensure the patient's safety and comfort. It is also essential to perform an in-depth diagnosis before prescribing herbs, much in the same way as one would for internal treatment.

References

Fan, G., Hyang, H., Lin, Y., et at. (2018). Herbal medicine foot bath for the treatment of diabetic peripheral neuropathy: protocol for a randomized, double-blind and controlled trial, PMC US National Library of Medicine, National Institutes of Health, Trials, BMC: Trials. 2018; 19: 483. Published online 2018 Sep 10. doi: 10.1186/s13063-018-2856-4. https://www.ncbi.nlm.nih.gov/pmc/articles/PMC6131772/

Fu, Q., Yang, Hui., Zhang, L., et al. (2020). Traditional Chinese medicine foot bath combined with acupoint massage for the treatment of diabetic peripheral neuropathy: A systematic review and meta-analysis of 31 RCTs, NIH, National Library of Medicine, National Center for Biotechnology Information: Meta-Analysis Diabetes Metab Res Rev 2020 Feb;36(2):e3218. doi: 10.1002/dmrr.3218. Epub 2019 Oct 29. https://pubmed.ncbi.nlm.nih.gov/31659861/

Zhang, Y., Yuan, H., Kang, J., et al (2020). Clinical study for external washing by traditional Chinese medicine in the treatment of multiple infectious wounds of diabetic foot. Study protocol clinical trial (SPIRIT compliant), Medicine: April 2020 - Volume 99 - Issue 17 - p e19841 doi: 10.1097/MD.0000000000019841. https://journals.lww.com/md-journal/fulltext/2020/04240/clinical_study_for_external_washing_by_traditional.45.aspx

Xiao, M., Liu, L.,Tumilty, S., et al. (2021). Efficacy and safety of Chinese herbal footbaths for the treatment of dysmenorrhea: Protocol for a systematic review and meta-analysis, PLoS One, Published: May 3, 2021. https://doi.org/10.1371/journal.pone.0250685. https://journals.plos.org/plosone/article?id=10.1371/journal.pone.0250685

Zhu, W., (2015). 速效足疗图典. Zhejiang Science and Technology Press; Hangzhou, China.

SECTION 8 - Appendices

Appendix 1. Case Study by Brian Grosam

Hot Flash Case Study by Brian Grosam

A 55-year-old female patient presented with severe hot flashes and night sweating for ten years. Accompanying symptoms included: problematic insomnia with frequent waking at night, elevated anxiety, irritability, high stress levels, brain fog, evening physical fatigue, minor abdominal bloating, good appetite, and normal bowel movements. The patient exercises regularly, eats a well-balanced low-carbohydrate diet, takes multivitamins, 2-3 alcohol drinks per week, worries about being slightly overweight, and is highly talkative with a history of headaches and vertigo, adult onset acne, and irregular periods that led to a hysterectomy three years prior.

Her pulse was moderate. Her tongue was slightly red with a dry-thin coating. The patient has taken the Chinese herbal formula Geng Nian An Pian in the past to quell her hot flashes. Upon our initial telephone conversation the patient was anxious and almost impatient to know which formula I would be prescribing and questioning how fast it would relieve her hot flashes and sleep issues. She agreed to receive acupuncture treatments twice weekly and listen to my expertise and take the herbal formulas I felt were best.

My original diagnosis was Kidney and Liver yin deficiency, with deficiency fire and hyperactive yang qi. I used my "excess hot flash acupuncture prescription": Baihui DU-20 , Shenting DU-24, Shenmen HE-7, Neiguan P-6, Hegu LI-4, Guanyuan REN-4, Neiting ST-44, Yinlingquan SP-9, Taixi KID-3, Taichong LIV-3, Yanglingquan GB-34 and added Rangu KID-2, Zhangmen LIV-13. I prescribed the herbal formulas Zuo Gui Wan and Jia Wei Xiao Yao San to strongly nourish the Kidney yin essence and to regulate the Liver and Spleen qi. The daytime hot flashes began to disappear, nighttime hot flashes began to lessen, and waking at night started to improve at the third treatment mark. The patient felt a 40% reduction in hot flashes while her stress and energy levels barely responded after eight acupuncture treatments.

For the next four treatments I began administering various herbal formulas trying to improve hot flash efficacy. Er Xian Tang, Huang Lian Jie Du Tang, and Tian Ma Gou Teng Yin proved to have a lesser effect than the original formulas with this patient. The lackluster effect of these formulas provided the necessary information that Kidney essence deficiency, excess fire, and ascending yang qi were not the main patho-mechanisms behind this particular hot flash environment, otherwise, the hot flashes would have continued to improve.

Kidney essence deficiency is a primary root pattern during menopausal transition. If the *zangfu* organ system is not functioning optimally, administered Kidney tonics will only be somewhat beneficial. Excess (stagnated) fire is often the 'branch' effect of an underlying 'root' cause. In certain situations, often seen in younger perimenopause patients, excess fire develops and takes over, where it becomes essential to drain. Ascendant yang qi can develop as the Kidney and Liver yin both gradually become deficient during menopausal transition.

Ascending yang qi can harass the brain affecting the thermoregulation ability of the hypothalamus. It can also disrupt the Heart qi and spirit, causing symptoms including hot flashes, insomnia, and anxiety. If the hot flash is not the direct result of excess fire or ascending yang qi, draining fire or sedating yang qi will be of little effect. I also changed the acupuncture strategy to a back acupuncture prescription: Dazhui DU-14, Zhiyang DU-9, Mingmen DU-4, Xinshu BL-15, Ganshu BL-18, and Shenshu BL-23 with modest, although temporary, improvement in quelling the hot flashes. Treating menopausal transition patients on the yang aspect of the body with yang qi stimulating points can produce profound efficacy. The theory is once yang qi is strong, only then can it support the regeneration of yin qi. The temporary and short-lived improvement with this technique proved something else was the root cause. I could now clearly see the true underlying patho-mechanism for this patient's hot flash environment.

Upon reevaluation it was clear the patient had much sustained and continued stress in her life including financial, work, and the death of her mother two years prior – all common scenarios in today's modern society. It was clear to me the patient was responding as well as her body would allow. However, her stress levels were maintaining a high level of Liver overactivity and a disturbed *shen* that did not allow for her body and *zangfu* organs to regenerate the necessary Blood and essence to regain internal yin-yang balance. I went back to my original acupuncture prescription, subtracted Taichong LIV-3 and added Xingjian LIV-2, Yongquan KID-1, and M-HN-3 Yintang. I also prescribed Long Dan Xie Gan Tang to drain stagnated Liver fire and Gan Mai Da Zao Tang to sedate the Heart so the patient could sleep. The patient underwent six additional acupuncture treatments with an 80% reduction in hot flashes with only 1-2 mild hot flashes per night, while the patient's sleep, stress and anxiety levels dramatically improved.

My conclusion is when the body naturally becomes deficient of blood, yin and yang, and its natural essence during menopausal transition – it logically needs to reproduce new supplies. However, when the body is under undue or sustained stressors, the internal *zangfu* organs are unable to regenerate the essential qi and blood the body requires to nourish the heart, brain, and body through this transition period. This patient's hot flash environment was created by an underlying deficiency of kidney and liver yin and blood, overconsumption qi and blood due to liver qi stagnation and liver fire, and heart *shen* disturbance. Only by cooling the liver and calming the spirit could her body begin to properly function and generate vital new qi and blood.

Appendix 2. A Practitioner's Toolkit for Managing the Menopause

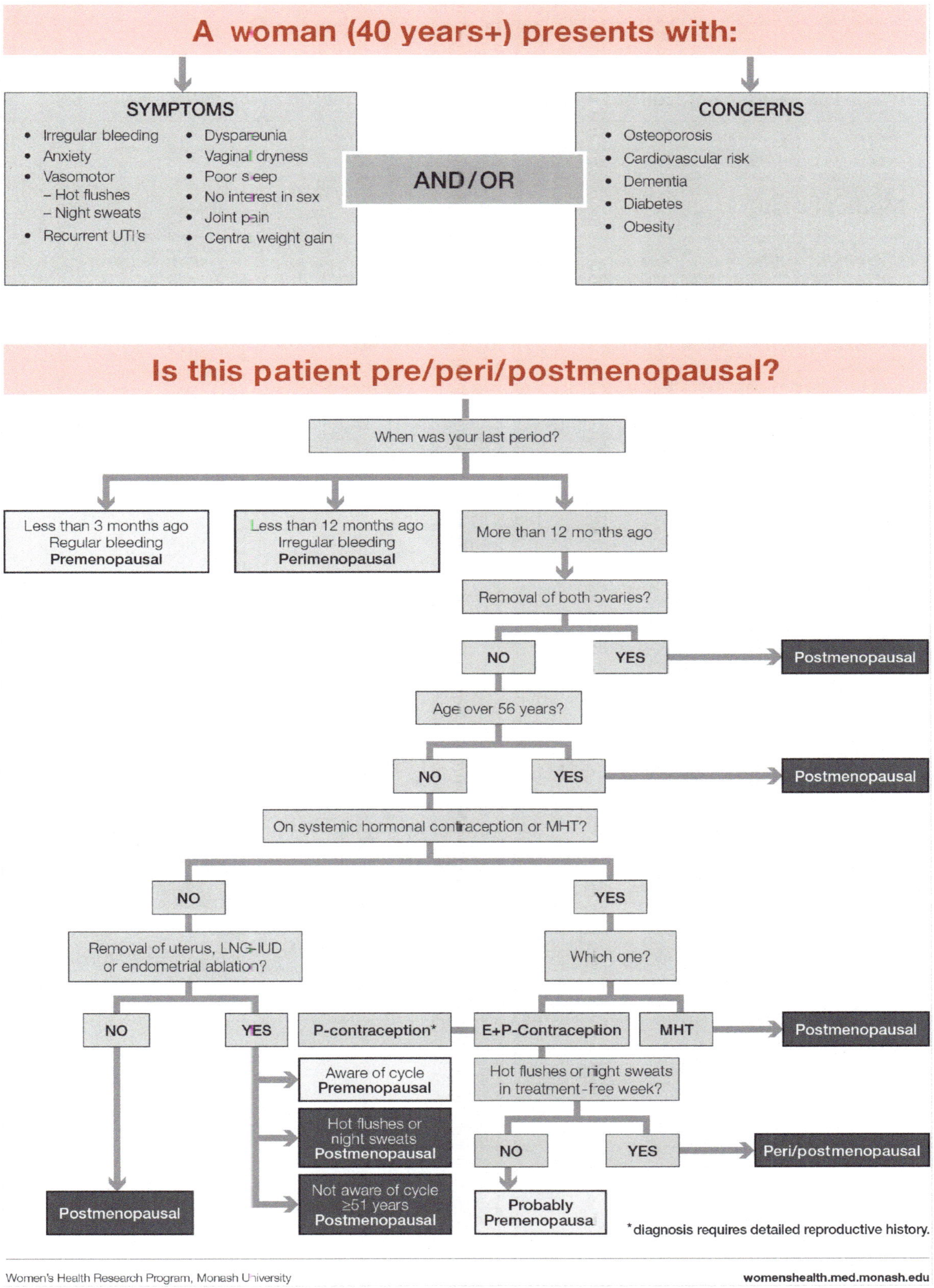

What do you need to know?

Full assessment required irrespective of presenting reason of the midlife woman

Medical history

Relevant gynecological facts:

- Bleeding pattern or LMP
- Past surgery eg hysterectomy/oophorectomy
- Current use of hormonal therapy
- +/- contraceptive needs

Major medical illnesses – consider:

- DVT/PE
- Breast cancer/endometrial cancer
- Thyroid disease
- Cardio/cerebrovascular disease inc HT
- Osteoporosis
- Diabetes
- Depression/anxiety/postnatal depression
- Recurrent UTI's
- Liver disease

Family history:

- Cardio/cerebrovascular disease
- Osteoporosis/fractures
- Dementia
- Cancer

Smoking/alcohol use

Current medication inc OTC medications

Social history

Examination

- Height and weight
- Blood pressure and cardiovascular system
- Pelvic examination (+/- Pap smear)
- Breast examination
- Thyroid examination

Investigations

FSH/estradiol

- Rarely needed
- Of no value in women on systemic hormonal contraception

Prog/LH/AMH levels of no diagnostic value

Midlife women (50 years) health assessment:

- Pap smear
- Mammogram
- Lipids
- FBG
- TSH
- Renal and liver function
- FBE/ferritin
- FOBT
- Vit D in at-risk women

What to consider

Premenopause

Peri- and early menopause

Postmenopause <60 years or within 10 years of menopause

- Health concerns including family history
- General health/disease management (lifestyle issues such as physical activity, diet, smoking, alcohol, obesity)

- Contraceptive needs

Management of:

- menopausal symptoms
- vulvovaginal atrophy
- prevention of osteoporosis
- sexual dysfunction

Menopausal hormonal treatment

Uterus intact

First-line management:

A. Combined transdermal (E+P) patch
B. Transdermal (E) patch or gel plus oral P or LNG-IUD
C. Oral E plus oral P or LNG-IUD
D. Tibolone
E. E plus SERM

Second-line management for persistent symptoms:

E implant* and P (LNG-IUD or oral P)

*Specialist referral

Post hysterectomy

First-line management:

A. Transdermal E patch or gel
B. Oral E
C. Tibolone

Second-line management for persistent symptoms:

E implant*

*Specialist referral

Perimenopausal treatment

E+P contraception	• Review contraindications to E+P contraception • Controls PMS/mastalgia/bleeding • Low dose and 17βE preferred
Oral E and LNG-IUD	Eliminates bleeding but not cyclical symptoms
Continuous E and cyclical P	• Irregular bleeding occurs • Cyclical symptoms • May suit some women

MHT dosing[1]

Estrogen

	Low dose	Moderate dose	High dose
CEE	0.3 – 0.45 mg/day	0.625 mg/day	1.25 mg/day
17β-estradiol	0.5 – 1.0 mg/day	1.5 – 2 mg/day	2 mg
Estradiol valerate	0.5 mg/day	1 mg/day	2 mg/day
Transdermal estradiol patch	25 – 37.5 μg/day	50 μg/day	75 – 100 μg/day
Estradiol hemihydrate gel	0.5 mg/day	1.0 mg/day	1.5 mg/day

Sequential P – daily dose for 14 days per month- lowest "safe" dose with:

	Low dose E	Moderate to high dose E
Dydrogesterone	5 mg	10 mg
Micronized progesterone	100 mg	200 mg
MPA	5 mg	5 – 10 mg
Norethisterone acetate (NETA)	1.25 mg	1.25 – 2.5 mg

Continuous P – daily dose – lowest "safe" dose with:

	Low dose E	Moderate to high dose E
Dydrogesterone	5 mg	5 – 10 mg
Drospirenone	0.5 mg	—
Micronized progesterone	100 mg	100 mg
MPA	2.5 mg	2.5 – 5 mg
Norethisterone acetate (NETA)	0.5 – 1.0 mg	>1.0 – 2.5 mg
LNG-IUD	device releasing 20 μg/24 hours	

Tibolone

Tibolone	2.5 mg daily

Evidence-based non-hormonal treatment[1] for vasomotor symptoms

Estrogen and SERM therapy

CEE 0.45 mg plus bazedoxifene	20 mg daily

SSRI or SSRI/SNRI– low dose (also treats menopausal mood disorder)	Venlafaxine 75mg, desvenlafaxine 50mg, escitalopram 10 mg, paroxetine 7.5 mg daily
Clonidine	100 μg daily
Gabapentin	300 – 900 mg daily
Pregabalin	75 – 150 mg twice a day
Hypnosis	
Cognitive behavior therapy	
Weight loss for obese women	
Stellate ganglion blockade*	Severe resistant VMS *specialist referral

[1] – Availability of hormonal/nonhormonal treatment and indications for use from regulatory bodies vary between countries.

Menopausal symptom management

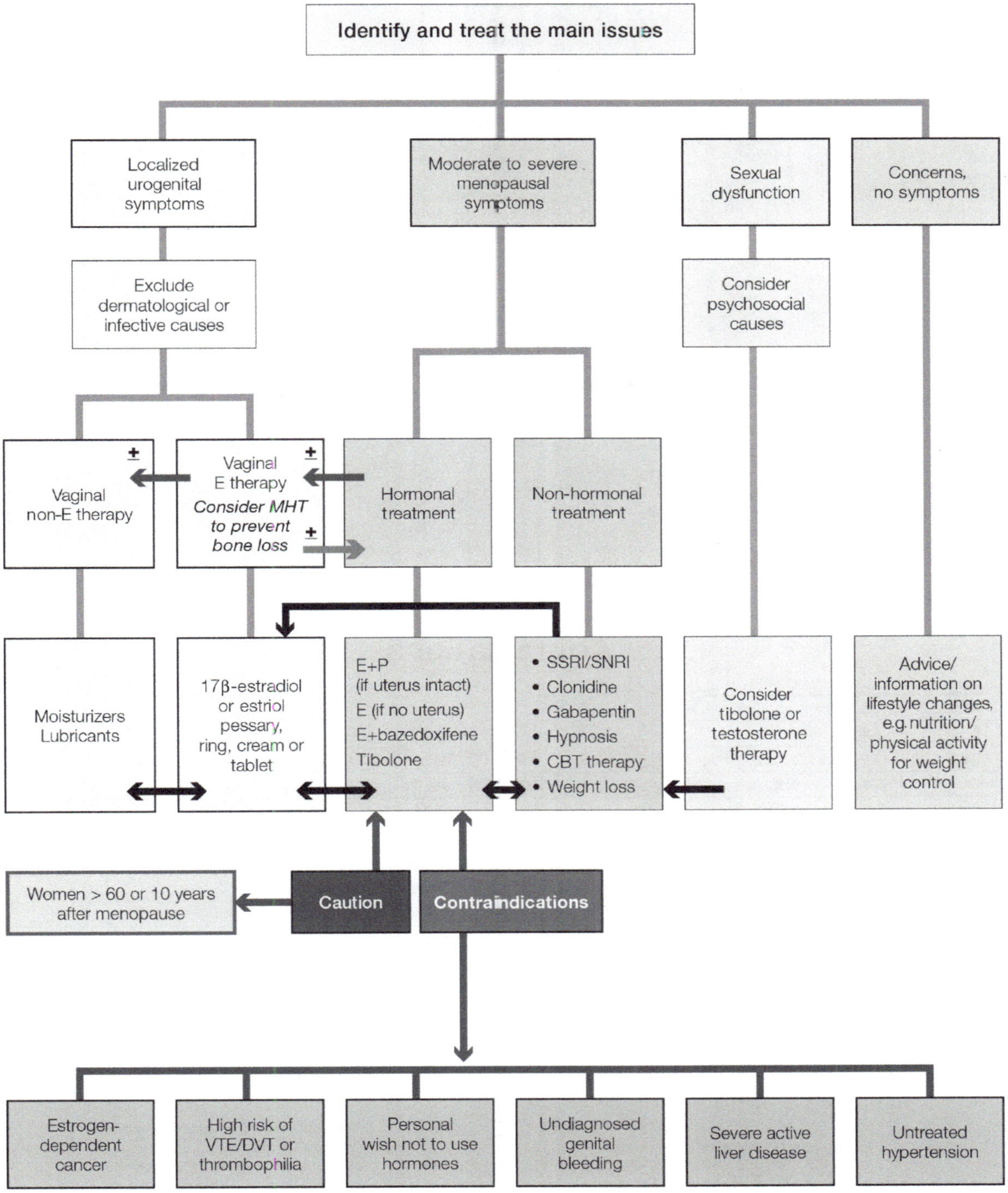

Review of treatment

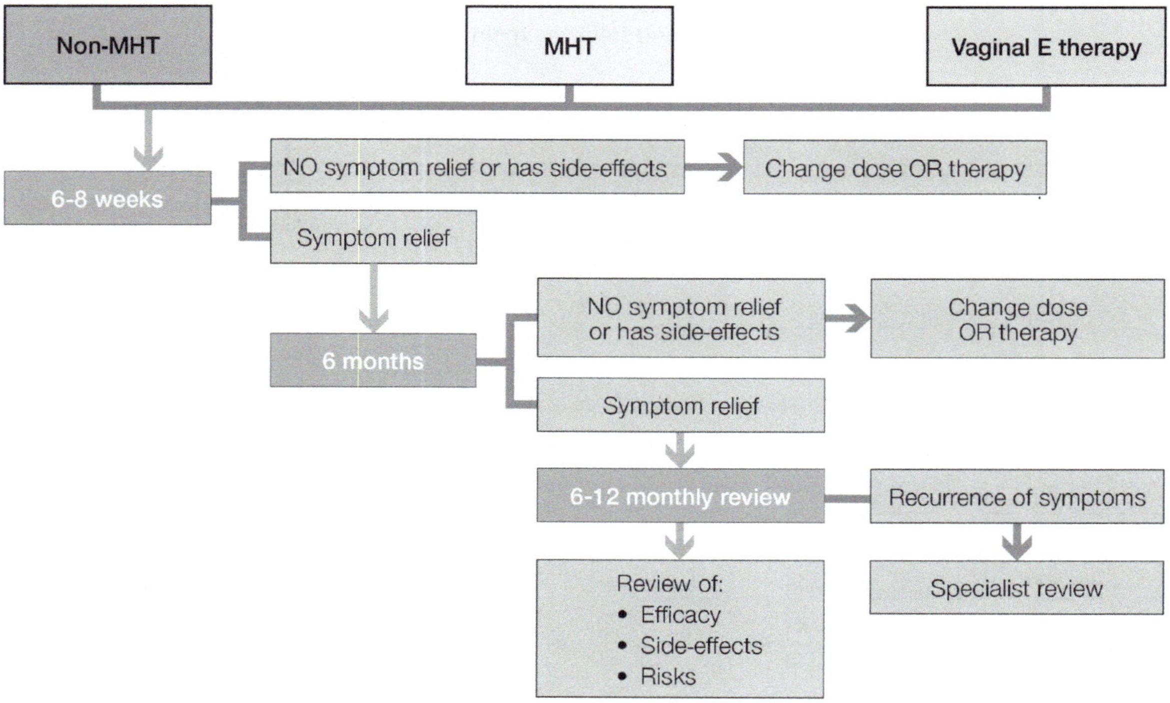

Abbreviations

AMH	Anti-Müllerian hormone
β	Beta
CEE	Conjugated equine estrogen
DVT	Deep vein thrombosis
E	Estrogen
FBE	Full blood examination
FBG	Deep venous thrombosis
FOBT	Fecal occult blood test
FSH	Follicle stimulating hormone
HT	Hypertension
inc	including
LH	Luteinizing hormone
LMP	Last menstrual period
LNG-IUD	Levonorgestrel intrauterine device
MHT	Menopausal hormone therapy

µg	microgram
mg	milligram
MPA	Medroxyprogesterone acetate
NETA	Norethisterone acetate
OCP	Oral contraceptive pill
OTC	Over the counter
P	Progestogen
Prog	Progesterone
SERM	Selective estrogen receptor modulator
SNRI	Selective noradrenaline reuptake inhibitor
SSRI	Selective serotonin reuptake inhibitor
TSH	Thyroid stimulating hormone
UTI	Urinary tract infection
VMS	Vasomotor symptoms
VTE	Venous thromboembolism

MONASH University
Medicine, Nursing and Health Sciences

Women's Health Research Program
Monash University
Alfred Centre, 99 Commercial Road
Melbourne Vic 3004, Australia
Tel: +61 (0)3 9903 0827
Fax: +61 (0)3 9903 0828
Email: womens.health@monash.edu

Appendix 3

EVIDENCE BASED

ACUPUNCTURE

EVIDENCE SUMMARY - MENOPAUSAL SYMPTOMS

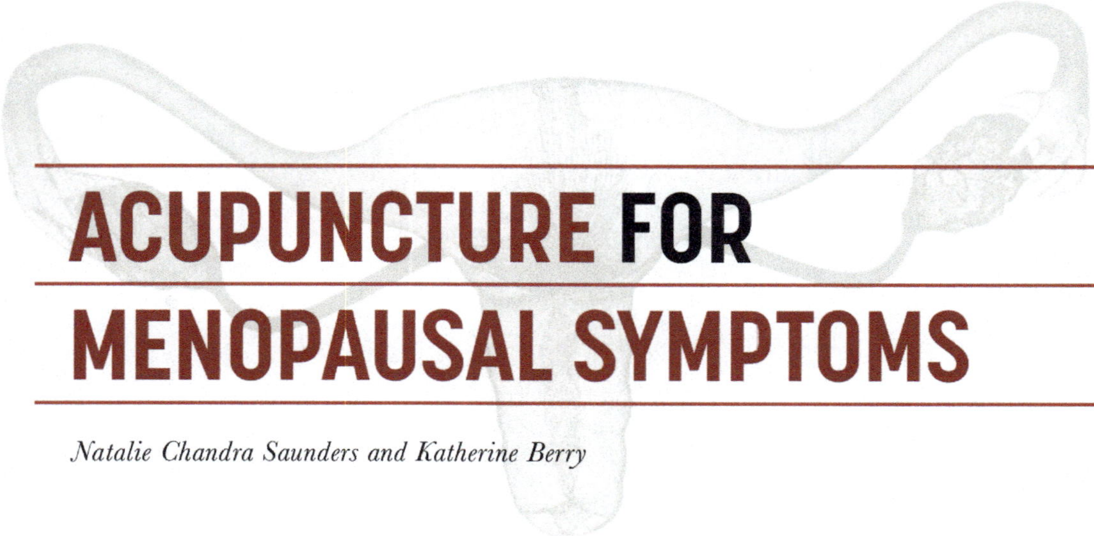

ACUPUNCTURE FOR MENOPAUSAL SYMPTOMS

Natalie Chandra Saunders and Katherine Berry

Menopause is a natural phenomenon and is defined as 12 consecutive months without a period. The average age of menopause in developed countries is 51 years.[1]

Although it is a natural process, the years preceding and succeeding the menopause can be associated with various symptoms, ranging in severity from mild to debilitating. The average duration of symptoms is seven years.[2]

Numerous factors influence the overall impact of menopause, including the age at which it occurs, ethnicity, culture, socio-economic background, general health and wellbeing. Whether menopause is surgically-induced or occurs naturally also plays a vital role. Furthermore, there are differences between women who have given birth to children versus those who have not, with the question of whether this was due to choice or circumstance further complicating the issue. For example, women who have been pregnant but never had children report having a more negative attitude toward menopause. However, women who have never had children are also less likely to report certain symptoms, such as hot flashes and vaginal dryness.[3,4]

Since the menopausal transition is such an individual and elongated process, tailored treatments such as those used in acupuncture may provide significant benefits.

Various studies have shown that acupuncture may offer relief from some of the most common menopausal symptoms. However, it is currently under-utilized in clinical practice.

VASOMOTOR SYMPTOMS

Vasomotor symptoms (VMS), including hot flashes and night sweats, are among the most common issues menopausal women experience. They affect approximately 70% of women in Western cultures. VMS are also one of the best-studied areas with regard to acupuncture and menopause.

A 2009 review by Alfhaily and Ewies[5] concluded that the majority of studies on acupuncture for VMS reported 50% reductions in hot flashes that lasted for up to six months. A 2015 meta-analysis by Chiu et al.[6] supports these results. It reviewed 12 studies with a total 869 participants, finding that acupuncture significantly reduced hot flash frequency and severity. It also found that acupuncture improved menopause-related psychological, somatic, and urogenital symptoms, as well as overall quality of life.

The results of these reviews suggest that acupuncture has significant benefits for women suffering from menopausal VMS.

DEPRESSION AND ANXIETY

Many menopausal women also suffer from mood disorders such as depression and anxiety. This is another area where acupuncture may help.

A 2013 review by Sniezek and Siddiqui[7] included six trials with a total of 605 female subjects aged 18-71. Of these studies, four were on depression (with three focusing on major depressive disorder), one was on anxiety, and one was on both conditions. One of the studies involved menopausal women with depression and VMS.

The authors of the study concluded that although the quality of the evidence was mixed, acupuncture was "promising" as a therapy for menopausal women with depression. They went on to say: "At this time, it is reasonable to use acupuncture as an adjunctive therapy for treating depression in postmenopausal women who have vasomotor symptoms."

An earlier 2007 review by Pilkington et al.[8] focused on acupuncture for anxiety. It included 12 controlled trials, 10 if which were RCTs. All of the trials reported positive outcomes.

SLEEP DISTURBANCE AND INSOMNIA

A 2015 review by Berezza et al.[9] included 12 studies on acupuncture for sleep disorders in post-menopausal women. The studies involved a wide range of treatment protocols, interventions, and durations. Overall, 75% reported improvements in sleep complaints following acupuncture treatment.

OSTEOPOROSIS

Osteoporosis is a common issue in post-menopausal women. Several large-scale reviews indicate that acupuncture could help.

A 2018 systematic review and meta-analysis by Pan et al.[10] included 35 studies and a total of 3014 participants. It found that, compared with pharmaceutical treatment alone, warm acupuncture increased bone mineral density (BMD) of the femur and lumbar spine. It also increased serum calcium and estradiol levels, reduced serum alkaline phosphatase, and relieved pain. Electroacupuncture also had positive effects on serum calcium, serum alkaline phosphatase, and pain.

A 2020 review by Xu et al.[11] supported these results. It included 13 systematic reviews and meta-analyses published between 2013 and 2018. They found high quality evidence that acupuncture and moxibustion can improve BMD in primary

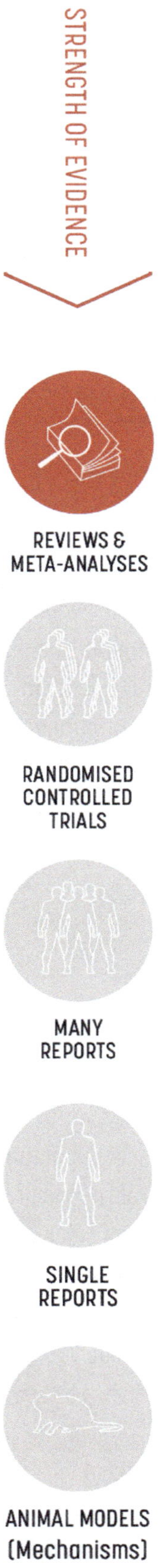

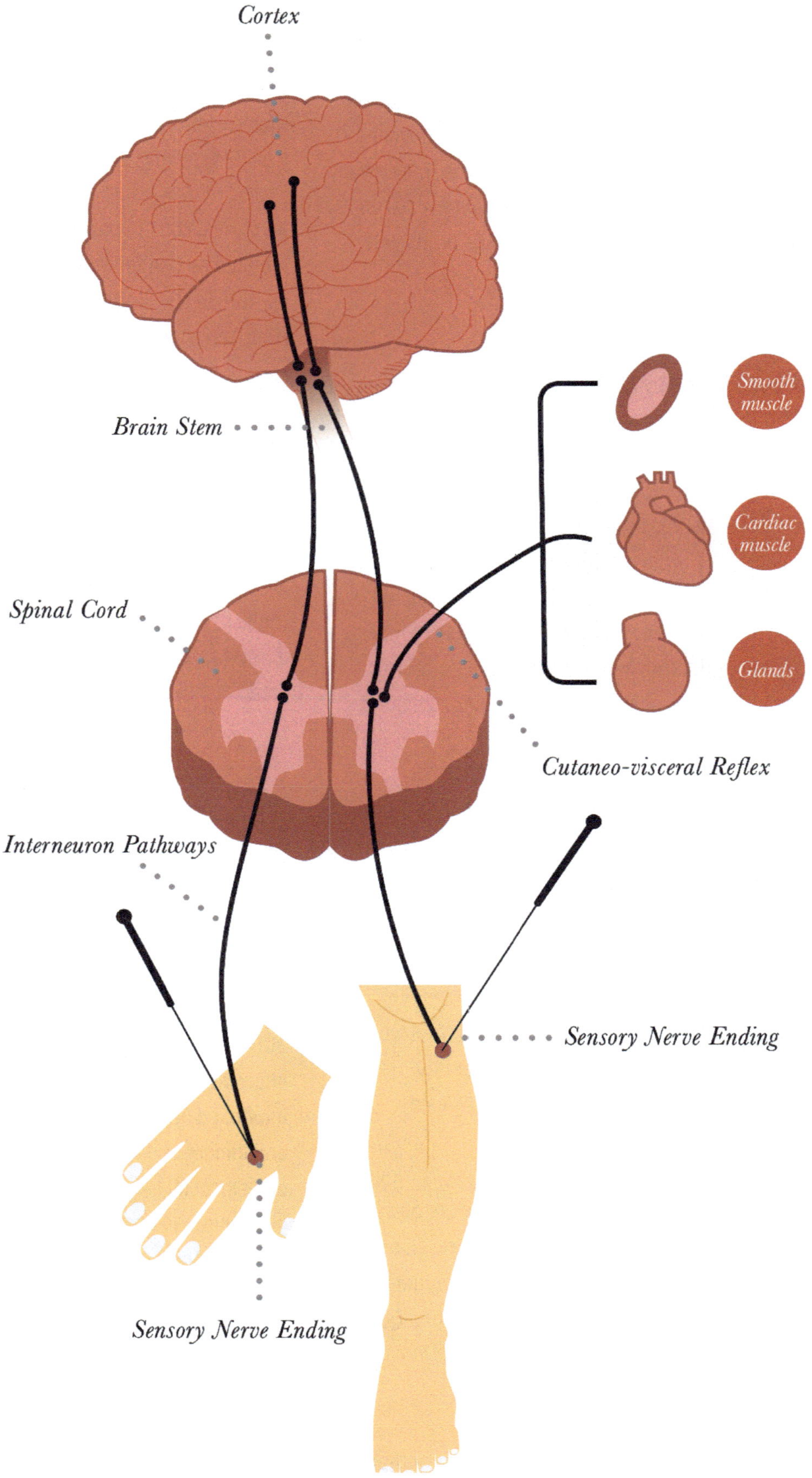

THE CENTRAL NERVOUS SYSTEM

osteoporosis. They also found that these therapies could benefit visual analog scale (VAS) pain scores, although the quality of the evidence was lower.

COGNITIVE DECLINE AND ALZHEIMER'S DISEASE

The risk of cognitive decline, including Alzheimer's disease (AD), also increases significantly following menopause. A 2019 systematic review and meta-analysis by Huang et al.[12] found that acupuncture provided some benefits. It included 13 studies comparing acupuncture with medication alone. The results showed that acupuncture had positive effects on Mini Mental State Examination scores, Ability of Daily Living Scale scores, AD Assessment Scale-Cognition scores, and a high clinical efficacy rate.

MECHANISMS

Acupuncture works via numerous physiological mechanisms, accounting for its diverse effects on the human body. One of the most critical of these is purinergic signaling, a system which utilizes adenosine triphosphate (ATP) as a signaling molecule in the regulation of a range of physiological functions. In the short-term, it plays a role in neurotransmission, neuromodulation, and secretion. In the longer-term, it influences proliferation, differentiation, migration, and death, thus directing the activity and fate of cells.[13]

Purinergic receptors have been investigated as potential therapeutic targets in a broad range of disorders, including many which affect peri and post-menopausal women. They include depression and anxiety, sleep disturbances, osteoporosis, endocrine disorders, cardiovascular, and neurodegenerative disease. In terms of VMS, studies have suggested that acupuncture influences the release of beta-endorphins.[7] These neurochemicals are thought to be involved in the pathophysiology of VMS, although this is still not clearly understood.

Acupuncture also appears to influence cortisol, cortisol metabolites, and DHEA levels.[10] Cortisol levels tend to increase following menopause, contributing to changes in mood, metabolism, bone density, and cognitive decline. It is, therefore, possible that the same underlying mechanisms play a role in the treatment of VMS, depression, anxiety, sleep disorders, abdominal obesity, osteoporosis, and dementia.

Further suggested mechanisms for acupuncture's effects on obesity include anti-inflammatory and antioxidant effects, regulating the endocrine system, promoting digestion, and influencing lipid metabolism.[14]

Meanwhile, animal studies have shown that acupuncture may offer some protection against osteoporosis by regulating the OPG/RANK/RANKL signaling pathways. All of these are involved in the protection of bone tissue.[15]

Finally, MRI studies on patients with AD or mild cognitive impairment have shown that acupuncture activates and deactivates several regions of the brain. They include the basal ganglia, cerebellum, cognitive, visual, and sensorimotor-related areas.[16]

MAINSTREAM APPROACH

Menopause is fast becoming a specialty area. In the past 40 years, our understanding of female endocrinology has improved greatly, expedited by the rapid growth of assisted reproductive therapy. This growth, coupled with women becoming more vocal about their experiences and seeking solutions, has brought menopause to the forefront of both medicine and the media.

The primary mainstream approach to treating menopausal symptoms is hormone replacement therapy (HRT), comprising either estrogen or progesterone monotherapy, or a combination of the two.

HRT has been controversial since the publication of the Women's Health Initiative[17], which suggested that its use increased the risk of breast cancer, stroke, and pulmonary embolism. However, industry-funded guidelines developed in partnership with clinical specialty groups have pointed to flaws in this study.

Current prescribing guidelines suggest that the benefits of HRT generally outweigh the risks for most women aged 60 or under, or within 10 years of menopause.[1] However, there is also evidence that these hormones can increase the risk of breast cancer and ovarian cancer. With so much conflicting information in circulation, the decision regarding whether or not to take HRT is a difficult one. Acupuncture, on the other hand, has a demonstrated track-record of safety and when performed by appropriately trained clinicians, has been found one of the safest treatments in modern medicine.[18]

Therefore, many women are now choosing other modalities, such as acupuncture, as a first-line treatment. Acupuncturists can also play a crucial therapeutic role by helping to inform and support women in adopting beneficial lifestyle changes.

REFERENCES

1. Jane FM, Davis SR. A Practitioner's Toolkit for Managing the Menopause.
Climacteric. 2014; 17(5): p.564-579.

2. Hillard T, Abernathy K, Hamoda H, et al.
British Menopause Society Management of the Menopause Sixth Edition 2017.

3. Thurston RC, Joffe H. Vasomotor Symptoms and Menopause: Findings from the Study of Women's Health across the Nation.
Obstetrics and Gynecology Clinics of North America. 2011; 38(3): p. 489-501.

4. Hess R, Olshansky E, Ness R, et al. Pregnancy and Birth History Influence Women's Experience of Menopause.
Menopause. 2008;15(3): p. 435-441.6.

5. Alfhaily F, Ewies AAA. Acupuncture in managing menopausal symptoms: hope or mirage?.
Climacteric. 2007; 10(5): p. 371-380.

6. Chiu HY, Pan CH, Shyu YK, Han BC, Tsai PS. Effects of acupuncture on menopause-related symptoms and quality of life in women in natural menopause: a meta-analysis of randomized controlled trials.
Menopause. 2015 Feb; 22(2): p. 234-244.

7. Sniezek DP, Siddiqui IJ. Acupuncture for Treating Anxiety and Depression in Women: A Clinical Systematic Review.
Medical Acupuncture. 2013; 25(3): p.164-172.

8. Pilkington K, Kirkwood G, Rampes H, Cummings M, Richardson J. Acupuncture for anxiety and anxiety disorders--a systematic literature review.
Acupuncture in Medicine. 2007; 25(1-2): p.1-10.

9. Bezerra AG, Pires GN, Andersen ML, Tufik S, Hachul H. Acupuncture to Treat Sleep Disorders in Postmenopausal Women: A Systematic Review.
Evidence-Based Complementary and Alternative Medicine. 2015; 2015:563236.

10. Pan H, Jin R, Li M, Liu Z, Xie Q, Wang P. The Effectiveness of Acupuncture for Osteoporosis: A Systematic Review and Meta-Analysis.
The American Journal of Chinese Medicine. 2018; 46(3): p.489-513.

11. Xu G, Xiao Q, Zhou J, et al. Acupuncture and moxibustion for primary osteoporosis: An overview of systematic review.
Medicine (Baltimore). 2020; 99(9): e19334.

12. Huang, Q., Luo, D., Chen, L. et al. Effectiveness of Acupuncture for Alzheimer's Disease: An Updated Systematic Review and Meta-analysis.
Current Medical Science. 2019; 39: p.500–511.

13. Burnstock G. Purinergic Signalling: Therapeutic Developments.
Frontiers in Pharmacology. 2017;8:661. Published 2017 Sep 25. doi:10.3389/fphar.2017.00661

14. Wang LH, Huang W, Wei D, et al. Mechanisms of Acupuncture Therapy for Simple Obesity: An Evidence-Based Review of Clinical and Animal Studies on Simple Obesity.
Evidence-Based Complementary and Alternative Medicine. 2019; 2019:5796381.

15. Huang F, Zhao S, Qiu M, et al. Acupuncture for primary osteoporosis: A network meta-analysis of randomized controlled trials protocol.
[published correction appears in Medicine (Baltimore). 2019 May;98(21): e15898]. Medicine (Baltimore). 2019;98(15):e15108.

16. Shan Y, Wang JJ, Wang ZQ, et al. Neuronal Specificity of Acupuncture in Alzheimer's Disease and Mild Cognitive Impairment Patients: A Functional MRI Study.
Evidence-Based Complementary and Alternative Medicine. 2018; 2018: 7619197

17. Manson JE, Chlebowski RT, Stefanick ML, et al. Menopausal hormone therapy and health outcomes during the intervention and extended poststopping phases of the Women's Health Initiative randomized trials.
JAMA. 2013; 310(13): p.1353-1368.

18. Linde, K., Streng, A., Hoppe, A., Jürgens, S., Weidenhammer, W., & Melchart, D. (2006). The programme for the evaluation of patient care with acupuncture (PEP-Ac) - a project sponsored by ten German social health insurance funds.
Acupuncture in Medicine, 24(Suppl), 25–32. https://doi.org/10.1136/aim.24.Suppl.25

EVIDENCE BASED ACUPUNCTURE

Saunders N. C. and Berry K. (2021).
Acupuncture for Menopausal Symptoms.
Evidence Based Acupuncture.
EDITION 1

Appendix 4. Evidence-Based Acupuncture Point Protocols

The following is a summary of studies conducted using various acupuncture point protocols. Although the selected points and methodologies are heterogeneous, the results are positive overall, suggesting that a diverse range of approaches may be valid when treating menopausal symptoms.

1. A Comparison of Acupuncture and Oral Estradiol Treatment of Vasomotor Symptoms in Postmenopausal Women[1].

Intervention

Electro-acupuncture vs. superficial needling vs. oral estradiol. Fourteen treatments were administered over a 12-week period, twice weekly for the first two weeks and once weekly thereafter.

Acupuncture Points

Xinshu BL-15 (bilateral)
Shenshu BL-23 (bilateral with electrical stimulation)
Ciliao BL-32 (bilateral with electrical stimulation)
Shenmen HT-7 (unilateral)
Sanyinjiao SP-6 (unilateral)
Yinlingquan SP-9 (unilateral)
Taichong LIV-3 (unilateral)
Neiguan P-6 (unilateral)
Baihui DU-20

Results

Prior to treatment, the number of hot flashes per 24 hours in the electro-acupuncture, superficial needling, and estradiol groups were 7.3, 8.1, 8.4, respectively. Following 12 weeks of treatment, these figures had reduced to 3.5, 3.8 and 0.8, respectively.

[1]Wyon, Y., Wijma, K., Nedstrand, E., (2004). A comparison of acupuncture and oral estradiol treatment of vasomotor symptoms in postmenopausal women, Taylor & Francis Online: Climacteric. 7(2): (pp.153-164). https://www.tandfonline.com/doi/10.1080/13697130410001713814.

2. A Randomized Controlled Pilot Study of Acupuncture for Postmenopausal Hot Flashes: Effect on Nocturnal Hot Flashes and Sleep Quality[2].

Intervention

Traditional acupuncture vs. sham acupuncture. Nine treatments were administered over a seven-week period, twice weekly for the first two weeks and once weekly thereafter. Three to six points were selected to address hot flashes and one to two points were selected to address secondary symptoms.

Acupuncture Points

Taixi KID-3
Sanyinjiao SP-6
Guanyuan REN-4
Shenshu BL-23

Primary Pattern

- Kidney yin deficiency with empty heat: replace Taixi KID-3 with Zhaohai KID-6, add Lieque LU-7.
- Liver yang rising: add Fengchi GB-20, Taichong LIV-3.
- Phlegm fire: add Fenglong ST-40, Quchi LI-11.
- If phlegm predominates, replace Guanyuan REN-4 with Zhongwan REN-12 and Shenshu BL-23 with Pishu BL-20.
- If heat predominates, add Xingjian LIV-2.
- Heart-Kidney disharmony: add Jiuwei REN-15, Yinxi HT-6.
- Qi stagnation/Blood stasis: add Gongsun SP-4, Neiguan P-6.
    - If stagnation predominates, add Taichong LIV-3, Hegu LI-4.
    - If stasis predominates add Xuehai SP-10.
- Kidney yin and yang deficiency: replace Guanyuan REN-4 with Qihai REN-6, add Zhishi BL-52, Fuliu KID-7.
- Spleen and Heart Blood deficiency: add Juque REN-14, Xinshu BL-15, Shenmen HT-7.

[2]Huang, MI., Nir, Y., Chen, B., et al. (2006). A randomized controlled pilot study of acupuncture for postmenopausal hot flashes: effect on nocturnal hot flashes and sleep quality, Elsevier, Journal Club Global – February 3, Fertility and Sterility: Reproductive Endocrinology| Volume 86, Issue 3, (pp 700-710), September 01, 2006
https://www.fertstert.org/article/S0015-0282(06)01005-3/fulltext

Secondary Pattern

- Spleen qi deficiency: Zhongwan REN-12, Pishu BL-20, Zusanli ST-36, Taibai SP-3.
- Liver Blood and Kidney yin deficiency: Ququan LIV-8, Yingu KID-10, Ganshu BL-18, Zhaohai KID-6 with Lieque LU-7.
- Heart qi deficiency: Tongli HT-5, Neiguan P-6, Qihai REN-6, Shanzong REN-17, Xinshu BL-15, Pishu BL-20.
- Kidney yang deficiency: Fuliu KID-7, Zhishi BL-52.
- Lung qi and yin deficiency: Zhongfu LU-1, Feishu BL-13, Lieque LU-7, Chize LU-5.
- Liver depression qi stagnation: Taichong LIV-3, Qimen LIV-14, Yanglingquan GB-34, Ganshu BL-18.

Additional Symptoms

- Profuse sweating due to pronounced yin deficiency: Fuliu KID-7, Taiyuan LU-9.
- Severe hot flashes due to replete heat: Dazhui DU-14.
- Night sweats due to pronounced yin deficiency: Fuliu KID-7 with Yinxi HT-6.
- Depression, anxiety, moodiness due to Liver depression qi stagnation: Taichong LIV-3 with Hegu LI-4 or Neiguan P-6.
- Poor concentration/lack of interest due to qi and yang deficiency: Baihui DU-20.
- Agitation, restlessness due to hyperactive Liver yang: Shenting DU-24 with Benshen GB-13, Daling P-7.
- Agitation, restlessness due to heart fire: Shaofu HT-8, Yinxi HT-6, Jiuwei REN-15.
- Rumination, obsessive thinking due to phlegm confounding: Chengling GB-18, Fenglong ST-40.
- Sleep disturbances: Jiuwei REN-15, Xinshu BL-15, Anmian M-HN-54, Sishencong M-HN-1 with Baihui DU-20.

Results

Women in the traditional acupuncture group experienced significantly greater reductions in nocturnal hot flash severity compared with the sham acupuncture group. Both groups experienced reductions in nocturnal hot flash frequency.

3. Acupuncture in Managing Menopausal Symptoms: Hope or Mirage?[3]

Intervention
Review of 17 English-language studies.

Acupuncture Points
Shenmai BL-62
Qimen LIV-14
Taixi KID-3
Shenmen HT-7
Zhigou SJ-6

Homeostatic Points
Sanyinjiao SP-6
Quchi LI-11
Zusanli ST-36

Sedative Points
Baihui DU-20
Hegu LI-4

Other Points
Taichong LIV-3
Fengchi GB-20
Yanglingquan GB-34
Guanyuan REN-4

Results
The authors conclude that the majority of women treated with acupuncture experience a 50% improvement in hot flashes that may continue as long as six months after treatment. However, most studies were of poor quality, small size, or lacking an adequate control group.

[3] Alfhaily, F., Ewies, AAA., (2007). Acupuncture in managing menopausal symptoms: hope or mirage? Taylor & Francis Online: Climacteric, 10(5): (pp. 371-380) https://www.tandfonline.com/doi/full/10.1080/13697130701612315.

4. A Pilot Randomized, Single-blind, Placebo-controlled Trial of Traditional Acupuncture for Vasomotor Symptoms and Mechanistic Pathways of Menopause[4]

Intervention

Traditional acupuncture vs. sham acupuncture vs. waitlist control. Treatment was performed three times per week for a total of 36 treatments, alternating between front and back point protocols.

Acupuncture Points

Front

Baihui DU-20
Neiguan P-6
Shenmen HT-7
Taichong LIV-3
Hegu LI-4
Quchi LI-11
Taixi KID-3
Sanyinjiao SP-6
Zusanli ST-36
Shanzhong REN-17
Qihai REN-6

Back

Dazhui DU-14
Xinshu BL-15
Ganshu BL-18
Pishu BL-20
Shenshu BL-23
Yanglingquan GB-34
Taixi KID-3

Results

Women in both traditional and sham acupuncture groups experienced reductions in vasomotor symptom frequency and severity as well as reporting improved quality of life. Women in the traditional acupuncture group had lower levels of DHEA and cortisol metabolites in comparison to those receiving sham treatment.

---

[4] Painovich, JM., Shufelt, CL., Azziz, R., et al. (2012). A Pilot Randomized, Single Blind, Placebo-Controlled Trial of Traditional Acupuncture for Vasomotor Symptoms and Mechanistic Pathways of Menopause. PMC US National Library of Medicine, National Institutes of Health, HHS Public Access, Author Manuscript: Menopause. Author manuscript; available in PMC 2013 Jan 1. Published in final edited form as: Menopause. 2012 Jan; 19(1): (pp 54–61).
doi: 10.1097/gme.0b013e31821f9171. https://www.ncbi.nlm.nih.gov/pmc/articles/PMC3246091/.

5. Efficacy of a Standardised Acupuncture Approach for Women with Bothersome Menopausal Symptoms: A Pragmatic Randomised Study in Primary Care[5]

Intervention

Western medical acupuncture with standardized point prescription vs. waitlist control. Treatment was performed weekly for five weeks.

Acupuncture Points

Zhongji REN-3
Guanyuan REN-4
Ququan LIV-8
Yinlingquan SP-9
Sanyinjiao SP-6

Results

Women in the acupuncture group experienced significant decreases in hot flashes, day and night sweats, general sweating, menopause-specific sleep problems, emotional symptoms, physical symptoms, and skin and hair symptoms at six-week follow-up.

[5] Lund, KS., Siersma, V., Broderson, J., et al. (2019). Efficacy of a standardised acupuncture approach for women with bothersome menopausal symptoms: a pragmatic randomised study in primary care (the ACOM study), BMJ Journals: BMJ Open, Volume 9, (issue 1). doi: 10.1136/bmjopen-2018-023637. https://bmjopen.bmj.com/content/9/1/e023637.

Appendix 5. TCEAM Formulas

The following formulas are listed in the order that they appear in the text.

Wu Zhu Yu Tang (吴茱萸汤, Evodia Decoction, Discussion of Cold Damage, c.220)	
Wu Zhu Yu (Evodiae Fructus) 9-12g Sheng Jiang (Zingiberis Rhizoma recens) 18g Ren Shen (Ginseng Radix) 9g Da Zao (Jujubae Fructus) 12 pieces	
Method	**Action**
Decoction. Dang Shen (Codonopsis Radix) may be substituted for Ren Shen at 2-3 times the dosage. Some practitioners use a lower dosage than stated above with only four pieces of Da Zao to prevent distension in the middle *jiao*.	Warm and tonify the Liver and Stomach, subdue rebellious qi, stop vomiting.

Zuo Jin Wan (左金丸, Left Metal Pill, Essential Teachings of [Zhu] Dan Xi, 1481)	
Huang Lian (Coptidis Rhizoma) 15-18g Wu Zhu Yu (Evodiae Fructus) 2-3g	
Method	**Action**
Prepare as a decoction.	Clear Liver heat, subdue rebellious qi, stop vomiting.

Wen Dan Tang **(温胆汤, Warm Gallbladder Decoction, Discussion of Illnesses, Patterns, and Formulas Related to the Unification of the Three Etiologies, 1174)**	
Zhu Ru (Bambusae Caulis in taeniam) 6g Zhi Shi (Aurantii Fructus immaturus) 6g Zhi Ban Xia (Pinelliae Rhizoma praeparatum) 6g Chen Pi (Citri reticulatae Pericarpium) 9g Fu Ling (Poria) 4.5g Zhi Gan Cao (Glycyrrhizae Radix praeparata) 3g	
Method	**Action**
Grind to powder and decoct 12g in one cup of water with five slices of Sheng Jiang (Zingiberis Rhizoma recens) and one piece of Da Zao (Jujubae Fructus). Strain and take as a draft before meals. Alternatively, prepare as a decoction.	Regulate qi, transform phlegm, clear the Gallbladder, harmonize the Stomach.

Bao He Wan **(保和丸, Preserve Harmony Pill, Essential Teachings of [Zhu] Dan Xi, 1481)**	
Shan Zha (Crataegi Fructus) 9-15g Shen Qu (Massa medicata fermentata) 9-12g Lai Fu Zi (Raphani Semen) 6-9g Chen Pi (Citri reticulatae Pericarpium) 6-9g Zhi Ban Xia (Pinelliae Rhizoma praeparatum) 9-12g Fu Ling (Poria) 9-12g Lian Qiao (Forsythiae Fructus) 3-6g	
Method	**Action**
Prepare as a decoction.	Regulate qi, transform phlegm, clear the Gallbladder, harmonize the Stomach.

***Zhi Bai Di Huang Wan* (知柏地黄丸, Anemarrhena, Phellodendron, and Rehmannia Pill, Investigations of Medical Formulas (1584)**	
Yan Chao Zhi Mu (salt-fried Anemarrhenae Rhizoma) 3-9g Yan Chao Huang Bai (salt-fried Phellodendri Cortex) 3-9g Shu Di Huang (Rehmanniae Radix preparata) 9-18g Shan Zhu Yu (Corni Fructus) 9g Shan Yao (Dioscoreae Rhizoma) 9g Fu Ling (Poria) 6-9g Mu Dan Pi (Moutan Cortex) 6g Ze Xie (Alismatis Rhizoma) 6g	
Method	**Action**
Prepare as a decoction.	Enrich yin, nourish the Kidney, drain excess heat.

***Zuo Gui Wan* (左归丸, Restore the Left Kidney Pill, Collected Treatises of [Zhang] Jing-Yue, 1624)**	
Shu Di Huang (Rehmanniae Radix preparata) 9-24g Chao Shan Yao (dry-fried Dioscoreae Rhizoma) 9g Gou Qi Zi (Lycii Fructus) 9g Shan Zhu Yu (Corni Fructus) 9g Jiu Chuan Niu Xi (wine-prepared Cyathulae Radix) 6g Tu Si Zi (Cuscutae Semen) 9g Lu Jiao Jiao (Cervi Cornus Colla) 9g Gui Ban Jiao (Testudinis Plastri Colla) 9g	
Method	**Action**
Prepare as a decoction.	Nourish yin, enrich the Kidneys, fill the essence, augment the marrow.

Jin Gui Shen Qi Wan (金匱肾气丸, Golden Cabinet Kidney Qi Pill, Essentials from the Golden Cabinet, c. 220)	
Sheng Di Huang (Rehmanniae Radix) 24g Shan Zhu Yu (Corni Fructus) 12g Shan Yao (Dioscoreae Radix) 12g Bao Fu Zi (baked Aconiti Radix lateralis) 3g Gui Zhi (Cinnamomi Ramulus) 3g Ze Xie (Alismatis Rhizoma) 9g Fu Ling (Poria) 9g Mu Dan Pi (Moutan Cortex) 9g	
Method	**Action**
Prepare as a decoction. Shu Di Huang may be substituted for Sheng Di Huang and Rou Gui for Gui Zhi.	Warm and tonify Kidney yang.

You Gui Wan (右归丸, Restore the Right Kidney Pill, Collected Treatises of [Zhang] Jing-Yue, 1624)	
Zhi Fu Zi (Aconiti Radix lateralis preparata) 3-9g Rou Gui (Cinnamomi Cortex) 3-9g Lu Jiao Jiao (Cervi Cornus Colla) 9g Shu Di Huang (Rehmanniae Radix preparata) 9-24g Shan Zhu Yu (Corni Fructus) 6g Chao Shan Yao (dry-fried Dioscoreae Rhizoma) 9g Chao Gou Qi Zi (dry-fried Lycii Fructus)9g Tu Si Zi (Cuscutae Semen) 9g Du Zhong (Eucommiae Cortex) 9g Dang Gui (Angelicae sinensis Radix) 6g	
Method	**Action**
Prepare as a decoction.	Warm and tonify Kidney yang, replenish essence, tonify Blood.

Tian Ma Gou Teng Yin (天麻钩藤饮, Gastrodia and Uncaria Drink, Deriving New Treatments for Patterns of Miscellaneous Disorders in Chinese Internal Medicine, 1958)	
Tian Ma (Gastrodiae Rhizoma) 9g Gou Teng (Uncariae Ramulaus cum Uncis) 12-15g Shi Jue Ming (Haliotidis Concha) 18-24g Zhi Zi (Gardeniae Fructus) 9g Huang Qin (Scutellariae Radix) 9g Yi Mu Cao (Leonuri Herba) 9-12g Chuan Niu Xi (Cyathulae Radix) 12g Du Zhong (Eucommiae Cortex) 9-12g Sang Ji Sheng (Taxilli Herba) 9-24g Ye Jiao Teng (Polygoni multiflori Caulis) 9-30g Fu Shen (Poriae Sclerotium pararadicis) 9-15g	
Method	**Action**
Prepare as a decoction, adding Shi Jue Ming first and Gou Teng near the end.	Calm the Liver, extinguish wind, clear heat, invigorate Blood, tonify the Liver and Kidney.

Huang Lian E Jiao Tang (黄连阿胶汤, Coptis and Ass-Hide Gelatin Decoction, Discussion of Cold Damage, c.220)	
Huang Lian (Coptidis Rhizoma) 12g Huang Qin (Scutellariae Radix) 6g E Jiao (Asini Corii Colla) 9g Shao Yao (Paeoniae Radix) 6g Ji Zi Huang (egg yolk) 2 yolks	
Method	**Action**
Prepare as a decoction, strain, and stir in the E Jiao and Ji Zi Huang when it has cooled slightly. Nowadays, the prefered form of Shao Yao is Bai Shao (Paeoniae Radix alba) and the Huang Lian dose is usually reduced by one-third to one-half.	Enrich yin, descend fire, eliminate irritability, calm the *shen*.

Qing Gu San (清骨散, Cool the Bones Powder, Indispensable Tools for Pattern Treatment, 1602)	
Yin Chai Hu (Stellariae Radix) 4.5g Zhi Mu (Anemarrhenae Rhizoma) 3g Hu Huang Lian (Picrorhizae Rhizoma) 3g Di Gu Pi (Lycii Cortex) 3g Qing Hao (Artemisiae annuae Herba) 3g Qin Jiao (Gentianae macrophyllae Radix) 3g Cu Chao Bie Jia (vinegar-fried Trionycis Carapax) 3g Gan Cao (Glycyrrhizae Radix) 1.5g	
Method	**Action**
The original text advises taking as a draft between meals. Alternatively, prepare as a decoction by doubling the dosage.	Clear deficiency heat, alleviate steaming bone disorder.

Bu Zhong Yi Qi Tang (补中益气汤, Tonify the Middle to Augment the Qi Decoction, Clarifying Doubts about Damage from Internal and External Causes, 1247)	
Huang Qi (Astragali Radix) 12-14g Ren Shen (Ginseng Radix 9-12g Bai Zhu (Atractylodis macrocephalae Rhizoma) 9-12g Zhi Gan Cao (Glycyrrhizae Radix praeparata) 3-6g Jiu Xi Dang Gui (wine-washed Angelicae sinensis Radix) 6-12g Chen Pi (Citri reticulatae Pericarpium) 6-9g Sheng Ma (Cimicifugae Rhizoma) 3-6g Chai Hu (Bupleuri Radix) 3-9g	
Method	**Action**
Prepare as a decoction. Dang Shen (Codonopsis Radix) is usually substituted for Ren Shen at 2 –3 times the dosage.	Tonify the middle *jiao*, augment qi, raise yang, lift the sunken.

Da Cheng Qi Tang (大承气汤, Major Order the Qi Decoction, Discussion on Cold Damage, c. 220)	
Da Huang (Rhei Radix et Rhizoma) 12g Mang Xiao (Natrii Sulfas) 9-12g Zhi Zhi Shi (prepared Aurantii Fructus immaturus) 5 pieces (12-15g) Zhi Hou Po (prepared Magnoliae officinalis Cortex) 24g	
Method	**Action**
The original text advises cooking the Zhi Zhi Shi and Hou Po in 10 cups of water until the liquid has reduced by half, then adding the Da Huang and cooking further until two cups remain. The Mang Xiao is mixed into the strained decoction. Nowadays, it is usually prepared as a decoction, adding the Da Huang towards the end of cooking and mixing the Mang Xiao into the strained decoction. Modern texts recommend reducing the Da Huang dosage to 6-12g and the Hou Po dosage to 12-15g unless there is severe abdominal distension. Discontinue use once loose stools have been induced.	Vigorously purge heat accumulation.

Qing Shu Yi Qi Tang (清暑益气汤, Clear Summer-Heat and Augment the Qi Decoction, Warp and Woof of Warm Febrile Diseases, 1852)	
Xi Yang Shen (Panacis quinquefolii Radix) 4.5-6g Xi Gua (Citrulli Exocarpium) 24-30g Lian Geng (Nelumbinis Caulis) 12-15g Shi Hu (Dendrobii Herba) 12-15g Mai Men Dong (Ophiopogonis Radix) 6-9g Dan Zhu Ye (Lophatheri Herba) 4.5-6g Zhi Mu (Anemarrhenae Rhizoma) 4.5-6g Huang Lian (Coptidis Rhizoma) 2-3g Gan Cao (Glycyrrhizae Radix) 2-3g Jing Mi (non-glutinous rice) 12-15g	
Method	**Action**
Prepare as a decoction.	Clear summer-heat, augment qi, nourish yin, generate fluids.

Xue Fu Zhu Yu Tang (血府逐瘀汤, Drive Out Stasis from the Mansion of Blood Decoction, Correction of Errors among Physicians, 1830)	
Tao Ren (Persicae Semen) 12g Hong Hua (Carthami Flos) 9g Dang Gui (Angelicae sinensis Radix) 9g Chuan Xiong (Chuanxiong Rhizoma) 4.5g Chi Shao (Paeoniae Radix rubra) 6g Niu Xi (Achyranthis bidentatae Radix) 9g Chai Hu (Bupleuri Radix) 3g Jie Geng (Platycodi Radix) 4.5g Zhi Ke (Aurantii Fructus) 6g Sheng Di Huang (Rehmanniae Radix) 9g Gan Cao (Glycyrrhizae Radix) 6g	
Method	**Action**
Prepare as a decoction. Chuan Niu Xi (Cyanthulae Radix) is often substituted for Niu Xi.	Invigorate Blood, dispel Blood stasis, spread Liver qi, unblock the channels.

Shao Fu Zhu Yu Tang (少腹逐瘀汤, Drive Out Stasis from the Lower Abdomen Decoction, Correction of Errors Among Physicians, 1830)	
Chao Xiao Hui Xiang (dry-fried Foeniculi Fructus) 1.5g Chao Gan Jiang (dry-fried Zingiberis Rhizoma) 0.6g Yan Hu Suo (Corydalis Rhizoma) 3g Dang Gui (Angelicae sinensis Radix) 9g Chuan Xiong (Chuanxiong Rhizoma) 3g Mo Yao (Myrrha) 6g Rou Gui (Cinnamomi Cortex) 3g Chi Shao (Paeoniae Radix rubra) 6g Pu Huang (Typhae Pollen) 9g Chao Wu Ling Zhi (dry-fried Trogopterori Feces) 6g	
Method	**Action**
Prepare as a decoction.	Invigorate Blood, dispel Blood stasis, warm the menses, alleviate pain.

Tao Hong Si Wu Tang (桃红四物汤, Four Substance Decoction with Safflower and Peach Pit, Supreme Commanders of the Medical Ramparts, 1291)	
Shu Di Huang (Rehmanniae Radix praeparata) 9-12g Bai Shao (Paeoniae Radix alba) 9-12g Dang Gui (Angelicae sinensis Radix) 9-12g Chuan Xiong (Chuanxiong Rhizoma) 3-6g Tao Ren (Persicae Semen) 3-6g Hong Hua (Carthami Flos) 3-6g	
Method	**Action**
Prepare as a decoction.	Tonify Blood, regulate the Liver, regulate the menses.

Wen Jing Tang (温经汤, Flow-Warming Decoction, Essentials from the Golden Cabinet, c.220)	
Wu Zhu Yu (Evodiae Fructus) 9g Gui Zhi (Cinnamomi Ramulus) 6g Dang Gui (Angelicae sinensis Radix) 6g Chuan Xiong (Chuanxiong Rhizoma) 6g Shao Yao (Paeoniae Radix) 6g E Jiao (Asini Corii Colla) 6g Mai Men Dong (Ophiopogonis Radix) 9g Mu Dan Pi (Moutan Cortex) 6g Ren Shen (Ginseng Radix) 6g Gan Cao (Glycyrrhizae Radix) 6g Sheng Jiang (Zingiberis Rhizoma recens) 6g Zhi Ban Xia (Pinelliae Rhizoma praeparatum) 6g	
Method	**Action**
Prepare as a decoction, adding the E Jiao to the strained liquid at the end. Nowadays, the prefered form of Shao Yao is Bai Shao (Paeoniae Radix alba) and Dang Shen (Codonopsis Radix) may be substituted for Ren Shen at 2-3 times the dosage.	Warm the vessels, dispel cold, nourish Blood, dispel Blood stasis.

Xiao Yao San (逍遥散, Rambling Powder, Formulary of the Pharmacy Service for Benefiting the People in the Taiping Era, 1107)	
Chai Hu (Bupleuri Radix) 9g Chao Dang Gui (dry-fried Angelicae sinensis Radix) 9g Bai Shao (Paeoniae Radix alba) 9g Bai Zhu (Atractylodis macrocephalae Rhizoma) 9g Fu Ling (Poria) (9g) Zhi Gan Cao (Glycyrrhizae Radix praeparata) 4.5g	
Method	**Action**
Prepare as a decoction.	Spread Liver qi, strengthen the Spleen, nourish the Blood.

Jia Wei Xiao Yao San (加味逍遥散, Augmented Rambling Powder, Summary of Internal Medicine, Ming Dynasty)	
Dang Gui (Angelicae sinensis Radix) 3g Shao Yao (Paeoniae Radix) 3g Fu Ling (Poria) 3g Chao Bai Zhu (dry-fried Atractylodis macrocephalae Rhizoma) 3g Chai Hu (Bupleuri Radix) 3g Mu Dan Pi (Moutan Cortex) 1.5g Chao Zhi Zi (dry-fried Gardeniae Fructus) 1.5g Zhi Gan Cao (Glycyrrhizae Radix preperata) 1.5g	
Method	**Action**
Prepare as a decoction with a small amount of Sheng Jiang (Zingiberis Rhizoma recens) and Bo He (Mentha haplocalycis Herba) added at the end.	Spread Liver qi, strengthen the Spleen, nourish Blood, clear heat.

Yue Ju Wan (越鞠丸, Escape Restraint Pill, Essential Teachings of [Zhu] Dan-Xi, 1481)	
Cang Zhu (Atractylodis Rhizoma) Chuan Xiong (Chuanxiong Rhizoma) Xiang Fu (Cyperi Rhizoma) Zhi Zi (Gardeniae Fructus) Shen Qu (Massa medicata fermentata)	
Method	**Action**
Grind equal amounts of ingredients to a powder and make water pills, or prepare as a decoction with 6–12g of each ingredient. Take 6–9g with warm water.	Promote movement of qi and release constraint.

Chai Hu Shu Gan San (柴胡疏肝散, Bupleurum Powder to Dredge the Liver, Indispensable Tools for Pattern Treatment, 1602)	
Cu Chao Chen Pi (vinegar-fried Citri reticulatae Pericarpium) 6g Chai Hu (Bupleuri Radix) 6g Chuan Xiong (Chuanxiong Rhizoma) 4.5g Chao Zhi Ke (dry-fried Aurantii Fructus) 4.5g Shao Yao (Paeoniae Radix) 4.5g Zhi Gan Cao (Glycyrrhizae Radix praeparata) 1.5g Xiang Fu (Cyperi Rhizoma) 4.5g	
Method	**Action**
Take in one dose before meals with two cups of water reduced to eight-tenths of a cup.	Spread Liver qi, harmonize Blood, alleviate pain.

Liu Wei Di Huang Wan (六味地黄丸, Six-Ingredient Pill with Rehmannia, Craft of Medicinal Treatment for Childhood Disease Patterns, 1119)	
Shu Di Huang (Rehmanniae Radix preparata) 18g Shan Zhu Yu (Corni Fructus) 9g Shan Yao (Dioscoreae Rhizoma) 9g Fu Ling (Poria) 6g Mu Dan Pi (Moutan Cortex) 6g Ze Xie (Alismatis Rhizoma) 6g	
Method	**Action**
Prepare as a decoction.	Enrich yin, nourish the Kidney.

Er Chen Tang (二陈汤, Two Aged Herb Decoction, Formulary of the Pharmacy Service for Benefiting the People in the Taiping Era, 1148)	
Zhi Ban Xia (Pinelliae Rhizoma preparatum) 15g Ju Hong (Citri reticulatae Exocarpium rubrum) 15g Fu Ling (Poria) 9g Zhi Gan Cao (Glycyrrhizae Radix preparata) 4.5g	
Method	**Action**
According to the original text, grind ingredients coarsely and take 12g as a draft with seven pieces of Sheng Jiang (Zingiberis Rhizoma recens) and one piece of Wu Mei (Mume Fructus). However, most modern texts omit these additions and substitute Chen Pi (Citri reticulatae Pericarpium) for Ju Hong. It is also possible to prepare the formula as a decoction, reducing the quantities of all ingredients by one-third.	Dry dampness, transform phlegm, regulate qi, harmonize the middle *jiao*.

Tian Wang Bu Xin Dan (天王补心丹, Emperor of Heaven's Special Pill to Tonify the Heart, Fine Formulas for Women with Annotations and Commentary, Ming Dynasty, 16th century)	
Sheng Di Huang (Rehmanniae Radix) 9g Ren Shen (Ginseng Radix) 4.5g Tian Men Dong (Asparagi Radix) 6g Mai Men Dong (Ophiopogonis Radix) 6g Xuan Shen (Scrophulariae Radix) 4.5g Dan Shen (Salviae Militorrhizae Radix) 4.5g Fu Ling (Poria) 4.5g Yuan Zhi (Polygalae Radix) 4.5g Jiu Xi Dang Gui (wine-washed Angelicae sinensis Radix) 6g Wu Wei Zi (Schisandrae Fructus) 6g Bai Zi Ren (Platycladi Semen) 6g Chao Suan Zao Ren (dry-fried Ziziphi spinosae Semen) 6g Jie Geng (Platycodi Radix) 4.5g Zhu Sha (Cinnabaris) 4.5g*	
Method	**Action**
Prepare as a decoction. Dang Shen (Codonopsis Radix) is usually substituted for Ren Shen at 2 –3 times the dosage.	Enrich yin, nourish Blood, clear heat, calm the *shen*.

* Zhu Sha is no longer used due to high levels of toxicity. Some formulas substitute with Shi Chang Pu (Acori tatarinowii Rhizoma), Huang Lian (Coptidis Rhizoma), Long Gu (Fossilia Ossis Mastodi), or Long Chi (Fossillia Dentis Mastodi).

Gan Mai Da Zao Tang (甘麦大枣汤, Licorice, Wheat, and Jujube Decoction, Essentials from the Golden Cabinet, c.220)	
Gan Cao (Glycyrrhizae Radix) 9g Xiao Mai (Triciti Fructus) 9-15g Da Zao (Jujubae Fructus) 10 pieces	
Method	**Action**
Prepare as a decoction. Many believe that long-term use will maximize the benefits of this formula.	Nourish the Heart, calm the *shen*, harmonize the middle *jiao*, relax muscle tension.

Suan Zao Ren Tang (酸枣仁汤, Sour Jujube Decoction, Essentials from the Golden Cabinet, c.220)	
Suan Zao Ren (Ziziphi spinosae Semen) 12-18g Fu Ling (Poria) 6g Zhi Mu (Anemarrhenae Rhizoma) 6g Chuan Xiong (Chuanxiong Rhizoma) 6g Gan Cao (Glycyrrhizae Radix) 3g	
Method	**Action**
Prepare as a decoction, crushing the Suan Zao Ren first. Some sources suggest decocting the Suan Zao Ren first, although this is no longer commonly done.	Nourish Blood, calm the *shen*, clear heat, eliminate irritability.

Gui Pi Tang (归脾汤, Restore the Spleen Decoction, Categorized Essentials for Normalizing the Structure, 1529)	
Ren Shen (Ginseng Radix) 3g (3-6g) Chao Huang Qi (dry-fried Astragali Radix) 3g (9-12g) Bai Zhu (Atractylodis macrocephalae Rhizoma) 3g (9-12g) Fu Ling (Poria) 3g (9-12g) Chao Suan Zao Ren (dry-fried Ziziphi spinosae Semen) 3g (9-12g) Long Yan Rou (Longan Arillus) 3g (6-9g) Mu Xiang (Aucklandiae Radix) 1.5g (3-6g) Zhi Gan Cao (Glycyrrhizae Radix praeprata) 0.9g (3-6g) Dang Gui (Angelicae sinensis Radix) 3g (6-9g) Zhi Yuan Zhi (processed Polygalae Radix) 3g (3-6g)	
Method	**Action**
Prepare as a decoction. The original text advises taking it with Sheng Jiang (Zingiberis Rhizoma recens) and Da Zao (Jujubae Fructus). Nowadays, it is usually prepared using the dosage in parentheses, with Dang Shen (Codonopsis Radix) substituted for Ren Shen at 2-3 times the dosage and Fu Shen (Poriae Sclerotium pararadicis) substituted for Fu Ling.	Augment qi, tonify Blood, strengthen the Spleen, Nourish the Heart.

Si Wu Tang (四物汤, Four-Substance Decoction, Secret Formulas to manage Trauma and Reconnect Fractures Received from an Immortal, c.846)	
Shu Di Huang (Rehmanniae Radix praeparata) 9-12g Bai Shao (Paeoniae Radix alba) 9-12g Dang Gui (Angelicae sinensis Radix) 9-12g Chuan Xiong (Chuanxiong Rhizoma) 3-6g	
Method	**Action**
The original text advises grinding equal amounts of each ingredient into a coarse powder and taking 9g as a draft before meals. Nowadays, it is usually prepared as a decoction using the doses specified above.	Tonify Blood, regulate the Liver.

Sheng Tie Luo Yin (生铁落饮, Iron Filings Drink, Awakening of the Mind in Medical Studies, 1732)	
Sheng Tie Luo (Ferri Frusta) 15-60g Dan Nan Xing (Arisaema cum Bile) 3g Bei Mu (Fritillariae Bulbus) 9g Xuan Shen (Scrophulariae Radix) 4.5g Tian Men Dong (Asparagi Radix) 9g Mai Men Dong (Ophiopogonis Radix) 9g Lian Qiao (Forsythiae Fructus) 3g Gou Teng (Uncariae Ramulus cum Uncis) 4.5g Dan Shen (Salviae miltiorrhizae Radix) 4.5g Fu Ling (Poria) 3g Fu Shen (Poriae Sclerotium pararadicis) 3g Chen Pi (Citri reticulatae Pericarpium) 3g Shi Chang Pu (Acori tatarinowii Rhizoma) 3g Yuan Zhi (Polygalae Radix) 3g Zhu Sha (Cinnabaris)*	
Method	**Action**
Prepare as a decoction, decocting the Shen Tie Luo first in five cups of water and reducing to three cups over three hours before adding the other ingredients.*	Sedate the Heart, eliminate phlegm, clear fire, calm the *shen*.

* Zhu Sha is no longer used due to high levels of toxicity. Some formulas substitute with other heavy and settling medicinals, such as Long Gu (Fossilia Ossis Mastodi) or Long Chi (Fossillia Dentis Mastodi).

Long Dan Xie Gan Tang (龙胆泻肝汤, Gentian Decoction to Drain the Liver, Precious Mirror of Health, Yuan Dynasty)	
Huang Qin (Scutellariae Radix) 4.5g Chai Hu (Bupleuri Radix) 6g Gan Cao (Glycyrrhizae Radix) 3g Ren Shen (Ginseng Radix) 3g Mai Men Dong (Ophiopogonis Radix) 6g Tian Men Dong (Asparagi Radix) 6g Huang Lian (Coptidis Rhizoma) 3g Zhi Mu (Anemarrhenae Rhizoma) 6g Long Dan Cao (Gentianae Radix) 3g Zhi Zi (Gardeniae Fructus) 3g Wu Wei Zi (Schisandrae Fructus) 10 pieces	
Method	**Action**
Prepare as a decoction.	Clear the Liver, drain fire, enrich yin, generate fluids.

Jin Suo Gu Jing Wan (金锁固精丸, Metal Lock Pill to Stabilize the Essence, Medical Formulas Collected and Analysed, 1682)	
Chao Sha Yuan Zi (dry-fried Astragali complanati Semen) 10g Qian Shi (Euryales Semen) 5g Lian Xu (Nelumbinis Stamen) 5g Duan Long Gu (calcined Fossilia Ossis Mastodi) 3g Duan Mu Li (calcined Ostreae Concha) 3g	
Method	**Action**
Prepare as a decoction.	Stabilize the Kidney, bind up *jing*.

<table>
<tr><th colspan="2">Ba Zhen Tang (八珍汤, Eight-Treasure Decoction, Experiential Formulas from the Auspicious Bamboo Hall, 1326)</th></tr>
<tr><td colspan="2">Ren Shen (Ginseng Radix) 6-9g
Bai Zhu (Atractylodis macrocephalae Rhizoma) 9-12g
Fu Ling (Poria) 12-15g
Zhi Gan Cao (Glycyrrhizae Radix praeparata) 3-6g
Shu Di Huang (Rehmanniae Radix praeparata) 15-18g
Bai Shao (Paeoniae Radix alba) 12-15g
Dang Gui (Angelicae sinensis Radix) 12-15g
Chuan Xiong (Chuanxiong Rhizoma) 6-9g</td></tr>
<tr><th>Method</th><th>Action</th></tr>
<tr><td>Prepare as a decoction. Dang Shen (Codonopsis Radix) may be substituted for Ren Shen at 2-3 times the dosage.</td><td>Tonify and augment Blood and qi.</td></tr>
</table>

<table>
<tr><th colspan="2">Zeng Ye Tang (增液汤, Increase the Fluids Decoction, Systematic Differentiation of Warm Pathogen Diseases)</th></tr>
<tr><td colspan="2">Xuan Shen (Scrophulariae Radix) 30g
Mai Men Dong (Ophiopogonis Radix) 24g
Sheng Di Huang (Rehmanniae Radix) 24g</td></tr>
<tr><th>Method</th><th>Action</th></tr>
<tr><td>Prepare as a decoction. The original text recommends using a single, large dose for acute conditions.</td><td>Generate fluids, moisten dryness, unblock the bowels.</td></tr>
</table>

Sha Shen Mai Men Dong Tang (沙参麦门冬汤, Glehnia and Ophiopogonis Decoction, Systematic Differentiation of Warm Pathogen Diseases, 1798)	
Sha Shen (Glehnia/Adenophorae Radix) 9g Mai Men Dong (Ophiopogonis Radix) 9g Yu Zhu (Polygonati odorati Rhizoma) 6g Sang Ye (Mori Folium) 4.5g Tian Hua Fen (Trichosanthis Radix) 4.5g Bian Dou (Lablab Semen album) 4.5g Gan Cao (Glycyrrhizae Radix) 3g	
Method	**Action**
Prepare as a decoction. The original text advises decocting in five cups of water and reducing until two cups remain.	Clear and nourish the Lung and Stomach, generate fluids, moisten dryness.

Qing Jing San (清经散, Clear the Menses Powder, Fu Qing Zhu's Women's Disorders, 17th Century)	
Mu Dan Pi (Moutan Cortex) 6g Bai Shao (Paeoniae Radix alba) 6g Shu Di Huang (Rehmanniae Radix praeparata) 6g Di Gu Pi (Lycii Cortex) 15g Qing Hao (Artemisiae annuae Herba) 6g Fu Ling (Poria) 3g Huang Bai (Phellodendri Cortex) 1.5g	
Method	**Action**
Prepare as a decoction.	Clear heat, cool Blood.

Gu Jing Wan (固经丸, Stabilize the Menses Pill, Essential Teachings from [Zhu] Dan-Xi, 1481)	
Zhi Gui Ban (prepared Testudinis Plastrum) 9g Chao Bai Shao (dry-fried Paeoniae Radix alba) 9g Chao Huang Qin (dry-fried Scutellariae Radix) 9g Chun Pi (Ailanthi Cortex) 6g Chao Huang Bai (dry-fried Phellodendri Cortex) 3g Xiang Fu (Cyperi Rhizoma) 4.5g	
Method	**Action**
Prepare as a decoction.	Enrich yin, clear heat, stop bleeding, stabilize the menses.

Dang Gui Bu Xue Tang (当归补血汤, Tangkuei Decoction to Tonify the Blood, Clarifying Doubts about Damage from Internal and External Causes, 1247)	
Huang Qi (Astragali Radix) 30g Jiu Xi Dang Gui (wine-washed Angelicae sinensis Radix) 6g	
Method	**Action**
The original text advises grinding to a coarse powder and preparing as a decoction.	Tonify qi, generate Blood.

Huang Lian Jie Du Tang (黄连解毒汤, Coptis Decoction to Resolve Toxicity, Arcane Essentials from the Imperial Library, 752)	
Huang Lian (Coptidis Rhizoma) 9g Huang Qin (Scutellariae Radix) 6g Huang Bai (Phellodendri Cortex) 6g Zhi Zi (Gardeniae Fructus) 6-12g	
Method	**Action**
Prepare as a decoction. Nowadays, the Huang Lian dosage is often reduced by one-half or two-thirds. Some Japanese sources recommend taking the decoction cool to enhance its cooling activity.	Drain fire, resolve toxicity.

Gui Zhi Tang (桂枝汤, Cinnamon Twig Decoction, Discussion of Cold Damage, c.200)	
Gui Zhi (Cinnamomi Ramulus) 9g Shao Yao (Paeoniae Radix) 9g Sheng Jiang (Zingiberis Rhizoma recens) 9g Da Zao (Jujubae Fructus) 12 pieces Zhi Gan Cao (Glycyrrhizae Radix praeparata) 6g	
Method	**Action**
The original text advises coarsely grinding and decocting over a low flame until seven cups of liquid reduces to three cups. One cup should be taken with rice congee to induce sweating. If no sweating occurs, take a second cup. If there is a little sweating, repeat once or twice, reducing the interval between doses. Alcohol and raw, cold, spicy, or greasy foods should be avoided during medication. Nowadays, it is usually prepared as a decoction, cooking for no longer than 20 minutes, and taken hot with the patient wrapped up to induce sweating. Stop administration once sweating occurs. The prefered form of Shao Yao is Bai Shao (Paeoniae Radix alba) and the Da Zao dosage is reduced to four pieces.	Release pathogenic factors from the muscle layer, regulate *ying* and *wei* qi.

Du Huo Ji Sheng Tang (独活寄生汤, Pubescent Angelica and Taxillus Decoction, Important Formulas Worth a Thousand Gold Pieces, 650)	
Du Huo (Angelicae pubescentis Radix) 9g Xi Xin (Asari Radix et Rhizoma) 6g Fang Feng (Saposhnikoviae Radix) 6g Qin Jiao (Gentianae macrophyllae Radix) 6g Sang Ji Sheng (Taxilli Herba) 6g Du Zhong (Eucommiae Cortex) 6g Niu Xi (Achyranthis bidentatae Radix) 6g Rou Gui (Cinnamomi Cortex) 6g Dang Gui (Angelicae sinensis Radix) 6g Chuan Xiong (Chuanxiong Rhizoma) 6g Sheng Di Huang (Rehmanniae Radix) 6g Bai Shao (Paeoniae Radix alba) 6g Ren Shen (Ginseng Radix) 6g Fu Ling (Poria) 6g Gan Cao (Glycyrrhizae Radix) 6g	
Method	**Action**
Prepare as a decoction. Nowadays, the Sang Ji Sheng dosage is usually 15-30g but Xu Duan (Dipsaci Radix) is often used as a substitute. Dang Shen (Codonopsis Radix) is usually substituted for Ren Shen at twice the dosage.	Expel wind-dampness, disperse painful obstruction, tonify deficiency.

Juan Bi Tang (蠲痹汤, Remove Painful Obstruction Decoction, Yang Family Formulas, 1178)	
Qiang Huo (Notopterygii Rhizoma seu Radix) 6g Jiang Huang (Curcumae longae Rhizoma) 6g Jiu Xi Dang Gui (wine-washed Angelicae sinensis Radix) 6g Mi Zhi Huang Qi (honey-prepared Astragali Radix) 6g Bai Shao (Paeoniae Radix alba) 6g Fang Feng (Saposhnikoviae Radix) 6g Zhi Gan Cao (Glycyrrhizae Radix praeparata) 4.5g	
Method	**Action**
Prepare as a decoction with 3g of Sheng Jiang Some practitioners substitute Bai Shao for Chi Shao (Paeoniae Radix rubra).	Tonify and harmonize *wei* and *ying* qi, dispel wind, eliminate dampness.

Xiao Huo Luo Dan (小活络丹, Minor Invigorate the Collaterals Special Pill, Formulary of the Pharmacy Service Benefiting the People in the Taiping Era, 1107)	
Zhi Cao Wu (Aconiti kusnezoffii Radix praeparata) 1.5-18g Zhi Chuan Wu (Aconiti Radix praeparata) 1.5-18g Zhi Tian Nan Xing (Arisaematis Rhizoma praeparatum) 9-18g Mo Yao (Myrrha) 6g Ru Xiang (Olibanum) 6g Di Long (Pheretima) 12g	
Method	**Action**
Prepare as a decoction.	Dispel wind, eliminate dampness, transform phlegm, invigorate Blood, unblock the collaterals, alleviate pain.

Wu Ji San (五积散, Five-Accumulation Powder, Secret Formulas to Manage Trauma and Reconnect Fractures Received from an Immortal, c.846)	
Ma Huang (Ephedrae Herba) 1.5-4.5g Bai Zhi (Angelicae dahuricae Radix) 1.5-4.5g Gan Jiang (Zingiberis Rhizoma) 1.5-4.5g Rou Gui (Cinnamomi Cortex) 1.5-4.5g Cang Zhu (Atractylodis Rhizoma) 3-9g Hou Po (Magnoliae officinalis Cortex) 1.5-4.5g Chen Pi (Citri reticulatae Pericarpium) 3-9g Zhi Ban Xia (Pinelliae Rhizoma praeparatum) 3-9g Fu Ling (Poria) 3-9g Jie Geng (Platycodi Radix) 3-9g Zhi Ke (Aurantii Fructus) 1.5-4.5g Dang Gui (Angelicae sinensis Radix) 1.5-4.5g Bai Shao (Paeoniae Radix alba) 1.5-4.5g Chuan Xiong (Chuanxiong Rhizoma) 1.5-4.5g Gan Cao (Glycyrrhizae Radix) 1.5-4.5g	
Method	**Action**
Prepare as a decoction.	Release the exterior, warm the interior, smooth qi flow, transform phlegm, invigorate Blood, reduce accumulation.

Xuan Bi Tang (宣痹汤, Disband Painful Obstruction Decoction, Systematic Differentiation of Warm Pathogen, 1798)	
Fang Ji (Stephaniae/Cocculi/etc. Radix) 15g Xing Ren (Armeniacae Semen) 15g Hua Shi (Talcum) 15g Lian Qiao (Forsythiae Fructus) 9g Zhi Zi (Gardeniae Fructus) 9g Yi Yi Ren (Coicis Semen) 15g Zhi Ban Xia (Pinelliae Rhizoma praeparatum) 9g Can Sha (Bombycis Feces) 9g Chi Xiao Dou (Phaseoli Semen) 9g	
Method	**Action**
Prepare as a decoction. Han Fang Ji (Stephaniae tetandrae Radix) is the most commonly used form of Fang Ji. The Chi Xiao Dou dosage is often doubled or tripled.	Clear and resolve damp-heat, unblock the channels, disband painful obstruction.

Gui Zhi Shao Yao Zhi Mu Tang (桂枝芍药知母汤, Cinnamon Twig, Peony, and Anemarrhena Decoction, Essentials from the Golden Cabinet, c.220)	
Gui Zhi (Cinnamomi Ramulus) 12g Ma Huang (Ephedrae Herba) 6g Bao Fu Zi (baked Aconiti Radix lateralis) 15g Zhi Mu (Anemarrhenae Rhizoma) 12g Shao Yao (Paeoniae Radix) 9g Bai Zhu (Atractylodis macrocephalae Rhizoma) 15g Fang Feng (Saposhnikoviae Radix) 12g Sheng Jiang (Zingiberis Rhizoma recens) 15g Gan Cao (Glycyrrhizae Radix) 6g	
Method	**Action**
Prepare as a decoction. The most commonly used form of Shao Yao is Bai Shao (Paeoniae Radix alba).	Unblocks yang qi, promotes movement, dispels wind, eliminates dampness, clears heat.

Shen Tong Zhu Yu Tang (身痛逐瘀汤, Drive Out Stasis from a Painful Body Decoction, Correction of Errors among Physicians, 1830)	
Qin Jiao (Gentianae macrophyllae Radix) 3g Chuan Xiong (Chuanxiong Rhizoma) 6g Tao Ren (Persicae Semen) 9g Hong Hua (Carthami Flos) 9g Gan Cao (Glycyrrhizae Radix) 6g Qiang Huo (Notopterygii Rhizoma seu Radix) 3g Mo Yao (Myrrha) 6g Dang Gui (Angelicae sinensis Radix) 9g Chao Wu Ling Zhi (dry-fried Trogopterori Feces) 6g Xiang Fu (Cyperi Rhizoma) 3g Chuan Niu Xi (Cyathulae Radix) 9g Di Long (Pheretima) 6g	
Method	**Action**
Prepare as a decoction.	Invigorate Blood, promote qi movement, dispel Blood stasis, unblock the collaterals, unblock painful obstruction, alleviate pain.

Huo Luo Xiao Ling Dan (活络效灵丹, Fantastically Effective Pill to Invigorate the Collaterals, Essays on Medicine Esteeming the Chinese and Respecting the Western, 1918-1934)	
Dang Gui (Angelicae sinensis Radix) 15g Dan Shen (Salviae miltiorrhizae Radix) 15g Ru Xiang (Olibanum) 15g Mo Yao (Myrrha) 15g	
Method	**Action**
Prepare as a decoction. Alternatively, grind to powder and divide into four equal portions to take with warm wine.	Invigorate Blood, dispel Blood stasis, unblock the collaterals, alleviate pain.

Gui Lu Er Xian Jiao (龟鹿二仙胶, Tortoise Shell and Deer Antler Two-Immortal Syrup, Concise Medicine, 1587)	
Lu Jiao (Cervi Cornu) 10-20g Gui Ban (Testudinis Plastrum) 5-10g Gou Qi Zi (Lycii Fructus) 3-6g Ren Shen (Ginseng Radix) 3-6g	
Method	**Action**
Prepare as a decoction.	Nourish and replenish yin, tonify *jing*, augment qi, tonify and strengthen yang.

Shu Jing Huo Xue Tang (舒经活血汤, Relax the Channels and Invigorate the Blood Decoction, Restoration of Health from the Myriad Diseases, 1587)	
Bai Shao (Paeoniae Radix alba) 4.5g Dang Gui (Angelicae sinensis Radix) 3.6g Chuan Xiong (Chuanxiong Rhizoma) 1.8g Sheng Di Huang (Rehmanniae Radix) 3g Tao Ren (Persicae Semen) 3g Cang Zhu (Atractylodis Rhizoma) 3g Fu Ling (Poria) 2.1g Niu Xi (Achyranthis bidentatae Radix) 3g Wei Ling Xian (Clematidis Radix) 3g Han Fang Ji (Stephaniae tetandrae Radix) 1.8g Qiang Huo (Notopterygii Rhizoma seu Radix) 1.8g Fang Feng (Saposhnikoviae Radix) 1.8g Long Dan Cao (Gentianae Radix) 1.8g Bai Zhi (Angelicae dahuricae Radix) 1.8g Chen Pi (Citri reticulatae Pericarpium) 3g Gan Cao (Glycyrrhizae Radix) 1.2g	
Method	**Action**
Prepare as a decoction with three pieces of Sheng Jiang (Zingiberis Rhizoma recens).	Unblock and relax the channels, invigorate Blood.

<table>
<tr><th colspan="2">Ping Wei San (平胃散, Calm the Stomach Powder, Concise Formulas to Aid the Multitudes, 1051)</th></tr>
<tr><td colspan="2">Chao Cang Zhu (dry-fried Atractylodis Rhizoma) 12-15g
Jiang Chao Hou Po (ginger-fried Magnoliae officinalis Cortex) 9-12g
Chen Pi (Citri reticulatae Pericarpium) 9-12g
Zhi Gan Cao (Glycyrrhizae Radix praeparata) 3-6g</td></tr>
<tr><th>Method</th><th>Action</th></tr>
<tr><td>Prepare as a decoction.</td><td>Dry dampness, improve the Spleen's trasportation function, move qi, harmonize the Stomach.</td></tr>
</table>

<table>
<tr><th colspan="2">Di Tan Tang (涤痰汤, Scour Out Phlegm Decoction, Fine Formulas of Wonderful Efficacy, 1470)</th></tr>
<tr><td colspan="2">Zhi Tian Nan Xing (Arisaematis Rhizoma praeparatum) 7.5g
Zhi Ban Xia (Pinelliae Rhizoma praeparatum) 7.5g
Fu Ling (Poria) 6g
Zhi Shi (Aurantii Fructus immaturus) 6g
Ju Hong (Citri reticulatae Exocarpium rubrum) 4.5g
Shi Chang Pu (Acori tatarinowii Rhizoma) 3g
Ren Shen (Ginseng Radix) 3g
Zhu Ru (Bambusae Caulis in taeniam) 2.1g
Gan Cao (Glycyrrhizae Radix) 2.1g</td></tr>
<tr><th>Method</th><th>Action</th></tr>
<tr><td>Prepare as a a decoction with 3-5 slices of Sheng Jiang (Zingiberis Rhizoma recens) and take after meals. The Ju Hong may be substituted with Chen Pi (Citri reticulatae Pericarpium).</td><td>Scour out phlegm, open the sensory orifices, tonify qi.</td></tr>
</table>

Tong Qiao Huo Xue Tang (通窍活血汤, Unblock the Orifices and Invigorate Blood Decoction, Correction of Errors Among Physicians, 1830)	
Chi Shao (Paeoniae Radix rubra) 3g Chuan Xiong (Chuanxiong Rhizoma) 3g Tao Ren (Persicae Semen) 9g Hong Hua (Carthami Flos) 9g Cong Bai (Allii fistulosi Bulbus) 3g Da Zao (Jujubae Fructus) 7 pieces Sheng Jiang (Zingiberis Rhizoma recens) 9g She Xiang (Moschus) 0.15g	
Method	**Action**
Prepare as a decoction, adding the She Xiang to the strained liquid with a small amount of Bai Jiu (Chinese white wine).	Invigorates Blood, dispels stasis, opens up the orifices.

Xiang Sha Liu Jun Zi Tang (香砂六君子汤, Six Gentlemen Decoction with Auklandia and Amomum, Discussion of Famous Physicians' Formulas Past and Present, 1675)	
Ren Shen (Ginseng Radix) 3g Bai Zhu (Atractylodis macrocephalae Rhizoma) 6g Fu Ling (Poria) 6g Zhi Gan Cao (Glycyrrhizae Rhizoma praeparata) 2.1g Chen Pi (Citri reticulatae Pericarpium) 2.4g Zhi Ban Xia (Pinelliae Rhizoma praeparata) 3g Sha Ren (Amomi Fructus) 2.4g Mu Xiang (Auklandiae Radix) 2.1g Sheng Jiang (Zingiberis Rhizoma recens) 6g	
Method	**Action**
Prepare as a decoction. Dang Shen (Codonopsis Radix) is usually substituted for Ren Shen at 2 –3 times the dosage.	Strengthen the Spleen, harmonize the Stomach, regulate qi, alleviate pain.

Fu Zi Li Zhong Wan **(附子理中丸, Aconite Accessory Root Pill to Regulate the Middle, Formulary of the Pharmacy Services for Benefiting the People in the Taiping Era, 1148)**	
Zhi Fu Zi (Aconitii Radix lateralis praeparata) 5-15g Pao Jiang (Zingiberis Rhizoma praeparatum) 3-15g Ren Shen (Ginseng Radix) 3-15g Bai Zhu (Atractylodis macrocephalae Rhizoma) 3-15g Zhi Gan Cao (Glycyrrhizae Radix praeparata) 3-9g	
Method	**Action**
Prepare as a decoction.	Warm yang, dispel cold, augment qi, strengthen the Spleen.

Ren Shen Yang Rong Tang **(人参养荣汤, Ginseng Decoction to Nourish Luxuriance, Discussion of Illnesses, Patterns, and Formulas Related to the Unification of the Three Etiologies, 1174)**	
Bai Shao (Paeoniae Radix alba) 9-18g Dang Gui (Angelicae sinensis Radix) 6-9g Chen Pi (Citri reticulatae Pericarpium) 4.5-6g Huang Qi (Astragali Radix) 6-9g Rou Gui (Cinnamomi Cortex) 3-6g Ren Shen (Ginseng Radix) 4.5-6g Bai Zhu (Atractylodis macrocephalae Rhizoma) 4.5-6g Zhi Gan Cao (Glycyrrhizae Radix praeparata) 3-6g Shu Di Huang (Rehmanniae Radix praeparata) 3-4.5g Wu Wei Zi (Schisandrae Fructus) 3-4.5g Fu Ling (Poria) 3-4.5g Chao Yuan Zhi (dry-fried Polygalae Radix) 3g	
Method	**Action**
Prepare as a decoction. Dang Shen (Codonopsis Radix) may be substituted for Ren Shen at 2-3 times the dosage.	Augment qi, tonify Blood, nourish the Heart, calm the *shen*.

Shou Xing Wan (寿星丸, God of Fertility Pill, Internal Medicine of Traditional Chinese Medicine, 2002)	
Huang Qi (Astragali Radix) 15g Bai Zhu (Atractylodi macrocephalae Rhizoma) 12g Fu Ling (Poria) 12g Dang Gui (Angelicae sinensis Radix) 9g Sheng Di Huang (Rehmanniae Radix) 9g Bai Shao (Paeoniae Radix alba) 9g Yuan Zhi (Polygalae Radix) 6g Ren Shen (Ginseng Radix) 6g Chen Pi (Citri reticulatae Pericarpium) 6g Zhi Tian Nan Xing (Arisaematis Rhizoma praeparatum) 6g Wu Wei Zi (Schisandrae Fructus) 6g Rou Gui (Cinnamomi Cortex) 3g Hu Po (Succinum) 3g	
Method	**Action**
Prepare as a decoction.	Tonify qi and Blood, strengthen the Spleen, dry dampness, expel phlegm, invigorate Blood, sedate the Heart, calm *shen*.

References

Scheid, V., Bensky, D., Ellis, A., Barolet, R., (2015). Chinese Herbal Medicine Formulas & Strategies, 2nd edition. Eastland Press : Seattle, USA.

Grosam, B., (2021). Understanding and Treating Hot Flashes in Menopause with Chinese Medicine. Singing Dragon: London and Philadelphia.

Wang, Y., Huang, Y., Xie, J., Hu, K., (2002). Internal Medicine of Chinese Medicine. Shanghai Chinese Medicine University Press : Shanghai, China

Appendix 6. Glossary of Traditional Chinese Medical Terms

Baomai (胞脉): The 'uterine vessels,' or 'uterine network vessels,' that connect the Heart and uterus, including parts of the *chongmai* and *renmai*. These vessels play a role in menstruation and nourishing the foetus during pregnancy.

Chongmai (冲脉): Also known as the Penetrating Vessel or Thoroughfare Vessel, this extraordinary vessel arises in the lower abdomen, emerges at the perineum, and travels along the Kidney channel to the chest, before ascending to the throat and face. Secondary branches connect with the sole of the foot and the *dumai* (Governing Vessel) This vessel is sometimes called the Sea of Blood and plays a crucial role in menstruation as well as regulating the twelve regular channels.

Dumai (督脉): Also known as the Governing Vessel, this extraordinary vessel arises in the lower abdomen, emerges at the perineum, and travels up the spine, traversing the head and terminating at the upper gum. Secondary branches connect with the Kidney, umbilicus, Heart, throat, and lower jaw. It is sometimes called the Sea of Yang and its primary function is regulating the six yang channels.

Guqi (谷气): Also known as 'grain qi,' this is the form of qi derived from food.

Jiao (焦) The three jiao, sometimes translated as 'three burning spaces' consist of the upper jiao (*shangjiao* -上焦 - the area above the diaphragm, housing the heart and lungs), the middle jiao (*zhongjiao* - 中焦 - the area between the diaphragm and the umbilicus, housing the liver, gallbladder, spleen, stomach, etc.), and the lower jiao (*xiajiao* - 下焦 - the area below the umbilicus, housing the kidney, bladder, intestines, etc.).

Jing (精): Usually translated as 'essence,' this vital substance is stored by the Kidney and is responsible for growth, development, reproduction, and aging. For further details, see Chapter 3.2 Seven Year Cycles of Jing.

Mingmen (命门): The 'Gate of Life' that is said to reside between the kidneys, or is attributed to the right kidney (while the left kidney is said to be the 'kidney proper'). It is the source of *yuanqi* (source qi), and houses fire and water, making up part of the ministerial fire, along with the Liver, Gallbladder, and Triple Burner.

Qi (气): Often translated as 'energy' or 'lifeforce,' qi is actually more accurately translated as 'gas,' 'air,' or 'breath.' In fact, its meaning can vary greatly depending on the context and whether it is used in combination with other characters. In TCEAM terms, it is most commonly used to refer to the vital substance responsible for warmth, movement, transformation, and containment (e.g. of the Blood).

Renmai (任脉): Also known as the Conception Vessel or Controlling Vessel, this extraordinary vessel arises in the lower abdomen, emerges at the perineum, and travels up the anterior midline to the mentolabial groove. A secondary branch connects with the eye, while another follows the course of the *chongmai* in front of the spine. This vessel is called the Sea of Yin and plays a role in menstruation and conception, as well as regulating the six yin channels.

Shaoyang (少阳): The 'lesser yang' channel, which corresponds to the Triple Burner and Gallbladder channels.

Shaoyin (少阴): The 'lesser yin' channel, which corresponds to the Heart and Kidney channels.

Shen (神): Usually translated as 'mind,' 'spirit,' or 'mind-spirit,' the shen is housed by the Heart and plays a role in consciousness, sleep, mental capacity, and emotion.

Taiyang (太阳) The 'greater yang' channel, which corresponds to the Small Intestine and Bladder channels.

Taiyin (太阴): The 'greater yin' channel, which corresponds to the Lung and Spleen channels.

Tiangui (天癸): Usually translated as 'heavenly water,' tiangui is responsible for fecundity and is often correlated with menstruation.

Weiqi (卫气): Also known as 'defensive qi,' this is the form of qi that circulates between the skin and flesh, controlling the opening and closing of the sweat ducts and preventing external pathogenic factors from penetrating the interior.

Yang (阳): The character 阳 depicts the sunny side of a mound or hill. As the complementary opposite to yin (阴), it represents daytime, light, warmth, activity, etc. In the body, it is associated with movement and functionality. Yang substances are relatively light, fast-moving, and intangible, for example, qi and *shen*.

Yangming (阳明): The 'yang brightness' channel, which corresponds to the Stomach and Large Intestine channels.

Yi (意): Usually translated as 'ideation,' this aspect of the cognitive function is stored by the Spleen.

Yin (阴): The character 阴 depicts the shady side of a mound or hill. As the complementary opposite to yang (阳), it represents night time, darkness, coolness, stillness, etc. In the body, it is associated with storage and nourishment. Yin substances are relatively dense, slow-moving, and material, for example, Blood, body fluids, and *jing*.

Yingqi (营气): Also known as 'nutritive qi' or 'construction qi,' this is the form of qi that generates Blood, circulating in the vessels and providing nourishment for the whole body.

Yuanqi (原气): Also known as 'source qi' or 'original qi,' this form of qi is generated by the Kidney and is the basis of all other forms of qi within the body. It is transported via the Triple Burner and can be accessed at the source points of the twelve channels.

Zangfu (脏腑): A general term for the five viscera and the six bowels. Zang (脏) refers to the Heart, Spleen, Lung, Kidney, and Liver (with the addition of the Pericardium in channel theory). Meanwhile, fu (腑) refers to the Small Intestine, Stomach, Large Intestine, Bladder, Gallbladder, and Triple Burner.

Zhi (志): Usually translated as 'will,' this aspect of cognitive function is stored by the Kidney.

References

Maciocia, G. (1989). The Foundations of Chinese Medicine. First edition. Churchill Livingston Elsevier, London, UK.

Wiseman, N., Feng, Y. (2014). A Practical Dictionary of Chinese Medicine. Third edition. Paradigm Publications, Taos, New Mexico, USA.

Index

B

D

E

F

G

H

I

J

K

L

M

Q

T

U

V

W

X

Y

Z